What People Are Saying About

Nursing Our Healer's Heart

Nursing Our Healer's Heart is radically revealing and beautifully unfolding in its healing message to all nurses. This work embraces a compassionate, philosophical, and scientific invitation and guide for nurses to face and disclose the shadows we carry in our healer's heart. While presenting the status of the trauma realities nurses endure, illustrating with data, which cannot be denied, Dr. Lorre Laws likewise opens space and paves the way forward for healing limitations. The straightforward writing and illustrations, combined with depth of scholarship, bring the work and world of nursing to a new global community of wisdom for heart-centered caring-healing. Every nurse can heal from just reading this book, being mentored back to one's healing heart.

Jean Watson, PhD, RN, AHN-BC, FAAN, LL (AAN), founder of the Watson Caring Science Institute

Dr. Lorre Laws' tender and wise book offers a clear path for nurses to receive the respect and nurture they need. Drawing on the emerging discoveries of relational neuroscience, she challenges the system to change in ways that can provide the support nurses need to thrive, and offers guidance for nurses to create communities of care as a sanctuary in the midst of so much pain and hard work. At this crucial juncture in healthcare, this is an indispensable book.

Bonnie Badenoch, author of *The Heart of Trauma: Healing the Embodied Brain in the Context of Relationships*

Here is a book for every nurse who feels over or on the edge of burnout, alone, traumatized, and exhausted, but at a loss as to exactly why or what to do about it. Dr. Lorre Laws sees you, and she has written from a depth of research, clinical experience, and caring to help you to recover your healer's heart. The book is thoroughly grounded in nursing theory along with the latest developments in the sciences of wholeness and neuroplasticity to guide nurses to nurture, nourish, heal, and thrive in all aspects of their bodymindessence. It is a brilliant and beautiful work of the heart, and I am delighted to recommend it not only to nurses but to anyone engaged in human caring and healing.

Janet F. Quinn, PhD, RN, FAAN

Institutions of medicine are hemorrhaging nurses while failing to adequately care for those who remain in the profession. While most discussions center around short-term hiring strategies to plug the holes of a sinking ship, *Nursing Our Healer's Heart* offers a long-term vision for healing the hardships and traumas of nursing. Dr. Lorre Laws has written a must-read book for those currently working as nurses, those who plan to become nurses, and those who were once nurses. Health care scholars will be captivated by an insider's honest reflections on the nursing profession.

Terrence D. Hill, PhD, Medical Sociologist at the University of Texas at San Antonio

In this thoughtful book, Dr. Lorre Laws assists us in understanding the role that unresolved trauma plays in chronic illness. Her book artfully explores complex layers of trauma, many often ignored or overlooked, and provides a vital resource for anyone treating or recovering from chronic illness. She presents us with different modalities which can be used successfully for healing, and her intelligent use of diagrams makes grasping complex concepts easy. I strongly endorse and recommend adding this book to the library of anyone who wishes for a deeper, more comprehensive understanding of trauma.

Mary Beth Ackerley, MD MD(H) ABIHM, co-founder of the International Society for Environmentally Acquired Illness

Nursing Our Healer's Heart

Nursing Our Healer's Heart

A Recovery Guide for
Nurse Trauma & Burnout

Lorre Laws, PhD RN

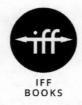

IFF
BOOKS

London, UK
Washington, DC, USA

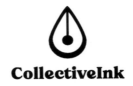

CollectiveInk

First published by iff Books, 2024
iff Books is an imprint of Collective Ink Ltd.,
Unit 11, Shepperton House, 89 Shepperton Road, London, N1 3DF
office@collectiveinkbooks.com
www.collectiveinkbooks.com
www.iff-books.com

For distributor details and how to order please visit the 'Ordering' section on our website.

Text copyright: Lorre Laws, PhD RN 2023

ISBN: 978 1 80341 378 5
978 1 80341 379 2 (ebook)
Library of Congress Control Number: 2023947323

A CIP catalogue record for this book is available from the British Library.

Design: Lapiz Digital Services

UK: Printed and bound by CPI Group (UK) Ltd, Croydon, CR0 4YY
Printed in North America by CPI GPS partners

The content of this book is for informational purposes only and is not intended to diagnose, treat, cure, or prevent any condition or disease. The reader understands that this book is not intended as a substitute for consultation with a licensed health practitioner. Please consult with your own healthcare specialist regarding the suggestions and recommendations made in this book. The use of this book implies your acceptance of this disclaimer.

We operate a distinctive and ethical publishing philosophy in all areas of our business, from our global network of authors to production and worldwide distribution.

For Katie & Ellie Mae DiBene and
our beautiful healing trinity.

Contents

Acknowledgements

Above all, I am grateful to Source, Creator, God, Elohim, Sophia, and all other names for the one divine being. My ancestors, guides, guardian angels, archangels, and all divine light beings, I thank you for your steadfast support and unconditional love. Thank you to the many spiritual teachers and ascended masters that support me in all that I do, including Louise Hay, Wayne Dyer, Kaia Ra, Lynn V. Andrews, Julia Cameron, Meilan Maurits, and most especially Eckhart Tolle, whose work and School of Awakening indelibly altered my life path, which culminated in writing this book and being of service to our global nursing community.

To my family, whom I love with all that I AM: parents Don and Sharon Laws, and my three incredible children — Katie, Ellie, and Cory, along with his wife Katy and daughters Sophie and Claire. You are my world. To the family I chose — my fellow healers, my tribe, my village, my everything: Cherie and Tai Jaques, Gail Christison, Dany Micheals, Shelby Clem, Theo and Annalisa Landy, Lisa Larsen, Justin Knoll, Michael Lawrience, Lyn O'Hara, Mary Johnson, Robin Doxey, Holly Fletcher, Britta Van Dun, Karin Zabriski, Tara Smith, and Lauren MacDonald. My heartfelt gratitude to Dr. Zubin Damania, whose *It's Not Burnout, It's Moral Injury* video compelled me to investigate burnout, moral injury, and ultimately nurse traumatization secondary to health system inadequacies.

My heart overflows with gratitude for those who directly supported me in writing this first book, which would not be here without the incredible support of my editor, mentor, and amazing human, Carolyn Crist, for whom I am grateful beyond measure. To the Hay House Writers Community & Authorpreneur community, including Reid Tracy, Kelly Notaras, Nancy Levin, and Charlie Griffin, I offer my most earnest gratitude for your support as I grow as a scientific writer into a mainstream author. I would have been lost without your leadership, guidance, and support. Thank you, thank you, thank you.

I am so very grateful to the people who loved and nurtured me as I grew in my personal and professional roles. Bonnie Badenoch, your tender, healing, and loving work ignited my own healing journey. There are no words to convey the magnitude of the contributions you made to my family. With my whole healer's heart, thank you. Jean Watson and Janet Quinn, my beloved and trusted nurse scholars and healers, thank you for your steadfast support as I encountered challenges and missteps. I am forever grateful for all you have done for me and our global nursing community. Terrence Hill, your mentorship and unwavering support of my work continues to inspire me. I appreciate you so, so much! Dr. Mary Ackerley, you are such a gifted visionary, physician, healer, and leader. Your extraordinary commitment to all you serve is beautiful to behold. Thank you for co-founding the International Society for Environmentally Acquired Illness and facilitating healing worldwide.

To my fellow nurses, scholars, scientists, and mentors — thank you for sharing in my scholarly journey. The road traveled was much richer with your friendship, companionship, and support. To my Pima Peeps, Mischala Grill (GOAT biology professor), Zoe Williams, Kelsey Coleman, Kelly Ruhlman, and Nick Densmore — we did the dang thing! Love and gratitude to my MEPN & PhD cohort members and my Wildcat Family at the University of Arizona's College of Nursing. I am so very grateful for the education and mentorship by all and most especially Drs. Leslie Ritter, Lois Loescher, Marylyn McEwen, Kim Shea, Sheila Gephart, Pam Reed, Stacey Nseir, Betty Parisek, and Connie Miller. Wildcats for Life!

A special thank you to the thousands of students I've had the privilege of educating. You are my professional everything. While I know you learned a lot during our time together, be assured that I learned and grew right along with you. Thank you for being my calling, my "why" for teaching. My heart is forever wrapped around yours.

Section I

Healing Is Possible

Introduction

This book was written for you, and it is about you, my most respected colleague, nurse, and healer. I, too, am a nurse. I wrote this book for nurses who have experienced or are experiencing trauma or burnout, or who do not feel safe, seen, heard, supported, and valued in practice. You and I are cut from the same cloth, for we, like all nurses, are healers. This means that we facilitate the healing of those in our care, even when curing isn't likely. As nurses, we are formal, licensed healers, with varying degrees of education and experience. Unique to each of us is our healer's heart. Remember the time when you first knew that you wanted to be a nurse? Can you recall your most fervent desire to help others in their most fragile and vulnerable times? Take a moment to remember and feel your healer's heart — the one that is or once was filled with empathy, compassion, and seemingly endless capacity to care. Can you feel the purity and innocence of your healer's heart before it got "ucked" up by the system? Feel the love, passion, and commitment you had for becoming and being a nurse.

It was your healer's heart and your highly intelligent mind that got you through the grueling prerequisites before you applied to nursing school. Do you remember completing your application, gathering your transcripts, writing a personal statement, taking an entrance exam, or interviewing for a seat — your seat — in a program that would formalize the intentions of your healer's heart? You did that. You persevered through a rigorous nursing school curriculum and clinical rotations. You studied for and passed your licensure exam. And then you both floundered and flourished during your transition into practice. Through grace, hard work, perseverance, and resilience, you grew into the incredible nurse that you are today. All because you answered the call of your healer's heart. You cared beyond

3

measure. It was palpable. But now, that once strong heartbeat and pulse of the healer's heart may be weak and thready. It is so difficult to nurture and protect that healer's heart while practicing in a system that does not. You, like many, may have had your heart crushed, broken, shattered, shredded, or steamrolled by a healthcare system that largely values profit or the spreadsheet over nurse safety and professional wellbeing that is a primary driver of safe, quality patient care.

Your practice and the nursing profession may look and feel different than what you envisioned and hoped for initially. You are a healer with scientific knowledge and clinical skills that are second to none. Your healer's heart must be conflicted as you practice in a healthcare system fraught with inadequacies and competing priorities. You may feel perplexed, overwhelmed, or frustrated by the healthcare system and the limitations it imposes on your ability to provide optimal care for your patients and wholly support your colleagues. Because of these constraints, you may feel like you're in restraints, unable to practice to the full scope of your license. Perhaps you, like me, feel defeated by a system that was not designed to fully facilitate healing and promote wellness but is, rather, a disease management system. Some days, it feels like a poorly crafted game of *Whack a Mole*. Nurses are literally running from one patient to the next, chronically understaffed, under-resourced, overworked, frequently marginalized, and often disenfranchised by a poorly designed system that requires you to *Suck. It. Up. Buttercup.* instead of prioritizing your safety and professional wellbeing, which flows into providing safe, high-quality care with optimal patient outcomes.

Perhaps you find yourself dreading your next tour or shift, knowing that the very best you can hope for is to leave each day thinking, "I did the best I could in a craptastic system." These words and experiences are mortal wounds to the healer's heart. We didn't come all this way — through rigorous education, training, transition to practice, and specialty training — to be experienced nurses who feel defeated by the system before we clock in each day. We do our best, but the system rarely provides the staffing, resources, and support for nurses to practice safely and fully within our professional scope.

You have seen and experienced a lot. Your healer's heart — your spirit — has probably felt broken and devastated on more than one occasion. You've cried in your car after work. You've put your head down on the table, in utter despair and frustration, during your lunch break. You have cared for and suffered along with your patients and their loved ones. You have given so much and asked for so little. You likely have experienced occupational trauma, compassion fatigue, moral distress or injury, resilience challenges, racism, ageism, genderism, secondary traumatic stress, presenteeism, or burnout . . . and the list goes on. You don't want to be hailed as a hero, endure one more free pizza lunch, or receive yet another disingenuous award or acknowledgment. You, like most nurses, want to be seen, heard, understood, valued, and treated like the invaluable professional that you are. You want to practice within the full scope of your license. There shouldn't be a "nursing school way" and a "real-world way" to practice. You shouldn't have your license held over your head when corporate or system demands require you to take more patients than is safe. You shouldn't have to fear a healthcare blame culture in response to seeing nurses be criminalized and punished for missteps secondary to a poorly designed healthcare system — one that often prioritizes financial gains over nurse and patient safety.

My Role as Your Guide and Mentor

Although I may not know you personally, I want you to know that through my role as a nursing scholar, I am listening. I compassionately see and hear you. As an empath and sensitive, I feel you and the suffering you have endured. Informed by all

I learned in my professional roles, I am here with a process and tools to facilitate your healing and support the realization of your goals. I am at the apex of my career, and I am sharing all the knowledge, science, and healing arts wisdom that I've accumulated over a lifetime of study and work.

I didn't start out as a university nursing professor. I, perhaps like you, come from difficult and humble beginnings. My first job, at 14 years old, was cleaning resident bathrooms in a skilled nursing facility. Shortly after my 15th birthday, I earned my certified nursing assistant credential and officially launched my nursing career. During the next three years, before I was old enough to vote, I cared for those experiencing their end-of-life transition. I was so humbled and honored by the privilege of caring for people in their fragility and vulnerability, all while celebrating their life and facilitating their transition with honor and dignity. These formative experiences were sacred. My healer's heart was curated and nurtured during these early years. My ability to see and be with others in these personal ways set the stage for what would become a long and meaningful career. I, like you, have cared for so many people, with compassion, honor, dignity, and respect. I witnessed and experienced miracles with my patients and colleagues.

Sadly, I've also had a front-row seat to the underbelly of the system inadequacies that deprioritize and marginalize the need for nurse safety and professional wellbeing. While performing my professional duties, I've experienced workplace violence by way of my patients or residents. I've been kicked, spat on, backhanded across the face, had my hair pulled, had food, drink, and excrement thrown at me, and have been called every profane word in the book. By a small number of coworkers, I've been bullied, gaslighted, marginalized, disenfranchised, and outright ignored. I'm betting you, too, are among the 44% of nurses who report physical violence and the 68% of nurses who have experienced verbal abuse. Healthcare workers, including nurses, are more likely to be assaulted than police officers or prison guards. Unlike police officers and prison guards, we are not trained to address the magnitude of workplace violence that is visited upon us — nor should we be. Health systems and organizations are responsible for providing occupational safety, and they fall short where nurse safety is concerned.

Perhaps you've also worked in settings where errors, near misses, and sentinel events occur, the vast majority of which are secondary to understaffing, limited resources, or leadership shortcomings. I've seen inequities and injustices visited upon our patients, ourselves, and our colleagues. I've observed rationing of care and unsafe staffing ratios. We've all seen and experienced it. Nurses frequently don't feel safe at work because *nurses are not safe at work*. We have done our best in a system that isn't at its best. These experiences — positive and negative — fueled my desire to be part of the change I wanted to see for myself, my fellow nurses, and the profession. We must shift the healthcare culture to one that prioritizes nurse safety and professional wellbeing. Our patients' safety, outcomes, and quality of care depend upon it.

These experiences inspired me to attain a Ph.D. in nursing so I could take my seat at the "grown-up's table" and make a difference commensurate with my ability to do so. With my role comes additional privileges and responsibilities, such as conducting research, developing and teaching curricula, and contributing to the knowledge and evidence base by publishing in professional journals and professional outlets. In preparation for these roles, this book, and the Haelan Academy & Community, I completed two integrative nursing fellowships. I am among the first faculty members in the US to develop and teach in an integrative, health-focused BSN program. My expertise is centered on nurse traumatization, healing, and integrative nursing. In my clinical practice, I serve as an integrative nurse coach and facilitate my clients in healing through nurse traumatization as they learn how to thrive instead of just survive in their practice. My personal passion centers on the intricacies of healing processes that are situated at the intersection of science and spirituality.

The topics in this book are those that contemporary nurse leader, Florence Nightingale, would hold dear. She lived and worked in a time that did not covet nor celebrate diversity, equity, or inclusion. During the historical context in which Florence lived, colonization, racism, slavery, and systemic oppression of women, indigenous persons, and other groups were prevalent. We are similarly navigating these social injustices today. Like Florence Nightingale, each of us are doing our very best to be a healing light in a world often fraught with darkness.

In Florence Nightingale's passionate plea, which speaks to her profound and earnest desire to improve the conditions in which nurses work, she said that she would "… rather, ten times die in the surf, heralding the way to a new world, than to stand idly on the shore." Her famous quote reflects the call of *my* healer's heart. I've been in the surf for more than a decade, looking for clues and a pathway to guide us from where we are as nurses to where we want to be — feeling safe, supported, and thriving in our practices. I'm simply showing up with my restored healer's heart and a framework to start the healing process, aimed at helping individual nurses who can translate their healing and wellness gains at the workplace. This pathway is intended to be a common healing language and actionable process that can aid us all in reaching our goals. I'm showing up to answer the call of *my* healer's heart. I'm being called to serve as a guide heralding the way to a new world of nursing — one that prioritizes nurse safety and professional wellbeing — lest I, too, stand idly and die on the shore. Within each of us resides the potential to heal, transcend, and come together as a global workforce that ushers in a new era of nursing. I hope you will join me and our like-hearted nurses.

The Road We're On: A Prolonged Nursing Crisis

We all want to do our best for our patients, but we arrive at work each day only to don the straitjacket of the poorly designed healthcare system, with too many patients and too few resources. We are caring for aging patients who are increasingly complex with multiple chronic conditions, and in the US, we have the most expensive healthcare system with the poorest outcomes on the planet. This is another mortal wound to the healer's heart, which my clients describe as feeling "in a bottomless pit" or "in a long tunnel with no light at the end of it." We feel defeated before we even see our first patient each day. We are tired, weary, overworked, traumatized, and burned out. Then, the pandemic landed in full force and profoundly exacerbated the existing healthcare system inadequacies.

The year 2020 was a complicated one in every sense of the word. We celebrated *The International Year of the Nurse and Midwife*, designated by the World Health Organization, to commemorate the 200th birthday of Florence Nightingale. This was intended to be the year where we celebrated the contributions of nurses and midwives to improve global health. It was a time to acknowledge and appreciate the nurse's role while addressing the challenging conditions in which we provide care. For some nurses, these celebrations were meaningful and appreciated. For others, the celebration fell short or was lost amid the pandemic. For most nurses, 2020 was also *The Year of Nurse Traumatization*, and we're still experiencing the ripple effects. We will for decades to come.

Prior to 2020, the world was already short of nearly 6 million nurses. The pandemic shook the world to its foundation in 2020, requiring those who were willing to take stock and redirect their course as needed. In 2021, the International Council of Nurses (ICN) reported that nurses were profoundly experiencing mass complex trauma that has devastating physical, mental, emotional, and existential consequences. The long-term effects

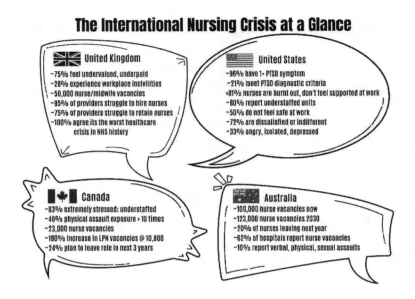

The International Nursing Crisis at a Glance

United Kingdom
- ~75% feel undervalued, underpaid
- ~28% experience workplace incivilities
- ~50,000 nurse/midwife vacancies
- ~95% of providers struggle to hire nurses
- ~75% of providers struggle to retain nurses
- ~100% agree its the worst healthcare crisis in NHS history

United States
- ~96% have 1+ PTSD symptom
- ~21% meet PTSD diagnostic criteria
- >81% nurses are burnt out, don't feel supported at work
- ~80% report understaffed units
- ~50% do not feel safe at work
- ~72% are dissatisfied or indifferent
- ~33% angry, isolated, depressed

Canada
- ~83% extremely stressed; understaffed
- ~46% physical assault exposure > 10 times
- ~23,000 nurse vacancies
- ~190% increase in LPN vacancies @ 10,800
- ~24% plan to leave role in next 3 years

Australia
- ~100,000 nurse vacancies now
- ~123,000 nurse vacancies 2030
- ~20% of nurses leaving next year
- ~62% of hospitals report nurse vacancies
- ~10% report verbal, physical, sexual assaults

of this mass trauma are manifesting now as nurses experience post-traumatic stress disorder (PTSD), depression, anxiety, and chronic physical and mental health challenges. Regardless of geographic location, nurses worldwide are experiencing similar traumas secondary to the systemic issues that persist in healthcare systems. These issues include poorly designed healthcare systems that prohibit nurses from fully practicing within the scope of their license, unmet professional wellbeing resources and supports, limited resources and toxic work cultures, workplace violence, understaffing, presenteeism, attrition, turnover . . . and the list continues. Given these and other factors, it is no wonder that the world is experiencing an international nursing crisis. In the image above, you can see how this crisis is playing out in countries across the world.

Nurses Do Not Necessarily Want to Leave

Nurses don't always want to leave, but they often feel they don't have a choice. According to a recent McKinsey & Co. report, 32% of US nurses are likely to leave their care positions. In

Elsevier Health's *Clinician of the Future* report, 75% of healthcare professionals will leave the profession in the not-too-distant future. The numbers aren't great for student nurses and early career nurses either. A recent study of Generation Z nursing students found that nearly 20% of third- and fourth-semester students are considering leaving the profession within two years of licensure. In addition, about 50% of first-year nurses are seriously thinking about leaving their organizations or the profession.

International healthcare leaders are making the need for healthcare and nursing workforce reforms known. At the 2023 Global Ministerial Summit on Patient Safety, World Health Organization (WHO) Director-General, Dr. Tedros Adhanom Ghebreyesus, proclaimed, "If it's not safe, it's not care." Safety isn't limited to patient safety. It includes safety for all healthcare professionals. Healthcare organizations protect and attempt to grow their bottom line by overworking and under resourcing their nurses. Medical doctor, Joseph Q. Jarvis, and Nurse Practitioner, Kindra Celani, similarly assert, "When nurses are not safe, patients are not safe." ICN President, Dr. Pamela Cipriano, reflected on the perspective of nurses worldwide in this statement, "As a profession, globally, we are asking for help. Because our nurses do not feel valued, they do not feel supported, and we know that over the course of time we need to grow our workforce supply and retain that supply, which is becoming a much more critical aspect when we look at the conditions affecting us right now."

The Great Nurse Resignation is upon us. Nurses are leaving direct care positions or the profession *en masse*. The public mistakenly thinks that nurses are leaving due to the pandemic's lingering impact. While this may be true for *some* nurses, the vast majority are leaving because of the longstanding system inadequacies that were magnified and exacerbated by the pandemic. Nurses across the globe summarize their feelings as

"We are tired, we are burned out, and we feel neglected and forgotten." They state that "Our voices aren't being heard. Our professional needs are not being met. We need consistently safe staffing ratios, as well as the resources and support to practice within our full scope." Nurses are now responding to their longstanding unmet needs with resignation letters.

But not every nurse *wants to leave*. In fact, most want to stay. We invest a lot of time, money, and energy in becoming a nurse, attaining specialties and board certifications, and training the next generation of nurses. We don't want to give up or leave the profession. We want to be safe, seen, heard, valued, and understood. We want a sustainable roadmap, community, and organizational support to attain professional wellbeing and fully engage in a safe nursing practice to the full scope of our license. However, that path can't be seen through the overgrown jungle of system inadequacies, trauma, burnout, and suffering. The point of impact, our individual and collective empowerment is now.

By 2030, the ICN predicts a global shortage of nearly 14 million nurses. This equates to roughly *half* of the current workforce. Imagine going to work and finding only half of your team there. Now project what that could mean for patient and nurse safety, as well as for quality of care and patient outcomes. We're already experiencing trauma, burnout, unsafe staffing ratios, limited resources, and moral injury. Under these conditions and at half-capacity, how are we going to safely care for our patients, let alone attend to our professional wellbeing? Nurses are already stretched to or beyond capacity. We're at the crossroads. Do we choose more of the same, more of being forsaken and sacrificed? Or do we choose the path that leads to healing, safety, and professional wellness? This is, as the idiom goes, where the rubber meets the road. We must choose which road we want to travel. Do we stay on pothole-laden

Traumatized & Burned-Out Alley or turn onto Professional Safety & Wellbeing Lane?

The Road We're Building — Nursing 2.0: Nurse Safety & Professional Wellbeing

Years ago, I traveled through these same crossroads and reached the same point of no return. I made my choice — I chose the road that leads to healing, professional wellbeing, and safety. I am committed to doing my part to guide you in doing the same. It is incumbent upon each of us, as individual nurses, healthcare professionals, and a global workforce, to break the cycle of nurse traumatization, burnout, and moral suffering. We can and must blaze the trail for our own healing. There is no such thing as "trickle down" healing. We must do our own personal and professional healing to partner with the larger efforts being made at the organizational, national, and international levels. We need to take our rightful place at the grown-up's

The Road to Nursing 2.0
The Nurse Safety & Professional Wellbeing Edition

Imagine the Possibilities

Avoidable Clinical Nurse Traumatization

Avoidable Student & Faculty Nurse Traumatization

Avoidable Community Nurse Traumatization

Nurses healing through traumas together

Thriving instead of surviving in practice

table and insist upon policy changes that prioritize nurse safety and professional wellbeing. To shift the nursing paradigm, we must work from our healed scars, together, with a grassroots, bottom-up approach, simultaneously with organizations as they engage in their top-down and other approaches. Sustainable change will emerge when the healing bridge built by us meets the organizational and policy bridges. This is how we partner together and usher in a new era of nursing, which I refer to as *Nursing 2.0: The Nurse Safety and Professional Wellbeing Edition*.

Nurses Do Not Intentionally Eat Their Young

An essential aspect of the healing process is to nurture our nursing students and early career nurses, who are particularly vulnerable to the existing healthcare culture that is embroiled within toxic workplaces and system insufficiencies. Over time, the unhealed compassion fatigue, moral injury, and trauma become embedded within the nursing cultural landscape only to further manifest as legacies of nurse marginalization, oppression, and unhealed-ness. Nurses often unknowingly and subconsciously transfer the unhealed-ness of it all to the next generation of nurses. This is what the phrase *nurses eating their young* describes. But nurses don't *intentionally* eat their young. This is occurring at the subconscious level, as the unhealed-ness that the established nurse experienced is implicitly passed down to the student and early career nurse. The legacies of embodied nurse traumas are *unintentionally* and *unknowingly* transmitted from one generation of nurses to the next. And the cycles of nurse oppression, marginalization, and traumatization continue, as they have done for more than 200 years.

For example, in today's context where a critical nursing shortage persists, students and transition-to-practice nurses are frequently supervised in clinical rotations by preceptor or supervising nurses with less than a year of experience. Nurse preceptors are often early career or mid-career nurses who are experiencing workplace traumatization, distress, and moral injury. My students report being advised by their clinical supervising nurses, with heartfelt compassion, to "get out [of nursing] now while you still can," "run, don't walk, from this profession," and "save your money, get out now." Student nurses are questioning their career choice in their assignments. This additional layer of uncertainty will compound the inherent transition-to-practice challenges that every nurse experiences. Currently, the majority of transition-to-practice and early career nurses face burnout within the first 6-12 months of practice. About half of them will leave their role or the profession.

Heralding Our Way to a New World of Nursing

So, if the tenured nurses are already leaving in droves or are experiencing presenteeism (being there, but unable to fully engage) and the new nurses aren't planning to stay, then we have a perfect storm of epoch proportion fast approaching on the horizon. This is why we can't wait for the system to fix itself. We can't wait for things to improve or go back to the hot mess that was pre-pandemic healthcare. We are at a tipping point. We either grab ourselves, one another, and the profession with both hands and do the immense healing and transformation that is before us, or we will be our own undoing ... by doing nothing. To paraphrase Florence Nightingale's quote, will we take the needed action to herald our way to a new world of nursing? Or will we stand idly and die on the shore?

It is true that nurses experience *unavoidable* occupational suffering that is inherent with the nursing role by caring for others in their most difficult and vulnerable moments. We show up with our whole healer's heart, our skillset, and evidence-based practice to deliver the highest quality of compassionate care. Unfortunately, most nurses experience *avoidable* occupational suffering, burnout, moral injury, compassion fatigue, and complex nurse traumatization. Nurses are telling me, "I just can't" ... and "Make it stop." Because of this, the nursing profession will soon be in an international crisis, which will deleteriously affect patient safety and quality of care. Leaders know that by 2030, the world will be short by nearly 14 million nurses. Much is being written and discussed regarding how to address the challenges surrounding the nurse workforce. All the usual strategies are being touted, such as improvements to work environments, nurse autonomy and recognition, and equitable distribution of resources, as well as fostering interprofessional relationships, redesigning workflow and leadership structures, creating safe nurse-patient staffing ratios and mandates, and rebuilding trust between nurses, administrators, and managers. These are all solid, evidence-informed strategies that absolutely have merit.

What is *also* needed, while the executives and policymakers attempt to correct the systemic issues, is to facilitate the healing of our nurses. We need to address their unmet needs *where and as they are now*. Nurse wellness, professional quality of life, job satisfaction, and retention are at an all-time low. Prioritizing nurse healing and wellbeing makes good sense given that nurses comprise 33–50% of all healthcare personnel. We need integrative approaches to facilitate healing for our weary, overworked, traumatized, or burned-out nurses. We must compassionately and ever so tenderly help one another to heal — heal the nurse within, heal the nurses beside us, and heal the profession. This is what is needed. There isn't time for us to wait for the system to figure itself out. The future of nursing is ours to forge together.

To do this, we must work from our healed scars instead of our open wounds to lead the prioritization of nurse safety and wellbeing. From there, we can heal and begin to thrive instead of just survive in our practices. We can self-empower, individually and collectively. We can answer the collective call of our healer's hearts — to lead ourselves and our patients — toward policies and practices that prioritize health and wellbeing over profit margins and seven-figure compensation packages for the C-suite executives. We must be intentional about bringing forth needed change. Without safe, healthy, well, and thriving nurses who support the foundation of the healthcare system, it will continue to implode.

"Working from our healed scars instead of our open wounds is the point of professional empowerment."

Lorre Laws, PhD RN

Where there are great challenges, there are great opportunities. This is our time, as a global profession, to rise strong and advocate for and insist upon the needed changes to optimize patient and nurse safety, quality of care, and patient outcomes. But how? We start by acknowledging our situation, assessing ourselves, and embarking on the healing process with and for one another. As whole, healthy, and connected nurses and nursing communities, we then partner with employing organizations and professional groups to prioritize nurse safety and wellbeing in the workplace. These are big ideas with lofty goals. But the alternative to self-empowering is to let the system continue to marginalize us into thinking we are nothing more than intervention technicians who are tethered to electronic health records.

The system isn't going to heal and transform nursing. We must do it, or we'll continue to experience trauma, burnout, moral distress and injury, compassion fatigue, lateral violence, turnover, and attrition. We get to choose. I choose healing. I am showing up for myself, my colleagues, and our profession in this way. According to the World Health Organization (WHO), "Achieving health for all will depend on there being sufficient numbers of well-trained and educated, regulated, and **well-supported nurses and midwives**, who receive pay and recognition commensurate with the services and quality of care that they provide." The key word here is "well-supported," which includes ending nurse traumatization and prioritizing nurse safety and professional wellbeing.

And So, Let Us Begin

I am doing my part to answer these calls for help from the ICN and WHO. I want you to know that you're not alone. There is light at the end of the tunnel. You're not stuck or broken in a bottomless pit. I'm climbing down to you with a ladder, flashlight, water, snacks, and an evidence-informed roadmap. I'll guide you from where you are to where you want to be in your professional wellbeing so you can thrive in your practice. I'm going to hold your healer's heart in mine, every step of the way. This book, written from my healer's heart, is a launching point for us to begin the healing process for ourselves, with others, and for our profession. It provides an integrative, whole-person-whole-system approach, strategies, and practices for us to embrace our similarities, celebrate our diversity, and come together as united professionals who stand ready to lead nurse safety and wellbeing efforts for ourselves, our patients, and our profession. This book is not a cure-all, one-size-fits-all, or quick-fix solution. It is a toolkit, grounded in nursing theories and relational neuroscience, that can be used to help you reconnect and rekindle your healer's heart and nursing practice.

This book can aid your recovery and wellness, which I'll call your *haelan* journey. *Haelan* is the Old English word for healing — to make whole, sound, and well. Your *haelan* process is unique unto you. Yet none of us are intended to heal alone, in a silo or cave. You'll also have the opportunity to connect, co-regulate, and heal together with other *Haelan Nurses* within our international, private, virtual *Haelan Academy & Community*. On my website at drlorrelaws.com, you'll find self-nurturing practices and resources to complement those offered in this book.

At the end of this book, you'll find tools and resources that can be shared with your nursing and organizational leaders as a framework to guide the difficult conversations and transitions ahead as we pave the road to prioritizing nurse safety and professional wellbeing. It is one brick in the long path of nursing history. We are at a nursing crossroads. Do we go back to the same-old-same-old patterns that didn't optimally support patients and the nurses who care for them? Or do we come together, in healed solidarity, and lead ourselves into *Nursing 2.0: The Nurse Safety and Professional Wellbeing Edition*? For me, there is no going back. The pandemic pushed us past the point of no return. Together, we must blaze a new trail in partnership with our healthcare organizations and systems. We must transform how the systems regard their nurses. We represent about one-half of the global healthcare workforce. We are the lynchpin of patient care. We can do this. It starts with you. And with me.

My hope is that this book will offer nurse healing and integrative approaches to guide how we can heal and engage in leading these change efforts. I stand ready to partner with you and all nurses as we co-facilitate healing with one another. I offer the teachings within this book from my love for our profession. From my healer's heart to yours, in unconditional love, I trust that you will embrace, modify, or abandon each teaching as best supports your needs, goals, beliefs, and values. I intend for you to have a rich and meaningful nursing practice and life — in whatever form that takes, as defined by you. As your teacher and guide, I gift these teachings to you. They are yours.

The profoundly meaningful relationship between the healer, the teacher, and the learner is eloquently described by Agnes Whistling Elk, as told by author Lynn V. Andrews:

As teachers, " ... we ARE the teaching. We don't stand up at a podium and lecture you about truth. We make you feel and breathe truth, become it. Every book is rewritten by the reader. If you read a book, it becomes your personal teacher. You bring to it what you are."

And so, let us begin.

Chapter 1

Nurse Trauma & Our Healer's Heart

Welcome to the next chapter of your career, where you will learn how to heal through all that has happened since your first day of nursing school to this very moment. I offer my heartfelt congratulations to you for taking this important step to prioritize *your needs, your healing,* and *your career.* If you haven't done so already, please read the Introduction so we all can experience this journey together, from the first word to the last word of this book.

It can be difficult to differentiate between burnout and traumatization symptoms. Most nurses report feeling burned out, but they may not be aware of how nurses are being traumatized in their professional roles, aside from vicarious or secondary trauma. As it turns out, there are several classifications of nurse-specific traumatization that you'll learn about soon. More studies are needed to fully differentiate nurse-specific traumatization from burnout syndrome and how that impacts you across all dimensions of your life. You, like millions of other nurses, may not realize that you have been affected by nurse trauma. You may be attributing what you are experiencing to burnout. The American Association of Colleges of Nursing recommends that we assume that *everyone* has experienced some type of trauma in their lives . . . including nurses. In this book, you'll learn about how nurses are traumatized in their practices and explore if and how you've been affected. Chances are that you've been affected, probably profoundly so.

Whatever you may be feeling, thinking, and embodying, please know these are natural responses to the hardships and traumas that you've endured. Your magnificent and highly evolved nervous system has kept you safe throughout it all. As you'll learn throughout our time together, much of what you're experiencing now is a result of how your nervous system adapted to keep you out of harm's way from your first breath to your current one. As you learn the language of your nervous system, how to navigate it, and how to partner with its wisdom, you'll experience healing in every aspect of your being. This is your safe space in which to feel, heal, co-heal, transcend, and remember or learn how to thrive in your practice and in life — independent of external circumstances and situations. Nurses from every corner of the globe will be with you, in healing support and solidarity. Each nurse brings with them their education, experience, and wisdom. Given the diversity in our worldwide nursing community, let's start with a few key terms to ground and connect everyone before we explore in more detail how your nervous system, thoughts, feelings, and behaviors adapted and responded to the challenging conditions in which you live and work.

Coming Together as a Global Community

Let's go back in time and explore our historical roots as healers — to a time when caregiving was done in the home, long before hospitals and healthcare systems. Back to a time when nursing was an unpaid calling, a familial or community endeavor. Long before nursing was an occupation and then a profession. Let's remember our calling and who we are as nurse-healers. Depending on where and when you attended nursing school, you may or may not have been taught aspects of the bigger picture of nursing, as a philosophy and discipline with deep roots in the healing traditions, arts, and sciences. As Florence Nightingale said, "The role of a nurse is to put her patient in the best position to be able to self-heal." To that I would add, "The role of a nurse is to also put *ourselves* in the best position for self- and co-healing while requiring safe working conditions that foster professional wellbeing."

To facilitate healing for our patients and ourselves, we draw upon the work of Dr. Jean Watson's *Philosophy and Theory of*

Transpersonal Caring and her rich body of work for inspiration and guidance. Just as we draw upon the unitary aspects of our consciousness while caring for our patients and facilitating their healing, we can do the same for ourselves. Together, we can restore our professional health and wellbeing in a holistic manner. As Dr. Watson reminds us, "We, as nurses and health professionals, know that when we step into the theories and philosophy of human caring, we step into a deep ethic of life, that connects us to the heart of our humanity, of healing the whole; it is here in this connection we touch the mystery of inner and outer space, that unites humanity across time and place around the world." It is from this deep connectedness with all of life that the seeds of the healer's heart are sown.

In these challenging times of misinformation, inequities, and social divisiveness, it can be difficult to stay connected to that which unites us all — love, caring, and compassion. Given the global nursing crisis and the need for us to come together as a global workforce to heal and usher in a new era of nursing, we can draw from the wisdom of nurse scholar, Dr. Janet Quinn, whose work profoundly inspired this book. Dr. Quinn describes how we improve patient outcomes by positioning them *in right relationship* for healing at or among one or more levels of the human experience. Similarly, as nurses, we can position ourselves — individually and collectively — *in right relationship* for healing and professional wellbeing. Note that we are not curing or fixing here. We are healing, which is a creative and unpredictable process with outcomes that will be unique to each person while contributing to the collective healing of our profession. Healing is always possible. And the time is now.

Our Shared Healing Terms
Let's start by exploring the word *heal*, which means to make sound or whole. The root word in Old English is *haelan,* or the

condition or state of being *hal*, or whole. For our purposes, we'll use *haelan* to describe the healing process as we move toward wholeness. As nurses who are coming together to lead needed changes, we'll describe this role as being a *Haelan Nurse*, defined as a nurse who, individually and collectively, is engaged in professional healing by reconnecting, regulating, and restoring the healer's heart and our profession to one that prioritizes nurse safety and professional wellbeing.

The healer's heart, your healer's heart, is your "why" — why you became a nurse. It's the beautiful amalgamation or mixture of all the reasons that you entered the nursing profession. Your healer's heart includes all the healers in your lineage, from the beginning of time to now. Within your healer's heart is the ancient healing wisdom and traditions that existed long before western medicine. Before there was medicine, there were healers — and there still are — despite the fact that integrative and complementary approaches aren't valued by a profit-driven system. So, nurses are truly licensed healers. Your healer's heart encompasses everything that has touched and moved you inside. What makes your eyes tear up or your throat thicken in response to another's plight. When your healer's heart is touched by another, every fiber of your being resonates with earnest compassion and a fervent desire to help, to facilitate healing. The healer's heart is what informs the *art of nursing*. Nursing philosophy, theory, and evidence-based practice informs the *science of nursing*. Nursing practice is informed by both the art and science of nursing.

"Haelan Nurse(s)" is the term, consistent with Quinn's healing perspectives, that we use to describe ourselves and the legacy of healers who have gone before us. We all are Haelan Nurses, in varying degrees and by virtue of our shared experience of being wounded and healing throughout life. As a result of our own healing, or the healing of a loved one, we experienced a shift. A spark ignited our healer's heart, and we

Healing-Centered Terms

hal, heal	To make sound or whole.
haelan, healing	The process of becoming *hal*, or whole.
Healer's Heart	Informs the *art of nursing* and the fact that all nurses are licensed healers. Includes all the healers in your lineage, from the beginning of time, before there were healthcare systems, to now. It encompasses everything that has touched and inspired us to become nurses. The healer's heart is our "why," informing why we nurse personally and professionally.
Haelan Nurse	One who, individually and collectively, is engaged in professional healing by reconnecting, regulating, and restoring the healer's heart and our profession to one that prioritizes nurse safety and professional wellbeing.

were called to help others with their healing process. Ultimately, we each answered the call from our healer's heart, which drew us to the prerequisite nursing courses, nursing school, and the profession of nursing. In the table above, you'll find terms that we'll reference often.

Throughout this book, you'll find Slow the Pace Speed Bumps that are designed for you to have an opportunity to pause, take a breath or two, reflect, or engage in a supportive healing practice. It would be a mistake to skip over the speed bumps, for doing so would mean skipping over the opportunity to receive and nurture yourself. And, with that, here's our first speed bump!

Slow the Pace Speed Bump

Reflect upon the terms hal-heal, haelan-healing, healer's heart, and Haelan Nurse. What feelings, sensations, perceptions, or thoughts do these terms conjure up? If you feel inspired to do so, grab a notebook or journal to capture your thoughts. Feeling creative? Use any medium of your choice, including artistic, musical, or nature-inspired ones to expand upon the meaning of these terms to you.

When you're done, settle into a contemplative moment and gently remember the time before you were a nurse. Think about all the people, circumstances, events, and situations that inspired you to become a nurse. Your healer's heart will help to answer these next questions.

What is your "why" for being a nurse?

How do you feel about the possibility of Haelan Nurses practicing in your workplace and around the globe?

As before, jot down or creatively express whatever comes through for you.

Want to connect with other Haelan Nurses? Head over to www.drlorrelaws.com to engage with a community of other like-hearted nurses!

Healing is possible.

Moving from Nurse Gaslighting to Thriving

Self-care has, in most cases, been reduced to a task list of attending to the externals of life: go to the gym, get a massage, buy healthy food, get on the yoga mat, and so on. Very little of what is typically perceived as self-care includes becoming aware of our inner world, attending to our nervous system, or aligning our deepest inner truths with our external world. Millions of nurses feel internally disconnected and stuck in their stress and trauma response patterns. Asking these nurses to just do better with their self-care or resilience development feels like a slap in the face. They *are* doing their very best with the tools at their disposal. What's needed are the right tools to support nurses to thrive despite the massive exposure to nurse-specific trauma they are experiencing every day. We'll discuss more on that topic in the sections below.

I've worked with thousands of students and nurses who consistently share the same response to the overuse and misuse of the terms *self-care* and *resilience*. And by response, I mean very strong feelings about being gaslighted when colleagues and leaders use these terms. For example, nearly every nurse eyerolls, heavy sighs, or otherwise shudders when the terms *self-care* and *resilience* are used in response to legitimate workplace concerns — like being able to hydrate, fuel, and relieve oneself during a shift. Or not being required to care for more patients than is safe and appropriate given the acuity and complexity of care needed. Ineffective or hostile management? Have you or a colleague made your needs known, advocated for better working conditions, or improved leadership only to have been gaslighted? Maybe you were told that it's important for you to engage in self-care or resilience-promoting activities but were not provided relief or opportunity to do so.

Let me be clear: *You are not responsible* for the healthcare system inadequacies that are beyond your purview or control. *You are not responsible* for the hostilities, incivilities, and violence that is inflicted upon you by others. *It is not a personal or professional weakness* or deficit that you need to attend to your most basic physiological needs during a 12+ hour shift. *It's not a personal or professional weakness* to take your earned, paid time-off according to your organization's policies. It is appropriate to defer responding to non-urgent emails or text messages until you're back on duty.

However, it *is* a professional and organizational weakness to gaslight nurses. Gaslighting, also known as institutional betrayal, describes how nurses who convey issues in the workplace are made to feel as though their complaints are insignificant or the issue isn't really happening. Gaslighting behavior creates a workplace culture of cognitive dissonance, doubt, lack of trust, and a deep sense of psychological and emotional damage. Nurse gaslighting can and often results in traumatization. So, to distance ourselves from the self-care, resilience, gaslighting arena, I will not be using those terms in this book or our community.

Our focus, as individuals and communities, is **nurturing, nourishing, and thriving**. Drawing from the work of nurse scholars Mary Ann Nemick, DNS, and Angela S. Prestia, PhD RN, NE-BC, let's explore their definitions for nurturing and nourishment, respectively, which I'll contextualize for us. **Nurturing**, for our purposes, is the process by which individuals and nursing communities engage their feelings, attitudes, behaviors, and substances that stimulate, foster, and support life and professional wellbeing. **Nourishment**, in the context of this book and community, goes beyond simply comforting. Nourishing oneself involves the active or passive act of providing sustenance to every aspect of one's being. Typically, you'll find the term body-mind-spirit used to describe the totality of the human experience, but it is not all encompassing as was once thought. Our goal is to nourish every aspect and dimension of our bodymindessence (defined below), from the mitochondria through the essence of who you are beyond the physical realm.

Bodymindessence is a term I use to expand upon the traditional body-mind-spirit perspective, which does not fully capture the essence of the human lived experience where trauma, healing, and right relationship are concerned. Bodymindessence is an umbrella term that encapsulates the totality of a person's unique and ever-changing lived experience in body (including the physical, etheric, astral, or other body dimensions with which you identify), mind, emotions, spirit, relationships, community, traumas, embodied trauma adaptations, implicit memories, legacies of suffering, and ancestral, generational, cultural, societal, gender, racial, ethnic, patriarchal, colonial abuses and oppressions.

Imagine the unlimited potential and possibilities that could emerge if you nurtured and nourished yourself with the same tender care that you would a newborn, a puppy, a kitten, or a seedling. What if you nourished every aspect of your bodymindessence with life-supporting perceptions, thoughts, decisions, feelings, behaviors, and relationships? Close your eyes, if that is comfortable for you, and take a moment to gently explore the possibilities. In your mind's eye, use your senses to tenderly imagine how you, in bodymindessence, would respond to being so authentically and genuinely nurtured and nourished. Your mind will probably rush in and tell you that it's not possible and that there's no way or no time. Thank your mind for producing whatever thoughts emerge and then release them so they may pass by, like harmless clouds in the sky. Just take a moment to be with yourself and the possibilities of nurturing and nourishing yourself to the fullest, most loving sense of the word.

Congratulations on sowing the very first Thriving-in-Practice-and-in-Life seed. You just had a glimpse of what possibilities await you. Let's add thriving, the ultimate goal, to our healing terms list. **Thriving** describes how we are vital and always open to learning in our personal and professional roles. It is based upon positive experiences, even those that emerge after overcoming adversity or hardship. Thriving is connected with improved health and wellbeing, and it is what many nurses yearn for but feel isn't possible in the current healthcare culture. That's because that viewpoint takes an "outside to inside" approach, whereby one allows external circumstances to dictate their inner health and wellbeing. The first step toward thriving is realizing that you have the power (in the empowerment sense of the word) to heal using an "inside to outside" approach, as you'll do throughout this book. Dr. Janet Quinn wrote about this in 2010, and her message is even more poignant today: "These are such challenging times, and so many people feel disempowered, as though there's nothing they can do, the problems are too big. We've also given away our sense of power, thinking that solutions come from outside of us, for example that 'the healthcare system' will take care of healing." But we can't transcend this sense of disempowerment if we are working from our open wounds (effects of nurse-specific traumatization) instead of healed scars (healing and integrating those traumas). So, we start healing from within and with one another as we move from unhealed and disempowered to empowered Haelan Nurses.

The practices in this book and in our community will give you a new language and approach to nurturing yourself personally and professionally so you can thrive in all dimensions of life. We'll take a deep dive into how we can thrive in practice and in life at the end of the book. For now, take a look at the following table and think about thriving as a state of vitality, openness, and learning that leads to better engagement, commitment, and wellbeing.

My treasured mentor, Dr. Bonnie Badenoch, whose healing work you will learn more about in upcoming chapters, highlights the importance of supporting and nurturing ourselves even when the workplace culture doesn't provide the time, resources, or space to do so. She states, "We are often so eager to support others, while our culture and even the conditions of our practices make it difficult to imagine or seek support for ourselves. We aren't meant to carry suffering alone." Bonnie's words, whether spoken or written, feel like poetry to me. We *aren't* meant to suffer in practice any more than we are meant to do so alone.

This is our time to imagine and seek support for ourselves — to nurture, nourish, heal, and thrive in all aspects of our

More Healing-Centered Terms

Nurture	Process by which individuals and nursing communities engage their feelings, attitudes, behaviors, and substances that stimulate, foster, and support life and professional wellbeing.
Nourish	The active or passive act of providing sustenance to every aspect of one's being or bodymindessence, from the mitochondria to the essence of who you are beyond the physical realm.
Bodymindessence	An umbrella term that encapsulates the totality of a person's unique and ever-changing lived experience in body (including the physical, etheric, astral, or other body dimensions with which you identify), mind, emotions, spirit, relationships, community, traumas, embodied trauma adaptations, implicit memories, legacies of suffering, and ancestral, generational, cultural, societal, gender, racial, ethnic, patriarchal, colonial abuses and oppressions.
Thrive	Describes how we are vital and always open to learning in our personal and professional roles. It is based upon positive experiences, even those that emerge after overcoming adversity or hardship. Thriving is connected to improved health and wellbeing across all dimensions of bodymindessence.

bodymindessence. We aren't waiting for healthcare to "heal us." Given that many healthcare systems are actually disease management systems, it is prudent for us to reclaim our power and leverage the innate potential for healing and wellness that resides within us all.

The Haelan Nursing Process

We all received education and training on how to use the nursing process, a systematic approach to providing client-centered care. Given the shortage of needed resources and high patient-to-nurse ratios, the five-step nursing process isn't optimally translated in practice. It's understandable and unfortunate, and yet here we are. Given our respective roles where this book is concerned, with me as the author/mentor/guide and you as the reader/colleague/client, I've grounded this book in the same nursing process that you learned about in school. As a refresher, the five steps of the nursing process include assessment, diagnosis, planning, implementation, and evaluation.

To ground this book in Quinn's perspectives on healing, I'm using a Haelan Nursing Process, which isn't a clinically-based process but rather a tender educational and self-discovery process where you can explore (assess) how you've been impacted by all that you've experienced (diagnosis). You'll learn about and decide which nurturing and nourishing steps you'd like to take to position yourself *in right relationship* for healing and professional wellbeing (plan). Through the exercises in this book and the Haelan Academy & Community, you'll put those plans into action by using Your Innate Care Plan (implementation). Throughout the book and beyond, you'll evaluate your progress and make any tweaks or adjustments as situations arise. Let's begin this process by exploring how you've been impacted by the stress, burnout, and/or traumatization you've experienced.

Impact to Oneself in the Broadest Sense

Below, in the Bodymindessence Impact Survey, you'll find some words to describe how you might be feeling in the physical, emotional, cognitive, behavioral, and existential dimensions of your bodymindessence. This may awaken some sensations, perceptions, memories, feelings, or thoughts about what you've experienced. If at any time you feel uncomfortable, anxious, or overwhelmed, simply pause and return to the Thriving-in-Practice-and-in-Life seed planting exercise you did earlier (also included below). Whatever you are feeling or experiencing is a natural response to extreme stress or trauma. If it feels like "too much" to take this survey right now, just skip right past it. You'll have an opportunity to explore later in the book. For now, listen to and honor your inner wisdom, knowing that for this survey, there's no score card, no tally, no results. Unlike clinical assessment, you're just gently looking within and considering how your stress, burnout, and/or traumatization has affected you.

Thriving-in-Practice-&-in-Life Seed Planting Exercise

Imagine the unlimited potential and possibilities that could emerge if you nurtured and nourished yourself with the same tender care that you would a newborn, a puppy, a kitten, or a seedling. What if you nourished every aspect of your bodymindessence with life-supporting perceptions, thoughts, decisions, feelings, behaviors, and relationships?

Close your eyes, if that is comfortable for you, and take a moment to gently explore the possibilities. In your mind's eye, use your senses to tenderly imagine how you, in bodymindessence, would respond to being so authentically and genuinely nurtured and nourished. Your mind will probably rush in and tell you that it's not possible and that there's no way or no time.

Thank your mind for producing whatever thoughts emerge and then release them so they may pass by, like harmless clouds in the sky. Just take a moment to be with yourself and the possibilities of nurturing and nourishing yourself, with others, to the fullest, most loving sense of the word.

Healing is possible.

Bodymindessence Impact Survey

Adapted from SAMHSA Trauma Informed Care in Behavioral Health Sciences.

Circle any terms below that describe your response, immediately or after any of the hardships you've endured. Just observe and notice — there's no score card or need to report anything to anyone. This is your safe space to explore your truth and experiences.

It's possible that you may be experiencing different sensations or having different perceptions, feelings, or thoughts after completing the Bodymindessence Impact exercise. If you're feeling unsettled, overwhelmed, or uncomfortable in any way, now is a good time to pause reading, and nurture and nourish yourself. What thoughts or behaviors would support your bodymindessence right now? Do you feel like moving? Then do whatever movement activity feels right for you. Feel like scrolling on your phone? If that's soothing to you, then go ahead. You can also engage your creative muse, your favorite music, or get into nature. If being still and contemplative feels good, engage in whatever practice feels right for now. If you

Bodymindessence: Physical Aspects

Nausea	Significant fatigue	Somatization, including increased focus or worry on bodily aches, pains, and symptoms	Lowered resistance to:
GI upset	Exhaustion		• colds
Sweating	Heightened startle responses		• flu
Shivering	Sleep disturbances		• infections
Lightheaded	Nightmares	Appetite changes	Long-term health effects such as
Faintness	Hyperarousal	Digestion changes	• liver
Shaking	Persistent fatigue		• heart
Muscle tremors	Increased cortisol levels		• autoimmune
Noticeable changes in:			• COPD
• heart rate			• among others
• respiration			
• blood pressure			

Note any additional observations here:

Bodymindessence: Emotional Aspects, Feelings

		Grief reactions	Emotional detachment
Numb	Anxious	Shame	from anything that requires
Detached	Generalized anxiety	Fragile	emotional reactions, such as:
Anxious	Phobias	Vulnerable	• significant, intimate, or family relationships
Severely afraid	Fear of recurrence	Irritable	• conversations about yourself
Guilt	Overwhelmed	Hostile	• discussion of traumatic events
Survivor guilt	Anger	Depressed	• reactions to traumatic events
Exhilaration because you survived	Rage	Mood swings	
	Sad	Disoriented	
	Helpless	In denial	
	Feeling "outside of your body" or otherwise unreal or depersonalized	Out of control	
		Constricted emotionally	

Note any additional observations here:

Bodymindessence: Cognitive Aspects

Concentration challenges	Strong identification with victims	Self-blame	Magical thinking about future trauma
Racing thoughts	Difficulty recalling aspects of an event	Preoccupation with event	Suicidal thinking
Ruminations	Exacerbation of prior trauma	Intrusive memories	In the US call 988
Things happening in slow motion	Belief that feelings or memories are dangerous	Flashbacks	In the UK call 116 123
Time-space distortions		Difficulty making decisions	In Canada call 988
Replaying events repeatedly		Generalization of trauma triggers	In Australia call 131114

Note any additional observations here:

Bodymindessence: Behavioral Aspects

Restlessness	Withdrawn	Increased use of alcohol, drugs, tobacco, or nicotine products	Social relationship disturbances
Startled reactions	Apathetic		Avoiding reminders of event
Sleep disturbances	Avoidant	Engaging in high-risk behaviors	Difficulty expressing myself
Decreased activity	Argumentative		
Appetite disturbances			

Note any additional observations here:

Bodymindessence: Existential Aspects

Intense use of prayer	Disruption of life assumptions	Loss of purpose	Reestablishing priorities
Restoration of faith in the goodness of others	• fairness	Renewed faith	Redefining the meaning of life
Loss of self-efficacy	• safety	Hopelessness	"They never told me it'd be like this."
Increased cynicism	• goodness	Disillusionment	"If I can survive this, I can survive anything."
Despair about humanity	• predictability of life	"I made a mistake about being a nurse."	
"This can't be what nursing is supposed to be, can it?"	Reworking life's assumptions to accommodate the event	Questioning "Why me?"	

Note any additional observations here:

weren't really affected by the Bodymindessence Impact exercise, that's OK, too. Wherever and however you are in this moment is perfect for you. When you're ready to read further, please do so. I'm with you now and through every word in this book!

Haelan Nursing Diagnosis

While I don't know you well enough to offer a personalized nursing diagnosis, I have worked with thousands of students and nurses and can offer a Haelan Nursing Diagnosis for our global nursing profession. In the US, where I practice, we use the North American Nursing Diagnosis Association (NANDA) guidelines to frame nursing diagnoses. Given where we find ourselves now as a nursing profession, my NANDA-ish nursing diagnosis for the nursing profession worldwide is this:

Haelan Nursing Diagnosis: "Disturbance in the performance of the nurse role related to avoidable nurse-specific trauma secondary to healthcare system inadequacies, as evidenced by nurse traumatization, burnout, attrition, presenteeism, and resilience challenges."

Lorre Laws, PhD RN

The Haelan Nursing Diagnosis considers and encompasses all your levels in the Maslow's Hierarchy of Needs. You are a whole person with a rich history and lived experiences. Nothing less than a comprehensive approach to moving from surviving to thriving will do. So, let's take a big picture glance knowing that you'll soon be curating your own innate care plan that will nurture and nourish you. As a super quick refresher, let's explore each of Maslow's levels overleaf, starting at the bottom of the pyramid and moving upward.

Psychological/Physiological level: The energetic, sub- and cellular levels, tissues, organs, and body systems and resources needed to nourish and nurture a person in bodymindessence.

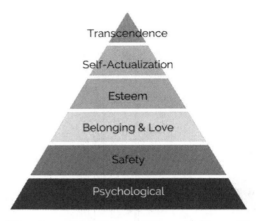

Maslow's Hierarchy of Needs

Safety level: Feeling and being safe and secure in one's environments and contexts, in personal and professional life.

Love and social belonging level: Feeling connected within and with others. Engaged in relationships that nourish, nurture, and support thriving in bodymindessence.

Esteem level: Feeling seen, heard, understood, worthy, accomplished, and respected by self and others.

Cognitive level: Being open, curious, and willing to explore and acquire knowledge, understanding, and meanings.

Aesthetic level: Experiencing balance, serenity, tranquility, meaning, and connection through the objects and systems within our personal and professional spaces.

Self-actualization level: Seeking personal growth opportunities, experiencing and realizing one's personal potential, self-fulfillment, and peak experiences. Living one's highest and best life, as they define it.

Transcendence level: Expanding and moving beyond one's self-conceived boundaries, both inwardly and outwardly where past and future senses of time are integrated into the present.

***

As you move through this book, you will heal, grow, and begin to thrive in all aspects of your bodymindessence and in all of Maslow's levels. We will do so with tender curiosity and great reverence for all you have seen, done, and experienced. Let's take a moment to reflect upon how you think, feel, and experience your personal and professional life right now. Please resist any temptation to skip over this exercise, for you will return to this exercise throughout the book.

Slow the Pace Speed Bump: The Four Questions

Over the years, I've found that two existential questions tend to emerge at this point of the journey which reflect our personal or professional crossroads. Let's take a moment to reflect upon these existential questions. Please note your responses by jotting them down in this book or in your journal or other convenient place so you can refer to them later. Go into as much detail as comfortable. If writing isn't your thing, use any medium of expression that resonates with you.

Two General Questions
1. Am I living life, or is life living me?
2. If life were my teacher, what would it have me learn?

Two Nursing Questions
1. Am I thriving in my practice or being drained by it?
2. If my practice were my teacher, what would it have me learn?

Healing is possible.

Good work in completing The Four Questions Reflection —
you'll be so pleased to see how your answers evolve throughout
this book. It's time for our first case story, where you can
relax while you learn about how other nurses are navigating
their experiences and how this book and practices are helping
them. Throughout the book, I will share case stories, which
are compilations of actual case studies from my practice and
professional experiences. These case stories do not pertain to
any one nurse or client, but rather, they are armchair syntheses
of experiences that nurses have bravely shared with me. I
use pseudonyms to ensure their privacy. I offer my heartfelt
gratitude to the nurses and students I have served over the
decades. As with them, I remain committed to nurturing you,
nourishing you, and facilitating your healing throughout our
time together. Our first case story is one that will resonate with
many of you, for it is the story of a new graduate, transition-
to-practice (TTP) nurse. We've all made that transition. It's a
doozy.

Jordan's Story

Jordan, an incredible young woman in her late 20s, was
referred to me by one of her mentors who had worked with me
during their own transition to practice. Like most TTP nurses,
Jordan was well-prepared to enter practice. Although she was
enthusiastic about beginning her practice, her feelings about
doing so ran the gamut from apprehensive to overwhelmed to
terrified. In her first nursing role, she was being mentored by
an incredible nurse with decades of experience — they worked
well together, and Jordan reported learning so much. She felt
very grateful to have an experienced mentor who really took the
time to train her and help her transition from new graduate to
TTP to early-career nurse.

Transitioning to practice is or was a very vulnerable time
for all of us. As the weeks passed and Jordan's time to practice

without a mentor grew near, she grew apprehensive, as most do. As she recalled in our first session several months later, it felt like she was being pushed off a cliff. And then came the betrayal. In her contract, it was stipulated that she would have "x" number of patients for the first six months, and then she would ramp up to "y" number of patients gradually during the rest of the year. The hiring manager and human resources representative assured Jordan throughout the hiring and onboarding process that they were committed to providing the best possible TTP experience for their new nurses.

But that's not what happened to Jordan. Within two weeks of starting her independent practice, she went from "x" to "y" number of patients — double the promised patient load. Jordan discussed this with her supervisor, who wrung her hands, said there was nothing she could do, and promised to help whenever she could. As Jordan later described it to me, "This is when the bottom fell out of my basket." She described herself as "not a quitter" and was determined to ride it out.

And then the unthinkable happened. On top of twice the number of patients that is prudent and safe for a TTP nurse, the organization required mandatory overtime as several nurses resigned. Jordan's supposed 8-hour shifts, 5 days a week, went to 12 to 14-hour shifts, 6 days per week. She went from a 40-hour workweek to a 78-hour workweek, along with an unsafe nurse-patient load for a new nurse. Jordan rolled up her sleeves and worked as hard and as best she could, but it took a huge toll on her health and wellbeing. Let's sit in on part of Jordan's session with me, so she can share her story with you.

***

Lorre: I'm so glad to meet with you today. You've taken a big step toward improving your situation. I've skimmed your Bodymindessence Impact Survey, and it looks like you have a lot going on. I'd love to hear your thoughts on what you're experiencing.

Jordan: Well, [exhales heavily, then speaks super quick] in a word, I'm burned out. I can't believe I'm burned out after only two months of practice, but I know I am. I have all the signs and symptoms that I learned about in nursing school.

Lorre: Oh, this must be so very difficult for you. Go on . . .

Jordan: [eyes water, a lone tear spilling over and trickling down her cheek] Um, so, I can't eat. I can't drink. I can't sleep. My mind won't turn off. I'm constantly thinking about work, my patients, what I need to do, what I wasn't able to do — I wake up thinking about it several times in the night. I can't sleep more than 1-2 hours at a time. I've lost over 20 pounds in two months, and I'm not trying to lose weight. I haven't exercised or done anything to take care of myself or my

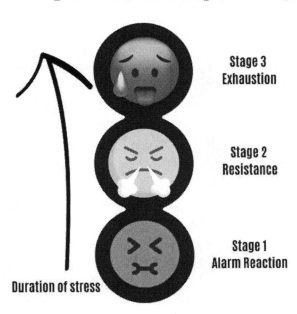

Selye's General Adaptation Syndrome

Stage 3
Exhaustion

Stage 2
Resistance

Stage 1
Alarm Reaction

Duration of stress

house, which is a disgusting mess. I haven't been able to see my kids in weeks. [She lets out a big sob and then quietly cries into the tissue I extend to her.]

Lorre: That's so much to experience in such a short amount of time. I can sense how exhausted, stressed, and burned out you are feeling. Let's unpack what's happening with you together, shall we?

Jordan: [nods while dabbing her eyes with the tissue]

Lorre: I'm not trying to go all nursing-school on you here, but for the sake of getting us together on the same page, do you remember learning about the General Adaptation Syndrome?

Jordan: [nods tentatively] I think so . . .

Lorre: Let's start with this handout to refresh your memory. [passes a clipboard to Jordan, who takes a moment to look it over]

Jordan: [sits upright, shoulders slumping less] Oh yes! I do remember this!

Lorre: Wonderful! Which stage — 1, 2, or 3 — best describes how you're feeling this week?

Jordan: I've been in Stage 3 for weeks now. I'm run down, and I've had two bad colds in two months. All I can do is lay on the couch with a work hangover after work and on my day off. Sometimes I just lay there with a blanket over my head, wanting it all to stop, end, go away . . .

Lorre: What you're experiencing is a very natural response to a very unnatural situation. When we're experiencing this kind of stress, it affects us right down to the mitochondria, which basically get stuck and don't have the capacity to make the ATP you need for energy.

Jordan: Really? How so?

Lorre: Well, you probably *didn't* learn about this in nursing school because this is a relatively new addition to the evidence base. I don't want to overwhelm you with too much information, but it has to do with Dr. Robert Naviaux's work in the field of the biological healing cycle, *salugenesis*. Looking at healing through the mission critical mitochondria functions, various stressors, all the usual suspects such as an acute injury or illness or chronic diseases, profoundly and adversely affect the mitochondria's ability to move through the three phases of healing known as the Cell Danger Response theory, or CDR. It explains how the mitochondria are impeded and can't make the programmatic transitions needed to complete the healing process. When this happens, the mitochondrial-to-organism signaling is impaired. And we don't want that. Our mitochondria are essential for salugenesis and energy production. But they protectively shut down to keep us safe when the stress levels exceed the cellular capacity to maintain homeostasis.

Jordan: [eyebrows raise with curiosity] I had no idea. What kind of stress can do that?

Lorre: Nearly every type of stress, in great excess or over a prolonged period of time, can impact us this way. Anything from biological threats like bacteria, viruses, fungi, or parasites to chemicals, like harmful chemicals in the air, soil, or water.

Cell Danger Response & Mitochondrial Dysfunction

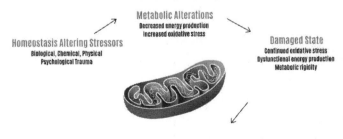

Metabolic Alterations
Decreased energy production
Increased oxidative stress

Homeostasis Altering Stressors
Biological, Chemical, Physical
Psychological Trauma

Damaged State
Continued oxidative stress
Dysfunctional energy production
Metabolic rigidity

Mitochondrial Dysfunction-Related Chronic Conditions

Migraines	Chronic Fatigue Syndrome	Alzheimer's & Parkinson's
Metabolic Syndrome	Cardiovascular disease	Autoimmune Disorders
Fibromyalgia	Autoimmune Disorders	Cancer, Autism, & others

Jordan: Fascinating. What about the kind of stress that I have? This burnout. Can it make my cells shut down?

Lorre: What you are experiencing is also psychological trauma and, yes, it can throw your system out of homeostasis, too, just like the other threats or stressors. If you flip to the next handout on the clipboard, you'll see how CDR works.

Jordan: [takes a moment to read the graphic, then sighs heavily] So, it's not me just being weak. Or lazy. [voice grows thicker as she speaks] Or not being a good nurse.

Lorre: Absolutely, it's not you. Your body is doing exactly what it is supposed to be doing under times of extreme stress. It is protecting you by shutting you down in multiple body systems, like your nervous system, right down to the cellular level and the mitochondria.

Jordan: [takes a deep breath, then exhales slowly in contemplation] Oh my God. I literally thought there was something wrong with me. Like I'm not strong enough or good enough to be a nurse. Everybody keeps telling me, "You need to do your self-care," and I'm like, "I can't even get off the couch." This makes so much sense. Thank you for taking the time to show this to me.

Lorre: It's an honor to help however I can. Your body is doing a brilliant job managing the inordinate amount of stress and psychological trauma you are experiencing. You are having a hard time getting off the couch because your mitochondria have been affected. You're not lazy or a bad nurse. You're a human being experiencing way too much stress and trauma. Your body initially compensated. But then it got overwhelmed because the stress and traumatization were too high, too much, for too long, so it protectively shut you down.

Jordan: I'm glad I met with you sooner rather than later. [glances at the worksheet again] I don't want any part of the chronic conditions that result from mitochondrial dysfunction! You've mentioned psychological trauma a few times. What do you mean by that?

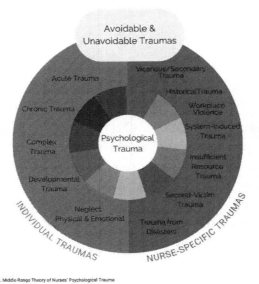

Adapted from Foli (2022). Middle-Range Theory of Nurses' Psychological Trauma

Lorre: [chuckles] We're literally on the same page — that's the next handout on the clipboard! Take a peek and we'll talk through it together. As we do, please put a checkmark next to any of the traumas you've experienced so you can get a big picture view of any traumas you may have experienced.

Avoidable and Unavoidable Trauma

We'll pause Jordan's session here, so I can describe what you're seeing in the image. As humans, we have similar neurobiology with the same cells and cell structures, which can be affected by traumatic events and experiences, as well as psychological trauma that requires healing and recovery. We can take those traumas and look at them from different angles — as individual traumas, such as adverse childhood experiences and other events that are unique to the individual-lived experience, or nurse-specific traumas, such as workplace violence and systemic factors. This is exactly what nurse scholar Dr. Karen Foli did in her *Middle-Range Theory of Nurses' Psychological Trauma* work and what I'm using to guide you through your healing process.

Broadly speaking, trauma is classified as either avoidable or unavoidable. In our profession, many nurses are leaving due to *avoidable traumas*, such as resource challenges, unsafe practice ratios, and toxic workplace environments. Sometimes, by the virtue of our work, there is also *unavoidable trauma* that we experience with our patients. Traumas are further classified as *individual traumas*, which are experienced in our personal lives, and *nurse-specific traumas*, which are experienced in our professional roles. Let's start with *individual traumas*.

Individual Traumas

As people, we are all subjected to traumas. Many, but not all, of which result in traumatization. We can be minimally or profoundly affected by the type, potency, frequency, and duration of the traumas that touch us. When not fully healed or integrated, trauma affects each of us differently across all

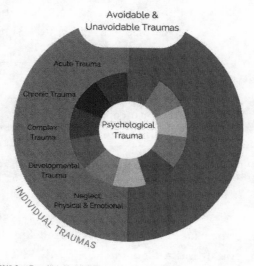

Adapted from Foli (2022). Middle-Range Theory of Nurses' Psychological Trauma

Individual Psychological Trauma

Types of Individual Trauma

Category	Description
Acute	Results from a single incident, such as a major car accident, sexual or physical assault, or a natural disaster.
Chronic	Results from repeated and prolonged distressing events over time, such as domestic violence or abuse or through environmentally acquired sources such as Lyme Disease or unknowingly living in a home with toxic mold.
Complex	Results from prolonged and repeated experiences of multiple types of trauma, often interpersonal in nature, which can lead to feeling trapped.
Developmental	Results from early childhood traumas, adverse childhood events (ACEs), chronic abuse, attachment and other disruptions in the child's significant relationships.
Neglect: physical, emotional	Results from a failure to meet a person's basic needs, including nurturance, affection, personal or medical care.

bodymindessence health and wellness domains. As you are reading about the types of individual traumas that may have touched you, do so with gentle reverence and great care. It might be uncomfortable or difficult reading for some people. Coming up, you'll find a *Slow the Pace Speed Bump*, where you can pause and nurture yourself.

You, like me, may have experienced or are experiencing one or more of these traumas. As we learned with many of our medication administration processes, *low and slow is the way to go*. That sage wisdom also applies to reading this book and becoming acquainted with how you have been touched by trauma. For some readers, it may be uncomfortable or distressing to learn — maybe for the first time — just how many workplace traumas we are exposed to every day. Some are inherent with patient care, and others result from healthcare system inadequacies. Should you notice any discomfort or unpleasant sensations, feelings, or thoughts, it will be helpful to take a break. We'll start this process as we approach a *Slow the Pace Speed Bump*.

Slow the Pace Speed Bump: Pausing to Nurture Yourself
Each of us has different lived experiences and responses to hardship and trauma. This is a great time to reflect and honor any sign that suggests that you might need to take a short break or share your feelings with a Haelan Nurse or trusted loved one.

You may find comfort in doing something that makes you feel safe, secure, and supported in the world. For me, sometimes that looks like making a hot beverage and snuggling a soft blanket while I connect with nature through my window or by sitting outside.

Other times, I need to move my body. I go for a walk, do my yoga or tai chi practice, do a shaking exercise, crank up the music and dance it out — anything goes!

Above all, honor and nurture yourself with compassionate, open, and loving care. Gentle self-inquiry and a willingness to heal is all that's needed.

Healing is happening.

Nurse-Specific Traumas

By virtue of going through nursing school and engaging in your nursing practice, you have already been exposed to various nurse-specific or nurse-patient traumas. Being exposed to these traumas doesn't necessarily mean that you were traumatized. However, many nurses *are* traumatized and may not know it. Many healthcare providers could easily attribute what you are experiencing to anxiety, depression, ADD/ADHD, chronic fatigue syndrome, fibromyalgia, and other conditions. Hence, the importance of learning the language of your nervous system and how to navigate it, which you are beginning to do now and will continue to do throughout this book. We'll continue our survey by discussing the seven types of nurse-specific traumas.

Vicarious or secondary trauma: occurs when witnessing someone else's trauma. In these instances, you're not experiencing the trauma, but you may develop symptoms related to the stress, as well as post-traumatic stress symptoms. For example, military nurses, or those who work with the military or veterans, can experience vicarious or secondary trauma when debriefing and living through the veterans' trauma or as a result of their horrific war experiences.

Workplace violence: can include verbal, written, or physical assault by patients, family members, or colleagues. Nurse-to-nurse lateral violence, disrespectful workplace behaviors, and incivilities can be particularly harmful. There are many work cultures with positive, respectful units where nurses thrive and support each other, as reflected by the terms *work family* or *work fam*. On the other hand, sadly, there are many nurses working in toxic work cultures, where workplace violence manifests as snide or rude comments, sarcastic remarks, gaslighting, favoritism, withholding support, unjust performance reviews, and holding grudges.

Historical or intergenerational trauma: as a professionally oppressed group, nurses experience the legacies of systemic

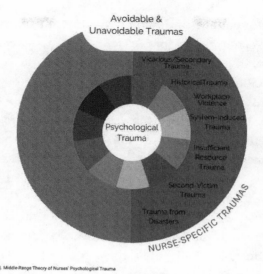

Avoidable &
Unavoidable Traumas

Vicarious/Secondary
Trauma

Historical Trauma

Workplace
Violence

System-induced
Trauma

Psychological
Trauma

Insufficient
Resource
Trauma

Second-Victim
Trauma

Trauma from
Disasters

NURSE-SPECIFIC TRAUMAS

Adapted from Foli (2022). Middle-Range Theory of Nurses' Psychological Trauma

Nurse-Specific Traumas

oppressions regularly. These legacies of historical and intergenerational trauma have been silently passed down through generations of nurses through the patriarchal, cultural, and social practices embedded within healthcare systems. Many nurses are unknowingly transmitting these unhealed, unresolved traumas to other nurses. The expression "Nurses eat their young" speaks to intergenerational professional trauma, which is frequently more substantial among underrepresented and marginalized groups.

System-induced trauma: for our purposes, includes exposure to traumatic healthcare systems or any other system that creates trauma (for example, having to testify in a court of law for a nursing-related situation or responding to a query from your licensure agency). This type of trauma can overlap with vicarious and secondary trauma. System-induced trauma is also known as treatment trauma if one's traumatic stress or traumatic experience occurs in response to a healthcare diagnosis or treatment. For instance, this can happen when caring for a patient undergoing treatment for severe burns, radiation, sexual trauma, or the isolation of patients dying alone in the hospital during the worst of the pandemic.

Insufficient resource trauma: this type of trauma is widespread across all sectors of healthcare delivery. It is a significant root cause of the *avoidable occupational suffering* experienced by nurses worldwide. Insufficient resource trauma describes how nurses are being denied time and/or resources to deliver safe, quality care to the full scope of their license. This type of trauma flies in the face of how we *should* care for patients. Nurses experiencing insufficient resource trauma are at very high risk for second-victim trauma (discussed below). Nurses who are leaving their roles cite insufficient resources such as staffing shortages, high patient-to-nurse ratios, and increasingly complex patients as the top reasons for leaving.

Second-victim trauma: describes how a nurse experiences psychological injury and traumatization after an adverse event or medical or medication administration error, often secondary to insufficient resources or being overworked. This type of trauma can cause major distress, even if the patient isn't harmed. The lingering effects of a medical error are complex and can result psychologically through shame, guilt, grief, anxiety, or depression. Cognitive nurse responses to second-victim trauma include compassion fatigue, burnout, and vicarious or secondary trauma. A host of physical manifestations and *emotional tsunamis* frequently result from second-victim trauma.

Disaster-related trauma: in itself, can represent a major source of distress and nurse-specific strain. Various types of natural disasters and climate-related catastrophes, such as droughts, wildfires, earthquakes, hurricanes, tornadoes, and tsunamis, are happening across the world, and they will only continue to escalate, with nurses there to help — often as first responders, placing them at risk for direct and secondary traumas.

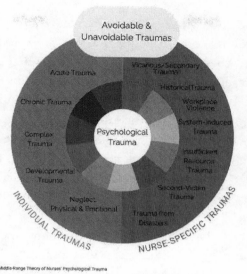

Adapted from Foli (2022). Middle-Range Theory of Nurses' Psychological Trauma

Avoidable & Unavoidable Traumas

Overall, nurses are exposed to many types of workplace traumas, which means a major culture shift needs to happen. As a nursing profession, we must require that we be provided with the resources we need to practice safely and ensure we aren't unnecessarily traumatized while caring for our patients. Ultimately, the nursing profession needs trauma-informed solutions. We simply can't wait for the system to solve this problem, given that (depending upon specialty) 33% to 48% of nurses report PTSD symptoms. Most nurses also experienced a global pandemic, which encompassed every individual and nurse-specific trauma listed above.

Nurse Traumatization: Who's Responsible for What?

Let's pause here for a moment to let all of that sink in. The ways in which nurses are exposed to workplace trauma can be significant and overwhelming. In the blame culture that exists within many healthcare organizations and systems, responsibility for *avoidable* nurse traumatization (workplace violence and incivilities, system-induced trauma, insufficient resource trauma, second-victim trauma) is wrongly attributed to nurses. It goes something like this, "If nurses took better care of themselves . . ." or "We need to provide resources for nurse self-care . . ." or "We should help nurses develop their resilience . . ." as if the healthcare system inadequacies driving the *avoidable* nurse traumatization are the nurses' fault.

Let me be very clear: **You are not responsible for the *avoidable* nurse-specific traumatization that you've experienced.** If your leadership suggests that you are responsible, or that you must have some self-care or resilience deficit, then they are engaging in gaslighting behaviors. **Healthcare organizations and systems are responsible for *avoidable* nurse-specific traumas.**

So, what are you responsible for? You are responsible for self-healing and co-healing with others. You are responsible for your health and wellness. You are responsible for deepening your awareness around how you've been affected by individual

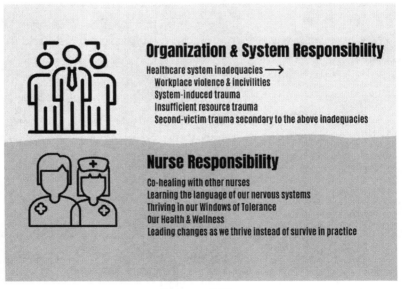

Responsibility

and nurse traumatization. You are responsible for learning the language of your nervous system so you can partner with it as you heal through traumatization and dysregulation and move toward healed, regulated wholeness and thriving in your Window of Tolerance. **You are responsible for you — your health, your wellness.** If, and when, you feel ready and willing to engage in or take a leadership role in shifting the nursing paradigm to *Nursing 2.0: The Nurse Safety and Professional Wellbeing Edition*, you will do so.

The Mass, Complex Trauma That Affected Everyone

The global pandemic added another layer to the avoidable and unavoidable traumas that touched us all in our personal and professional lives. Nobody escaped the pandemic, which brought forth additional layers of trauma for everyone to navigate. Using the pandemic as the shared trauma we experienced together, we'll explore the phases that we went through. You'll return to and work with these phases later in the book. For now, just explore these phases and contemplate

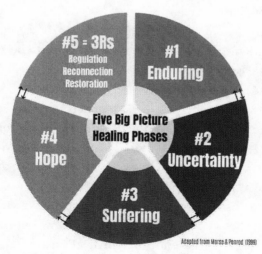

Adapted from Morse & Penrod (1999)

The Five Big Picture Phases of Haelan

if and how you experienced them. Nurse scholars, Janice Morse and Janice Penrod, have described these phases as *enduring, uncertainty, suffering, hope,* and *The Three R's* (originally the reformulated self) of regulation, reconnection, and restoration of the healer's heart and bodymindessence homeostasis.

Phase 1: Enduring

When you were in the initial *enduring* phase of the pandemic, you were likely in a state of disbelief as you tried to determine what to do. Like how to develop strategies to protect yourself from infection and learn how to manage yourself individually and as part of the nursing profession. Your survival instincts kicked in. You experienced a lot in a very short amount of time. Lockdowns. Masks or no masks? If masks, which ones were safest? Where's the PPE? You may have been asked to work outside of your expertise. You may have considered how to work without putting your loved ones in harm's way. In the enduring phase, the collective focus was on making it through the situation while trying to remain in control. For example, people were stockpiling toilet paper and resources in case the distribution channels went down.

Consistent with the enduring phase, there was no real goal other than staying alive and figuring out what to do next. There wasn't a clear and visible route toward that goal yet. Humanity was suspended in a present-oriented state of being. Insert your favorite movie reference here — mine is *Groundhog Day.* People were aware of what was happening, but we couldn't forecast beyond it just yet. We were tethered to our devices and the media. It's all we talked about, which is consistent with the appropriate "motormouth" behavior for this phase. We contemplated all the if/then scenarios. These are all natural responses to adversity or trauma in the enduring phase. As our awareness grew, we began to recognize the enormity of it all, a transitional space before entering the uncertainty phase.

Phase 2: Uncertainty

People then moved into the next phase of *uncertainty* as they realized the enormity of what was happening. Individual and collective goal(s) started to emerge. The first goal was to realize that people couldn't be in lockdown forever, lest our society crumble to irreparable levels. But society didn't yet know how to go about resuming daily life. The goals emerged (people need to get back to daily living), but their routes (how to go about it) did not. People didn't have all the information they needed to fully weigh up the pros and cons. The conflicting messages in the news, public health, and political narratives didn't help. Many felt stuck, suspended, or frozen. This degree of uncertainty can paralyze hope. As people endured, they were in a state of suspended emotions, a hallmark characteristic of this phase. It was like being a track athlete. We were at the starting blocks but didn't know if we were running a 100-yard dash or a marathon. The level of knowing had moved from Phase 1's awareness of the difficult event to Phase 2's acknowledgment of it. Humanity had to navigate the pandemic, even if the needed information to inform the route was not yet clear.

Phase 3: Suffering

Over time, as the layers of Phase 2's uncertainty mounted, the allostatic load exceeded people's capacity to manage — an expected process that leads to Phase 3's active *suffering*. This is experienced as an emotional tsunami where normal stress management techniques no longer work. In Phase 3, the suspended state of emotions from Phases 1 and 2 come crashing down like a tsunami wave. This is the most emotional of the phases and the one where most people need additional and/or professional support.

During this phase, people understood that the pandemic was happening and that it was real. This acknowledgment impacted how they perceived the past and their uninvited, indelibly changed future. Feeling emotionally overwhelmed by the magnitude of the pandemic, many of the goals set in Phase 2 got obliterated by Phase 3's emotional tsunami of suffering. People described Phase 3 as feeling like they were drowning, stuck in quicksand, at the bottom of a dark pit, or in a long tunnel with no light at the end. Many felt buffeted by the event, like the hits just kept coming, over and over again. Every time they'd stand up and start moving forward, they'd get bowled over by another wave of the emotional tsunami. It's hard to see it at the time, but Phase 3's suffering and tsunamis are actually processes of deep repair.

Phase 4: Hope

Through the process of suffering, which is also a process of repair, reality begins to seep in, and there's a glimpse of a new future. During the pandemic, individually and collectively, people started to see beyond their despair and sought to commiserate with others. As the new reality of a prolonged pandemic was pieced together, people grew increasingly focused. The perception of time progressed from the past (from before the onset of the pandemic) to the present (emotional tsunami and suffering) to the future (hope-informed goals and their routes emerging). During Phase 4, many people moved toward perceiving a hopeful future, while others returned to Phase 1, 2 or 3. It's a dynamic, non-linear process that is unique to every individual — just as a cancer patient experiences these phases after receiving a diagnosis. Two steps forward, three steps back is a very natural rhythm for some, while for others a lightning round once through each phase is *their* natural rhythm. This journey is not a one-size-fits-all process. Some people are not well-equipped to do the emotional work of suffering. This is where we, as nurses, facilitate healing.

Over time, Phase 4's hope leads to a deeper level of acceptance. With this fuller acceptance, people more deeply realize the significance of the difficult events of their past, their altered present, and their irrevocably changed future. Hope is an expectation with a nonspecific outcome where emotions are consciously held in check while bracing for negative outcomes. People hold their hope and future plans in balance while also attempting to mitigate negative outcomes.

In addition, people realistically evaluate personal and external resources and strive to form supportive relationships with those who are similarly aligned. These relationships are extensions of the social commiseration experienced in the earlier phases. They are bolstering and reinforcing each other's hope. As they move beyond the catastrophe of the initial difficult event, they emerge from suffering and are firmly rooted in hope. People continually monitor for evidence, signs, signals, or feedback that signifies that the route chosen is the right one. They adapt and pivot as needed, coming to understand that they have become wiser people with an expanded appreciation of life. At the end of the hope phase is a renewed perspective on life.

Phase 5: The 3 R's

The 3 R's, as you'll soon learn, make up part of the formula guiding Your Innate Care Plan: *Regulation* in your nervous system, *Reconnection* within and with others, and *Restoration* of bodymindessence homeostasis and your healer's heart. From this more healed perspective, you'll grow wiser. You'll have accepted the past, endured, and transcended uncertainty. You'll come to understand that while you suffered, you also experienced a profound process of repair. You'll find acceptance and hope. You'll be ready to be open to the uninvited future before you and live it fully. You'll have shifted from a state of inner turmoil, brokenness, or disconnection to a more connected, whole, and healthy self.

Chapter Wrap-Up

This was an important first chapter in which you came together as a global nursing community. You learned about important terms like hal, heal, haelan, healing, your healer's heart, and what it means to be a Haelan Nurse. You learned how, in this book, we're moving away from the frequently misused terms of "self-care" and "resilience" so we can embrace nurturing, nourishing, and thriving in our wholeness — in bodymindessence. You explored how you have been affected by the stress, burnout, and traumatization you've experienced. Through Jordan's story, you reconnected with that time when you were a TTP nurse. You refreshed your memory or learned new information regarding the GAS and CDR theory and discovered how you may be at risk for mitochondrial dysfunction and its related manifestations. Importantly, you learned about the individual traumas that can affect anyone, along with the avoidable and unavoidable nurse-specific traumas that can additionally affect you in your professional role. As you reflected upon the pandemic, you learned about the Five Phases through which everyone travels on their healing journey: Phase 1 Enduring, Phase 2 Uncertainty, Phase 3 Suffering, Phase 4 Hope, and Phase 5 The 3R's of regulation, reconnection, and restoration.

You did it! Congratulations! That was a lot to take in, and you're now prepared to learn how to partner with the wisdom of your nervous system — the system that is ever vigilant in keeping us safe and protected. You'll learn the language of your nervous system and how to navigate it. This will inform how you, by engaging with this book, will curate Your Innate Care Plan to ensure you thrive in practice and in life. At the end of each chapter, you'll find Haelan Nurse Activities where you'll personalize and enrich your reading and healing experiences. For those interested in taking a deeper dive into the topics discussed, you'll find Deeper Dive Resources at the end of each chapter and on my website at drlorrelaws.com.

Haelan Nurse Activities

Activity #1: Expanding Upon the Four Questions

Expand on the four questions that you may have reflected upon, journaled about, or creatively expressed around earlier:

Two General Questions

1. Am I living life, or is life living me?
2. If life were my teacher, what would it have me learn?

Two Nursing Questions

1. Am I thriving in my practice or being drained by it?
2. If my practice were my teacher, what would it have me learn?

Then, consider these follow-up questions to each response above:

1. Independent of circumstances and the influence of others, what does my healer's heart need for me to be, know, do, or change?
2. If I had a magic wand, how would I use it to improve my situation, feeling, or experience?

Activity #2: Your Journey to the 3 Rs

Reflect upon a time that you were presented with a hardship or traumatic experience. Notice any perceptions, sensations, or thoughts that emerge and pause at any time to soothe and nurture yourself. You've been through so much. You survived it all. Now is the time to be soft, gentle, and tender with yourself. After you've completed your reflection below, share your experience with trusted loved ones and other Haelan Nurses. No one heals in a silo, all alone. We are hardwired to co-heal with others. Let your story and your truth be seen, heard, supported, and nurtured.

Haelan Phases Activity

My journey was that time when ...

Phase of the Journey	Phase characteristics	What I/we sensed, felt, or experienced
Enduring	Awareness Holding on Present-focused Deer in headlights No goals No route to goals	
Uncertainty	Recognition Beginning to comprehend Need more information Goals emerge No routes to goal yet	
Suffering	Acknowledgement Emotional tsunami Overwhelms goals No route to goals Stuck, broken, drowning Process of repair	
Hope	Acceptance Future-oriented Goals and their routes emerge Holding emotions in check Bracing for negative outcomes Commiserating with others	

Reformulated Self as the 3Rs: regulation reconnection and restoration	Wiser, "better person" because of the experience
	More inner connectedness than disconnectedness
	Realizing gains from healing work completed in the preceding phases

Deeper Dive Resources

Conti-O'Hare, M. (2002). *The nurse as wounded healer: From trauma to transcendence.* Jones & Bartlett Learning.

Foli, K. J. (2022). "A middle-range theory of nurses' psychological trauma" in *Advances in Nursing Science,* 45(1), pp.86-98. https://doi.org/10.1097/ANS.0000000000000388.

Page, R. L., Peltzer, J. N., Burdette, A. M., & Hill, T. D. (2020). "Religiosity and health: A holistic biopsychosocial perspective" in *Journal of Holistic Nursing,* 38(1), pp.89-101. https://doi.org/10.1177/0898010118783502.

Quinn, J. F. (n.d.). *Quinn, on healing.* Saint Anselm College. https://www.anselm.edu/sites/default/files/Documents/Academics/Department/Nursing%20Cont%20Education/Handouts/6Healing_Quinn's_model.pdf.

Sitzman, K., & Watson, J. (2014). *Caring science, mindful practice.* Springer Publishing Company.

Chapter 2

Our Brains & Trauma

Now knowing that healing, *haelan,* is to make whole or move toward healing, it's important to consider healing in the context of trauma and how our nervous system responds and adapts. As nurses who live in various continents and countries, we experience(d) heterogeneity in our nursing school curricula. It's possible that we didn't learn about or have long since forgotten about these topics: (a) recent advances in neuroscience and transpersonal neurobiology; (b) how we transform, self-regulate, co-regulate, and shape the development of our nervous systems *with one another;* (c) trauma-informed self-nurturance and nourishment in bodymindessence, and; (d) how our parents' attachment patterns tend to influence our own attachment styles, thereby propagating legacies of disruptive attachment patterns.

Given the differences in our educational and practice backgrounds, it seems prudent to review nurse trauma through the lens of Drs. Bonnie Badenoch, Daniel J. Siegel, Gabor Mate, Stephen Porges, Bessel Van Der Kolk, Bruce D. Perry, Peter A. Levine, and other trauma and neuroscience experts. Although all nurses are educated and trained regarding the anatomy, physiology, and pathophysiology of the nervous system, not all nurses are trauma-informed nurses and fewer still know how to translate that knowledge into the foundation of self-nurturing practices. Over the course of millions of years, something like 500 million years, your brain and nervous system evolved into the intricate system that governs nearly everything, including your physical safety. The brain and nervous system embody wisdom that transcends what the mind can fully conceive. It makes good sense to partner with the wisdom of your brain and nervous system instead of fighting against it. So, in a very simplified manner, I'll walk you through the highlights, knowing that for some of you it will be a review. For others, it will be new information. For all of us, it's an opportunity to come together as a trauma-informed, healing-centric nursing profession as we discover how we've been affected by trauma and how we can facilitate our healing with one another.

Your Brain & Trauma

As we unpack how your brain, nervous system and other bodily systems are affected by trauma, I'll use basic language. The reason for this is two-fold: (1) nurses from all parts of the world are coming together with different educational backgrounds, and (2) as you'll see in the sections ahead, it is important for you to stay as balanced in a whole brain state as possible. I can support you in this by not going into full-throttle physiology in these sections, though we're all very capable to do so. That said, let's start by using Dr. Dan Siegel's Hand Model of the Brain and Dr. Annie Hopper's framework for the limbic system's structures and abbreviated functions.

If you bend your elbow so your fingers point upwards, and make a relaxed fist with your thumb tucked under your fingers, as shown in the image below, you can visualize how your brain functions when it's in a regulated state. Your forearm represents the spinal cord, your wrist represents the brain stem, and your thumb is the amygdala, which is connected to your palm, which represents the other limbic system structures. The lower two-thirds of your fingers represent the cerebral cortex while the tips of your fingers represent the prefrontal cortex.

Siegel's Hand Model of the Brain

Now, to make sure you're not feeling like you're in nursing school again (!), let's refresh your memory regarding the brain structures and their functions in an abbreviated manner.

Hand Model of the Brain

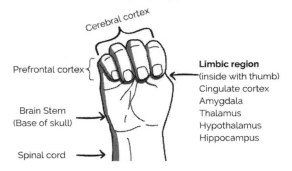

The **brainstem** is responsible for autonomic functions, such as breathing, heart rate, balance, reflexes, and appetite, among others. It initiates the fight-or-flight response during times of real or perceived danger. The **limbic system** is involved with sensory, emotional, and behavioral survival responses. There are many roles performed by the limbic system components, which Dr. Hopper describes as (a) **The Director**: the cingulate cortex calls the shots; (b) **The Reactor**: the amygdala responds to real or perceived threats; (c) **The Messenger**: the thalamus is a command central clearinghouse for the body's information system; (d) **The Chemist**: the hypothalamus is in charge of homeostasis and profoundly influences the endocrine system's release of DOSE hormones during times of safety (dopamine, oxytocin, serotonin, endorphins) or CAN hormones when safety is threatened (cortisol, adrenaline, norepinephrine); and (e) **The Memory Keeper**: the hippocampus drives learning and memory processes. The rest of the hand model structures are the **prefrontal cortex**, which is the chief in charge of thinking and decision making, along with the **cerebral cortex**, which governs complex functions such as thinking, reasoning, emotions, and language.

Thinking about the Hand Model of the Brain using an upstairs and downstairs approach, as shown in the next image, the upstairs brain would include the frontal and prefrontal

Abbreviated Brain Structures and General Functions

Structures	General Functions
Brainstem	Autonomic functions such as breathing, heart rate, balance, reflexes, appetite, among others. Initiates fight or flight response during times of real or perceived danger.
Limbic System	Involved with sensory, emotional and behavioral survival responses. Limbic System structures and functions: Director: Cingulate cortex Reactor: Amygdala Messenger: Thalamus Chemist: Hypothalamus Memory Keeper: Hippocampus
Prefrontal cortex	Executive thinking and decision making. This part of your brain is in the driver's seat until there's a threat (real, perceived, past, or present) that activates the limbic system, which then gets into the driver's seat to address the threat.
Cerebral cortex	Complex functions — language, reasoning, thought, emotions, memory.

Hand model of the brain adapted from Siegel (2010); Limbic system structures and functions adapted from Hopper (2014).

cortices and the downstairs brain would include the limbic system and brainstem.

To highlight the relationship between the upstairs and downstairs brains, imagine a time when you were much, much younger. Imagine that you stubbed your big toe on the nightstand badly. Like, it took your breath away. You doubled over in pain, and it hurt for weeks afterwards. You recovered from the experience and moved on while your hippocampus, the memory keeper, retained that information in the archives for future reference.

Upstairs & Downstairs Brains

Fast forward to a few years later when you clumsily *almost* stub your toe again. This time, your Threat Detector (Chief in Charge of Neuroception, who you'll meet in the next sections) and cingulate cortex engaged and your amygdala, the reactor, came to your rescue. Then, the hypothalamus signaled for the release of cortisol so you could use the fight-or-flight response to get away from that potential threat as quickly as possible. The downstairs brain did its job brilliantly, all faster than you could blink your eyes.

It was then time for the upstairs brain to do its job. The cortex, or thinking brain, assessed the situation. The prefrontal cortex did the deeper analysis to determine whether the downstairs brain's signal of threat and the corresponding physiological and emotional responses were warranted. If they were, you would have completed the fight-or-flight sequence. If not, you would have quickly returned to your pre-nightstand state. Your

Upstairs & Downstairs Brains

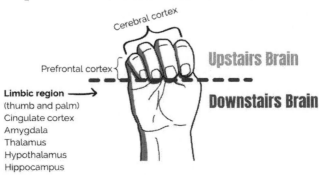

Cerebral cortex

Prefrontal cortex

Limbic region ⟶
(thumb and palm)
Cingulate cortex
Amygdala
Thalamus
Hypothalamus
Hippocampus

Upstairs Brain

Downstairs Brain

upstairs and downstairs brains, in this example, collaborated effectively.

But the upstairs and downstairs brains don't always collaborate effectively. For example, let's say that you — like most people — experienced very early childhood attachment disruptions. Or that you experienced early childhood trauma, chronic or toxic stress experiences, and/or any number of the individual traumas — the unintegrated aspects of which were stored in the body and mind over time. These artifacts can, and often do, impede effective collaboration between the upstairs and downstairs brains. Trauma overwhelms or blocks access to the upstairs brain. The staircase that ordinarily connects the upstairs and downstairs brains is not accessible. The upstairs and downstairs brains are temporarily disconnected, rendering the upstairs brain offline. In short, the upstairs brain "flips its lid," as shown in the image below:

The Upstairs Brain Flips Its Lid
When the upstairs brain flips its lid, your upstairs brain is no longer in the driver's seat. This means that your ability to

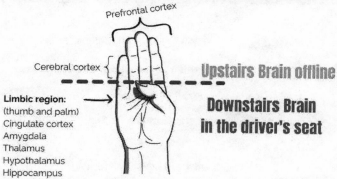

Disconnected
Upstairs & Downstairs Brains

Prefrontal cortex

Cerebral cortex

Upstairs Brain offline

Limbic region:
(thumb and palm)
Cingulate cortex
Amygdala
Thalamus
Hypothalamus
Hippocampus

Downstairs Brain
in the driver's seat

assess and evaluate the real or perceived threat through the higher-level brain centers goes temporarily offline. Therefore, the limbic system is promoted to the driver's seat for the time being. The limbic system is running amuck and isn't governed by the upstairs brain — the one in charge of deeper analysis and modulated emotions, thoughts, and behaviors. You can't be as effective with your communication, control, or emotions. Logic and reason are lost on you now. The limbic system can't hear or respond to any of it until the upstairs brain comes back. It feels like you've got a front row seat on the Hot Mess Express.

Although it may feel and look like you're on the Hot Mess Express, it is important to note that when the upstairs brain flips its lid, *it is not a conscious choice or decision.* You're not stuck. You're not broken. You are adaptive. What you are experiencing is an adaptive response from your highly evolved nervous and limbic systems, contextualized and informed by the entirety of your lived experiences. So, if you've ever felt embarrassed, ashamed, or any kind of way, please extend a lot of grace, compassion, forgiveness, and nurturance to yourself. Your limbic system was in the driver's seat for a bit. It's a perfectly natural response

Flipping Our Lid is Not a
Conscious Choice – It's an Adaptation

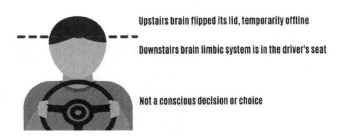

Upstairs brain flipped its lid, temporarily offline

Downstairs brain limbic system is in the driver's seat

Not a conscious decision or choice

We are not stuck. We are not broken. We are adaptive.
We just need to learn the language of and how to navigate our nervous systems.

that happens to everyone. Now that you have completed the refresher about how your brain operates during times of real or perceived danger, let's explore how your nervous system is involved in this process so you can understand in more detail how these adaptations and responses work.

The Hemispheres and Their Collaborative Worldviews

How our brain develops in early childhood is a complex topic where trauma is concerned. Drawing from the work of Dr. Iain McGilchrist, let's quickly explore how the two hemispheres of our brain work together. The following explanation covers an extremely abbreviated overview of an extraordinarily complex topic. For those interested in taking a deeper dive, please enjoy Dr. McGilchrist's book, which is referenced at the end of the chapter.

Ideally, the skull brain's left and right hemispheres collaborate with each other so we can fully integrate the feels and our lived experiences, including traumas. Contrary to what you may have learned in nursing school, scientists are reporting that both hemispheres *fire together* via a complex wiring diagram known as a connectome. But the right and left hemispheres view the world differently while collaborating in an integrated balance, as shown in the corresponding image.

The Right Hemisphere

The right hemisphere (RH) worldview values our uniqueness as individuals and the subjective, "juicy" stuff. The RH uses emotions and intuition. It thinks simultaneously and freely in pictures. It is the hemisphere that sees the bigger picture, our contexts, our relationships, and the complexity of our nonlinear world. It helps us to relate to the world around us and understand it as a whole. The RH takes in new information, including unhealed bits of wisdom, and has tremendous capacity for mindfulness and present moment connection. This

Hemispheric World Views

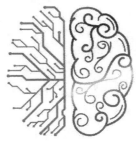

Left Hemisphere

Logic, reason
Thinks in words
Ordered, sequential
Non-emotional

Right Hemisphere

Emotion, intuition
Thinks in pictures
Deals in wholes
Relationships

is the hemisphere of relationship vibes. The RH is an open, highly receptive space that is foundational to and essential for a positive relational life. It is not concerned with tasks or judgements, logic or reason. It's all about the juicy, subjective feels — in no structured order. The RH is where much of the hardwiring and processing occurs to maintain the social relationships that are integral to our survival. When it gets wounded or traumatized, it impedes the process.

The Left Hemisphere

The left hemisphere (LH) is also essential, and its worldview values logic, reason, and constructing a story, process, or system from the subjective, juicy RH information. It thinks in words and deals with the parts rather than the whole. It identifies with the individual versus the RH's identification with the group. The LH's primary objective is to manipulate things — to bring order and create systems from the information garnered from the RH. Without the stabilizing nature of the LH, we'd live in the fluid, unstructured RH information in a state of utter disarray and chaos.

The LH isn't concerned with the juicy feels of the subjective realm. It values tasks, behaviors, judgments, goals, success, knowledge, accomplishments, and non-feeling outcomes. The LH filters out all the relational aspects of the information it

Right & Left Hemisphere Collaboration

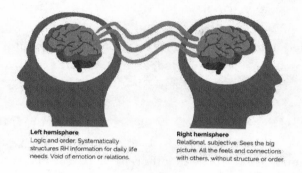

Left hemisphere
Logic and order. Systematically structures RH information for daily life needs. Void of emotion or relations.

Right hemisphere
Relational, subjective. Sees the big picture. All the feels and connections with others, without structure or order.

receives, rendering the juicy, feeling, relational information dead on arrival. The LH is the depersonalized, "either-or" judgment hemisphere that always wants more — more knowledge, more goals, more success, more accomplishments. There is no relational "we" experience in the LH. This can be a very sad thing for people who are left-shifted in their hemispheric collaboration.

Now that you're acquainted with the hemispheres, it's important to note that the LH is not "superior" to the RH. This outdated view of the role of the hemispheres has been replaced by the importance of both hemispheres firing together harmoniously. If anything, through the lens of Dr. McGilchrist's work, the RH is naturally the "master," while the LH — in all its indispensable glory — is really an emissary or diplomat in service to the RH. To function optimally, we need the RH master and the LH emissary to seamlessly integrate and collaborate with each other.

I like to use a puzzle analogy to describe the relationship between the RH and LH. The RH is all the puzzle pieces — in different shapes, sizes, and colors — that come out of the puzzle box in no particular order. The LH organizes the heap of jumbled RH puzzle pieces into piles, with one for the puzzle border and the other piles organized by color or theme. Then, through organizing the patterns and using logic and reason, the puzzle comes together. Without the puzzle pieces in their various shapes, colors, and sizes from the RH, there would be no puzzle. Similarly, without the LH, there'd never be a completed puzzle because we'd never be able to put it together. Both hemispheres are needed, as are their differing worldviews. Integration is key for LH and RH collaboration.

Disruptions to Hemispheric Collaboration

Trauma of all types, ACEs, disrupted early childhood attachment systems, and other hardships can interfere with your right-left hemispheric collaboration. Current trauma or past unintegrated trauma emerges first through the RH and right limbic system. Depending upon a myriad of factors, it is possible and sometimes likely that the RH will get wounded in the process. When your RH is wounded, you adapt by shifting further into the LH. By doing so, your hemispheres no longer collaborate effectively.

When your hemispheres aren't able to collaborate optimally, it feels like an inner split or tug-of-war. It feels like you're split into parts such as the RH, LH, and RH-associated bodily neural streams and circuits. It goes something like this: The Threat Detector picks up a cue in your inner or outer environment

Trauma Disrupts Hemispheric Collaboration

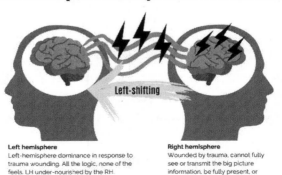

Left hemisphere
Left-hemisphere dominance in response to trauma wounding. All the logic, none of the feels. LH under-nourished by the RH.

Right hemisphere
Wounded by trauma, cannot fully see or transmit the big picture information, be fully present, or make good connections with others.

that is perceived as a potential or real threat. As part of its 24/7 surveillance protocol, it cross-checks the stimuli with everything in Your Repository (the meta database where every lived experience is stored — you'll learn more below), including your unintegrated traumas, which are stored within your body's neural circuits and connected to your eyes, ears, nose, skin, muscles, gut, heart, and others. When unintegrated traumas emerge, they move up through the RH circuit. Depending upon how your nervous system adapted to prior trauma, it could cause your upstairs brain to flip its lid and the limbic system to run unchecked. Or, you may have wounds in the RH itself as a result of prior trauma, thereby thwarting RH-LH collaboration.

Under ideal circumstances, the seemingly opposing needs of the hemispheres work in harmony together. The RH wants connection, subjectivity, and relationship with others. The LH wants a depersonalized sense of order, structure, and process. So how do these two seemingly opposing hemispheres work together? By using an iterative right-left-right hemispheric collaboration process. I use the analogy of putting new laces into my shoes. I insert one lace into the right hole, another into the left. If the integration between the right and left shoelaces stopped there, my foot wouldn't be in that shoe after the first step. So, I continue lacing — the right to the left, the left to the right, and so forth until my shoelaces are fully integrated with the shoe. From our nervous system's point of view, this right-left-right iterative and ongoing conversation between our hemispheres brings hemispheric stability, thereby enriching our lived experiences.

Left-Shift Adaptation to Trauma

But this right-left-right collaboration isn't always possible in the wake of trauma. In response to the traumas you are exposed to personally and professionally, you further adapt by protecting the sensitive RH by desensitizing. RH desensitization means shifting away from the "feels" of the RH toward the depersonalized, distant, and analytical LH. As with the other circuits and their hybrid responses, this is not a conscious choice, but rather an adaptive response. Presented with trauma that exceeded your ability to manage internally and relationally, your RH adapted for the purpose of emotional survival. By virtue of this shift to the LH, you can be pulled away from the RH's capacity for giving and receiving connection, compassion, and relations. This adaptive RH response has potential to further traumatize as the sense of connection within and with others takes its toll over time. It's how you can sit among your most treasured loved ones and still feel utterly alone. That's how left-shiftedness feels.

Left-Shiftedness Is a Societal Adaptation

Scientists have reported that most of us — about 75% — have become left-shifted in our hemispheres since the industrial age. This is compounded by the overwhelming amount of information that we must process in modern society. As our inner and outer experiences become increasingly unmanageable in response to all that we have and continue to experience, we collectively and adaptively shift to LH dominance. As we move from the RH to the LH, our relational capacities and needs go partially or largely unmet. We feel cut off from ourselves and others. We long for a felt sense of connection that seems just out of our reach in the context of our unhealed traumas. We long for happiness and meaning beyond what the LH values in terms of recognition, accomplishment, and success.

Evidence of societal left-shifting is evident across many dimensions, including recent studies that examined accelerated declines in empathetic capacity and a corresponding rise in narcissism. We see evidence of left-shifting in healthcare systems, with algorithm-driven healthcare, fee-for-service health systems, fiscal outcomes that are preferred to whole-person healing, spreadsheets that emphasize bottom lines, and policies that stretch nurses to or beyond capacity.

Nowhere in these left-shifted processes do we find the RH value for relational aspects of nursing, caring, healing traditions, and patterns of knowing that are central to positioning our patients *in right relationship* for healing. The system is focused on how many patients you can take, how quickly and efficiently you can attend to their needs, and how many interventions or medications you can administer. Patients enter the healthcare system with legitimate needs to connect and have a meaningful relationship with their nurses, in service to their healing. But our left-shifted healthcare culture can't see past LH values of logic, productivity, and success. We find ourselves on a slippery slope, which will likely be compounded by artificial intelligence challenges in the decades to come.

As Dr. McGilchrist reminds us, "Einstein said that the rational mind (LH) is a faithful servant, but the intuitive mind (RH) is a precious gift . . . we live in a world that has honored the servant but has forgotten the gift." This is, in part, how healthcare systems and the collective minds that contributed to their development found themselves taking a reductive, mechanistic approach to healthcare delivery. Systems are designed to prioritize LH worldviews at the expense of RH ones. Left unchecked, Dr. McGilchrist astutely asserts that the LH will continue to dominate the mind and reshape the world that is healthy for neither the planet nor its inhabitants. This is a good time to slow the pace and integrate what you've read in the next Slow the Pace Speed Bump.

Slow the Pace Speed Bump: Bonnie's Body Scan & Collaborating Hemispheres or Left-Shifting Reflection

Let's pause for a moment to let the information you just read be felt, experienced, processed, and structured by your hemispheres. In this reflection activity, start by compassionately supporting your nervous system as it settles. You might find Bonnie's Body Scan appealing. While breathing comfortably, visualize feet to earth, then connect through your feet to the star at the center of the earth. Visualize and observe sensations next from earth to feet, feet to lower legs, lower legs to upper legs, upper legs to belly, belly to heart, and heart to the skies above.

Let's take a few moments to observe in gentle, self-compassion. Notice any sensations, thoughts, or feelings. Then, notice how you respond to them. Do you gesture and invite your sensations in, or is there an impulse to push them down, aside, or away? Just notice, free of self-judgment, how your nervous system adapted and responds.

Bring your attention to how your skull brain is attending to the sensations, thoughts, or feelings. Do you allow time, space, and gentle, open curiosity around the subjective and whole picture RH worldview? Is there time and inner supportive space for the LH to fully receive that which comes from the RH? Or do you notice a left-shifting adaptation that takes you straight to problem-solving, sense-making, or task-doing? Just notice and observe if and how you may be experiencing left-shifting.

There's no right or wrong in this practice. You're just creating time, inner space, and receptivity to explore how you may have adapted in response to the traumas that touched you in some way. Observe your bodily sensations and feelings. Notice how your mind responds to them.

You are becoming better acquainted with your nervous system and its adaptive wisdom. Refer to this practice frequently to notice the richness of your felt bodily sensations and your hemispheric responses. What does it feel like when your RH and LH are collaborating? In agreement? In disagreement or conflict?

If you observe left-shifting, circle back to Bonnie's Body Scan to reconnect with the bodily neural streams that bring information to the RH. Just notice, gesture inclusion to what is emerging, and embrace radical self-acceptance as you partner with the ever-adapting wisdom of your nervous system.

Healing is happening.

Whole Brain Healing

It makes logical sense to have all brain systems work harmoniously and collaborate effectively. When the RH and LH are collaborating effectively, they support connectedness between your upstairs and downstairs brains. Whole brain healing supports coherency between the hemispheres so information and data can seamlessly flow in the RH-LH-RH endless and harmonious communication loop.

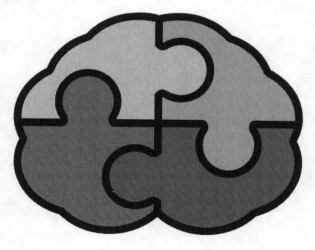

Ruptures & Repairs

Where human relationships and interactions are concerned, it is important to note that we don't always align, see, hear, understand, or meet each other's needs. I'm reminded of Ron Siegel, PhD's quote, "At some level, we're all broken-hearted. At some level, we've all got disappointments. We've all got pain, and we all have difficulties. In our lives it's really by opening to those experiences that we connect to ourselves, that we can connect to one another."

As social beings, connection is required for survival. At first glance, you'd think that we'd connect 100% right, 100% of the time. But when we peel back the layers of connection, studies suggest that about 33% of the time, we get it "right" with one another on the first try — meaning that we really connect, see, hear, value, understand, and meet the other's needs. The other 66% of the time, we don't fully connect or get it right. When this happens, minor or major ruptures occur.

It is so helpful to know this information. Although ruptures are often difficult or painful, they are normal interpersonal phenomena. Knowing that I will get it right 33% of the time, and that others will get it right with me 33% of the time, evokes a strong sense of compassion, empathy, patience, and forgiveness . . . of myself and others. We all meet one another with the best of intentions, and it isn't a defect or flaw when we don't get it wholly right. It's as though life has presented us with the opportunity to extend grace, compassion, and forgiveness to one another at least 66% of the time. It also means that we should expect roughly two ruptures for every one time we get it right with each other.

Essentially, we are engaged with repairing and healing ruptures more than half of the time. It is a natural part of life. And yet, so many of us resist it — for a number of adaptive reasons that we'll discuss in more detail later. For now, extend tender compassion and forgiveness to yourself and others for the ruptures that were unintentionally visited upon you and those that you unintentionally caused in others. Honor the inherent opportunity to learn and grow through relationships, for that is how humans are hardwired, relationally speaking.

Chapter Wrap-Up

In this chapter, you learned about your upstairs and downstairs brains and how flipping one's lid is not so much a conscious choice as it is an adaptation. You learned about the seemingly competing worldviews of the RH and LH and came to understand that you need both hemispheres to collaborate effectively. You also learned how trauma can disrupt your RH-LH collaboration, which can leave you feeling left-shifted and disconnected within and with others. All of this highlighted the importance of taking a whole brain healing approach for recovery and wellness. Throughout this book, you'll learn how to support neuroplasticity, bodymindessence alignment, and balance harmonization, as well as recovery practices to optimize your whole brain healing and wellness. Now that we've taken a big picture review of how trauma affects the brain, let's take a little time to explore further in your Haelan Activities below. Give yourself a little more time to process and integrate all that you've learned so far. Then, you'll be ready to learn how to navigate your nervous system in the next chapter.

Haelan Nurse Activities

To get a sense of how we flip our lids and both give and receive ruptures in life, in service to our growth and development, let's take a moment to gently explore. These activities can be done first individually through journaling or your favorite creative expression medium. Then, to facilitate co-healing, share your stories with other Haelan Nurses and trusted loved ones. Notice how good it feels to honor the ruptures and repairs you've

Upstairs & Downstairs Brains

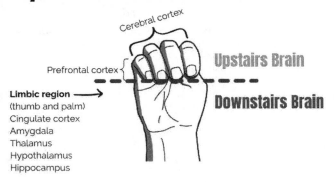

Cerebral cortex

Prefrontal cortex

Upstairs Brain

Limbic region ⟶
(thumb and palm)
Cingulate cortex
Amygdala
Thalamus
Hypothalamus
Hippocampus

Downstairs Brain

experienced while being compassionately seen, heard, valued, and supported by others. **Healing is happening.**

Who's in the Driver's Seat?
In this activity, you'll refresh your limbic system knowledge and then do a sorting exercise to see who is in the driver's seat.

Limbic System Refresher
Using Dr. Dan Siegel's Hand Model of the Brain, review the general structures and functions, starting with the brainstem and ending with the cerebral cortex.

Who's in the Driver's Seat?
Generally speaking, the prefrontal and cerebral cortices are in the driver's seat as you move through your day. But, in response to a threat (past, present, real, or perceived), the prefrontal cortex and limbic system (amygdala) disconnect, referred to as how we "flip our lids." The prefrontal cortex goes offline and is no longer in the driver's seat. To address the threat, the limbic system gets in the driver's seat and calls the shots.

Over the next several days or weeks, observe when it feels like your upstairs brain or downstairs brain (limbic system) is in the driver's seat. For example, when your upstairs brain is

Abbreviated Brain Structures and General Functions

Structures	General Functions
Brainstem	Autonomic functions such as breathing, heart rate, balance, reflexes, appetite, among others. Initiates fight or flight response during times of real or perceived danger.
Limbic System	Involved with sensory, emotional and behavioral survival responses. Limbic System structures and functions: Director: Cingulate cortex Reactor: Amygdala Messenger: Thalamus Chemist: Hypothalamus Memory Keeper: Hippocampus
Prefrontal cortex	Executive thinking and decision making. This part of your brain is in the driver's seat until there's a threat (real, perceived, past, or present) that activates the limbic system, which then gets into the driver's seat to address the threat.
Cerebral cortex	Complex functions — language, reasoning, thought, emotions, memory.

Hand model of the brain adapted from Siegel (2010); Limbic system structures and functions adapted from Hopper (2014).

in the driver's seat, you're able to address life's stressors and return to homeostasis after the stressor abates. Your stress response is measured and commensurate with the magnitude of the stressor. For example, if a car cuts you off in traffic and you nearly get in an accident, you swerve or brake, vocalize or gesture your frustration, and resume a normal driving pattern.

Disconnected
Upstairs & Downstairs Brains

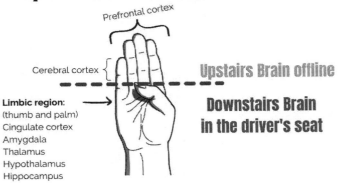

The Upstairs Brain Flipping Its Lid

When your upstairs and downstairs brains disconnect (upstairs brain flips its lid), then the downstairs limbic system brain is in the driver's seat. Imagine the same scenario of a car suddenly cutting you off in traffic and you nearly avoiding an accident. You may overreact, shut down, or get stuck in the stress response. When our limbic system is in the driver's seat, there is a discrepancy between our perception of the threat (including the neuroendocrine dysregulation cascade) and the external reality. In short, there's a mismatch between what is happening in our external environment and how we respond to it internally, which then may manifest as maladaptive behavioral responses. So, if you get cut off in traffic and the limbic system responds, it will do so disproportionately — using the horn repeatedly after the offending vehicle has left, rolling down the window and yelling, getting out of the car to make a scene, and so on.

With all this in mind, just notice who's in the driver's seat in response to life's daily stressors and note your observations in the table.

Who's in the Driver's Seat?

Daily Life Stressor	My Response when the Upstairs Brain is in the Driver's Seat	My Response when the Downstairs Brain Limbic System is in the Driver's Seat
Example: Getting cut off in traffic, almost in an accident.	I brake and swerve, then verbalize what an idiot move that was. I'm mad, but I get over it and move on with my day. I don't give it much, if any, thought.	I brake and swerve, then sound the horn for as long as I can. I'm pissed off! I drive up next to the other car, roll down my window, and use gestures and profanity. When I get to my destination, I tell everyone about the incident and post the details on social media. I'm mad all day and my body feels tight and clenched. I hate bad drivers!

Rupture & Repair Reflection or Conversation

Recall that we, as social beings, only wholly connect with one another about 33% of the time. The rest of the time (about 66%), we experience ruptures or unintentionally create ruptures in others. There is no shame or blame where life's inherent and necessary ruptures and repairs are concerned, for they inform how we grow and become ever more resilient. Knowing that helps somewhat, but no matter what side of the rupture we are on, they still sting, hurt, and resonate until we embrace and address the healing opportunity embedded within them. By addressing the prompts below, you can gently explore how you have affected others and how they have affected you. Should any unpleasant sensations emerge, take a break to nurture

Rupture I Experienced

Prompt	Your Notes
Describe a time you experienced a rupture at home or at work.	
How did this rupture feel, generally speaking? Describe any felt sensations from then or now.	
How did this rupture affect the relationship between your upstairs and downstairs brains? Did your limbic system get in the driver's seat? If so or if not, describe whatever sensations, perceptions, or emotions that emerged.	
How did this rupture affect the relationship collaboration between your RH-LH? Did you left-shift at all? If so or if not, describe whatever sensations, perceptions, or emotions that emerged.	
What remains unrepaired or unhealed in response to this rupture?	
What do you need, in any aspect of your bodymindessence, to continue healing through the rupture?	
If you can nurture your rupture to support your healing process, please take a break and do so now.	
For self-nurturing that can't be done now, please schedule a date with yourself (and others, as desired) to support your healing process.	
Note any lingering thoughts, feelings, or sensations here. Healing is happening.	

Rupture I Caused in Another

Prompt	Your Notes
Describe a time you unintentionally created a rupture for someone else, at home or at work.	
How did this rupture feel, generally speaking? Describe any felt sensations from then or now.	
How did this rupture affect the relationship between your upstairs and downstairs brains? Did your limbic system get in the driver's seat? If so or if not, describe whatever sensations, perceptions, or emotions that emerged.	
How did this rupture affect the relationship collaboration between your RH-LH? Did you left-shift at all? If so or if not, describe whatever sensations, perceptions, or emotions that emerged.	
What remains unrepaired or unhealed in response to this rupture?	
What do you need, in any aspect of your bodymindessence, to continue healing through the rupture?	
If you can nurture your rupture to support your healing process, please take a break and do so now.	
For self-nurturing that can't be done now, please schedule a date with yourself (and others, as desired) to support your healing process.	
Note any lingering thoughts, feelings, or sensations here. Healing is happening.	

yourself. You can flip back to the previous Slow the Pace Speed Bump: Bonnie's Body Scan & Collaborating Hemispheres or Left-Shifting? exercise at any time.

Deeper Dive Resources

Badenoch, B. (2017). *The heart of trauma: Healing the embodied brain in the context of relationship*s (Norton Series on Interpersonal Neurobiology). W.W. Norton & Company.

McGilchrist, I. (2019). *The master and his emissary: The divided brain and the making of the western world.* Yale University Press.

Perry, B. D., & Winfrey, O. (2021). *What happened to you?: Conversations on trauma, resilience, and healing.* Flatiron Books.

Siegel, D. J., & Bryson, T. P. (2021). *The power of showing up: How parental presence shapes who our kids become and how their brains get wired.* Ballantine Books.

Chapter 3

Navigating Our Nervous Systems

In a lightning round review, recall that the nervous system consists of two subdivisions, the central nervous system (brain and spinal cord) and the peripheral nervous system (autonomic and somatic systems). The autonomic nervous system (ANS) has three distinct hierarchical nervous system divisions: sympathetic (SNS), parasympathetic, and enteric. There is a hierarchy to the ANS which, evolutionarily speaking, consists of three components that help keep us safe: the SNS, and the parasympathetic division's dorsal and ventral vagal aspects of the vagus nerve (cranial nerve 10). Throughout the book, I will use the term *nervous system* (NS) for the autonomic nervous system, noting that the entire NS works in concert within its vast networks, circuits, plexuses, and all body systems. No one needs to get bogged down in terminology, so we'll keep it simple to support balanced hemispheric collaboration.

The Three Circuits

With huge gratitude for the work of Dr. Stephen Porges, whose Polyvagal Theory has revolutionized trauma-informed care, I'll introduce the three circuits or hierarchical states that come online in response to the ever-changing internal and external conditions. At the top of the hierarchical ladder is the **Ventral Vagal *I am and we are safe* Circuit**. This circuit is involved with social engagement, motion, emotion, and communication. When it comes online, it provides a neural foundation for evoking or re-engaging the *I am and we are safe* mechanisms, including being able to see the "big picture" of the situation, feelings of trust, and the ability to co-regulate with others.

When the ventral vagal circuit is online, you feel calm, cool, collected, and connected.

In response to real or perceived danger, the **SNS** *All-Hands-On-Deck* **Circuit** will come online. This is an active protection process, which mobilizes all physiological energy resources so we can engage in a fight-or-flight response. When this circuit comes online, you are in a **hyper**aroused state. Depending upon internal and external conditions, you may move towards the stimuli with anger or rage, etc. Or you may move away from the stimuli while experiencing worry or anxiety, etc. All the expected physiological responses engage, such as increased heart rate, blood pressure, and CAN hormones (cortisol, adrenaline, norepinephrine). In addition, blood is shunted to vital organs, fuel is made readily available to the muscles, and your bronchi dilate. Physiological functions that are not directly related to fight or flight, such as relational ability, digestion, and immune responses, temporarily decrease in deference to addressing the threat.

In the face of life-threatening danger where fight or flight are not likely to be successful, the **Dorsal Vagal** *No-Hands-On-Deck* **Circuit** comes online. This is your passive protection circuit that results in partial or total immobilization. Here, energy resources are paused to put you in a **hypo**aroused state. Evolutionarily speaking, you are behaviorally shut down and dissociated mentally in an attempt to appear inanimate so a predator or threat (say, a saber-toothed tiger) won't recognize you. Or, if it does recognize you, you will be spared a lot of pain and suffering should you be meeting your demise. When your dorsal vagal circuit comes online in today's context, you may feel dread, numb, trapped, and partially or totally shut down.

The three circuits are hierarchical, as shown by the ladder and the bidirectional arrows in the Circuits of the Autonomic Nervous System image. What this means is that these circuits

Vagus Nerve &
Circuits of the Autonomic Nervous System

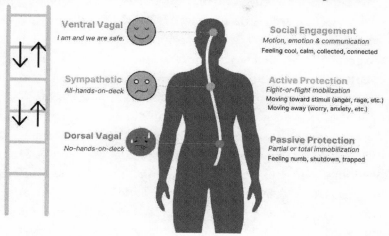

Ventral Vagal
I am and we are safe.

Social Engagement
Motion, emotion & communication
Feeling cool, calm, collected, connected

Sympathetic
All-hands-on-deck

Active Protection
Fight-or-flight mobilization
Moving toward stimuli (anger, rage, etc.)
Moving away (worry, anxiety, etc.)

Dorsal Vagal
No-hands-on-deck

Passive Protection
Partial or total immobilization
Feeling numb, shutdown, trapped

come online in sequential order. If the ventral vagal circuit is online when a life-threatening event occurs, the sympathetic circuit comes online to attempt to address the threat. If the SNS response can't resolve the threat, *then* the dorsal vagal circuit comes online. Conversely, if your dorsal vagal circuit is online, you can't just skip the middle rung of the ladder to get ventral vagal to come online. Your NS will move through the SNS circuit en route to the ventral vagal circuit as conditions become progressively safer.

The three circuits (ventral vagal, sympathetic, and dorsal vagal) can come online wholly or in part, and in various combinations. These hybrids will be discussed below, followed by how your Threat Detector and Your Repository also function to keep you safe.

The Four Hybrids

There are four hybrid combinations that emerge when the circuits come together in response to internal and external conditions.

You'll learn more about the mixology and how to navigate the hybrids throughout the book. For now, I'll introduce the four hybrids: **play, stillness, fawn, and freeze**, which are depicted in the Circuits & Hybrids image. Please note that some experts classify fawn and freeze as part of the SNS response. For our purposes, since each fawn and freeze contain more than one circuit, I'm classifying them as hybrids. For example, in the **play hybrid**, we need a mixture of ventral vagal and SNS to get us up and moving so we can enjoy leisure activities, play with our children, and be creative in the kitchen. In the play hybrid, we are relaxed yet energized, ready to explore, engaged with our loved ones, and connected with the community and within ourselves.

The **stillness hybrid** consists of a mixture of dorsal and ventral vagal to support us when it's time to be safe and still, without the fear. When we're in the stillness hybrid, we can readily engage in stillness activities like meditation or holding noble, contemplative silence. Sometimes, certain types of tantric and intimate partner activities fall in the stillness hybrid, as can yin yoga, slow tai chi, or qigong practices. As your SNS circuit comes online, you may find it increasingly difficult or downright impossible to engage in stillness activities.

The **fawn, or "please & appease," hybrid** is a mixture of ventral and dorsal vagal with some SNS. It is a complicated hybrid that is frequently associated with people who have experienced ACEs and complex traumas. In response to your internal and external conditions, your Threat Detector determines that the best strategy for survival is compliance in the form of pleasing or appeasing the person(s) who is/are perceived as a threat or danger. When you're in the fawn response, all three circuits are online. It feels like your NS is slamming the gas and brake pedals to the car floor at the same time, while turning up the radio to please the threat. Dr. Stephen Porges describes the fawning or "please & appease" response as a highly effective synergism of our social engagement system. The SNS engagement provides enough energy to give the impression that we are on board with the aggressor or predator so they'll trust us (and not harm us), while the dorsal vagal is signaling for us to disconnect within to help us sell this survival ruse. It's a complex hybrid that feels like a lot to manage when it's online.

The **freeze hybrid** is often confused with the dorsal vagal circuit *no-hands-on-deck,* so it's important to differentiate them. Like all circuits and hybrids, the freeze response is an involuntary response. It is not a cognitive choice but rather an adaptive response when fighting, fleeing, or fawning are not possible. Both the SNS (hyperarousal) and dorsal vagal (hypoarousal) circuits come online. The freeze response is one where you are bursting with **hyper**arousal energy but can't discharge or release it because the dorsal vagal is coming online to shut you down to a **hypo**aroused state. Throughout this book, you'll learn how to nurture your NS as the circuits and hybrids go online and offline. For now, explore the image that depicts how the Threat Detector signals to the circuits and their hybrids to come online to keep you safe in any situation you may encounter.

Circuits & Hybrids

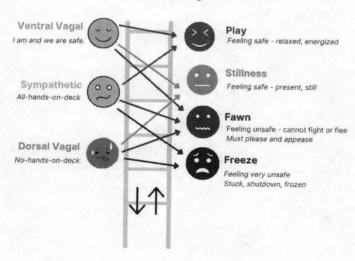

The Threat Detector

Dr. Stephen Porges coined the term *neuroception* to describe how your neural circuits, below the level of consciousness, function to differentiate between internal and external cues of safety, danger, or life-threatening danger. In other words, within each of us is a Threat Detector that is tasked with 24/7 surveillance. Its job is to keep us safe, in partnership with the three circuits and their hybrids described above. The Threat Detector decodes and interprets the external environment, including people, animals, and inanimate objects, and then signals to the NS, which brings the appropriate circuit(s) online. The Threat Detector also conducts 24/7 surveillance on the inside of your body. It decodes and interprets the internal environment (such as sensations or visceral feelings), including everything contained within Your Repository. In short, the Threat Detector surveys, decodes, and interprets your inner and outer worlds — including any unhealed bits (sometimes called old parts or adaptive parts) from prior trauma. For our purposes, we'll use the term **unhealed bits of wisdom** or simply **unhealed bits** to describe any unintegrated trauma that you embody either directly through your own lived experiences or indirectly through the legacies of ancestral or generational trauma.

Slow the Pace Speed Bump: Healing-Centered Language & Reflection

Let's take a moment to come together in awareness to acknowledge how difficult life can be, and how each person can be so profoundly affected by what they have experienced directly or through ancestral legacies.

Much has been written and discussed about difficult experiences in traditional and social media outlets. Some of it is not very inclusive or compassionate. Needed is a softening of the perception and the language around trauma and trauma healing.

What happened to you/me/us/them?

Given that our focus is healing, nurturing, nourishing, and thriving, we'll take a *What Happened to You/Me/Us/Them?* approach, which is consistent with the work of Dr. Bruce Perry. Please tenderly refrain from asking, *What is wrong with you/me/us/them?*, for doing so could be perceived by the Threat Detector as a concerning sign. Instead, please ask in a heartfelt, compassionate manner, *What happened to you/me/us/them?* This healing-centered approach keeps us all on the same, inclusive, nurturing page — for everyone has experienced some form of trauma.

Triggers are out

In this book, I purposely and compassionately refrain from the use of the word *trigger* to describe the stimulus that is perceived by the Threat Detector as a past or present danger, including the unhealed bits of wisdom in Your Repository. Instead of triggers, we'll use the more compassionate, less aggressive *stimulus* or *stimuli* to describe these inputs.

Unhealed bits of wisdom (unhealed bits)

Instead of unintegrated trauma that is embodied or stuck in the body's tissues, organs, joints, neural circuits, and plexuses, we'll use the term *unhealed bits of wisdom* or simply *unhealed bits* to compassionately describe the embodied trauma artifacts that patiently await healing and integration.

When conditions are more favorable for healing, as assessed by your Threat Detector and NS, the unhealed bits of wisdom in Your Repository will emerge for healing. When they emerge in their own perfect time (which is not always convenient), they are always in service to your healing and growth, even though unpleasant or uncomfortable sensations or feelings may accompany them. Unhealed bits of wisdom. They are a beauty to behold and sometimes a little tricky to navigate. You'll be an expert in caring for your unhealed bits soon.

Reflection, Journaling, or Creative Expression

As you reflect upon these terms, explore how they feel when you speak, write, or creatively express them. To contextualize this exercise, recall a situation or event that was very difficult for you. And by very difficult, on a scale from 0-10, go with something in the 1-5 range so as not to signal a potential danger to the Threat Detector. Then, ask yourself these questions and notice any sensations, thoughts, or feelings that emerge during the next 30-60 seconds, or longer.

1. What is wrong with me?
2. What happened to me?
3. I am triggered.
4. I am experiencing a stimulus.
5. Within me, there are unintegrated traumas.
6. Within me, there are unhealed bits of wisdom.

Take home message: The Threat Detector is on duty 24/7, in service to your survival. Choose thoughts and words that signal safety to the Threat Detector. This will support the ventral vagal circuit to come or remain online in its *I* *am and we are safe* mode. By doing so, you'll spend more time feeling calm, cool, collected, and connected.

Healing is happening.

Your Repository

Your Repository contains the totality of all lived experiences from this lifetime and those of your ancestors by virtue of your genetic coding. Each of us embodies the remnants or artifacts of trauma that were not able to be fully healed, processed, or integrated at the time it occurred — our unhealed bits of wisdom. As you'll learn more about shortly, this is often because we didn't have the person or people we perceived that we needed at that time. Or, because the people we needed weren't equipped to fully address the trauma, or they were unavailable physically, mentally, emotionally, spiritually, or situationally. When this happens, whatever part of the traumatic experience that didn't heal or integrate gets stored in bodily organs like muscles, fascia, and the gut (among others). Or it gets stored within our systems, such as the neural plexuses, circuits, and networks that influence bodily functions.

Your Repository contains the entire database of unhealed bits that remained in your ancestral lines and are encoded in your DNA. Your Repository also contains all the unhealed bits from this lifetime. If and when conditions are more favorable to heal, process, and integrate these trauma remnants, your unhealed bits will emerge. You, in bodymindessence, are always striving for homeostasis and optimal wellness. Liberating yourself from the embodied unhealed bits is healing of the highest order that has positive ripple effects through every dimension of life. You'll learn, throughout this book, how to recognize, welcome, and address your unhealed bits as they emerge.

Your Repository
Threat Detector & Circuits

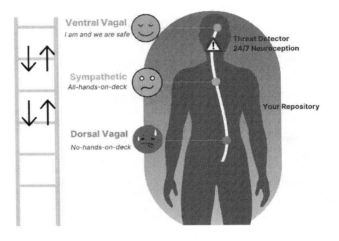

In summary, the Threat Detector, with its ever-vigilant surveillance, triangulates the data in your inner and external environments along with the unhealed bits contained within Your Repository. The Threat Detector considers *all* data (external, internal, Your Repository, and unhealed bits) in its assessment. It will then signal which of your three circuits needs to come online and to what degree. The highly individualized nature of the Threat Detector is one of the reasons why two or more people can share the same stressful event or situation and come away with very different NS responses. Your Threat Detector and Your Repository are as unique as you are. Both are, and always have been, in service to your survival. Just as the evolutionary need to be in families, communities, and societies is in service to your survival.

Jordan's Story Continues
Let's return to Jordan's case story and observe how she is being impacted in her NS and other dimensions of her bodymindessence. In Chapter 1, Jordan learned about the

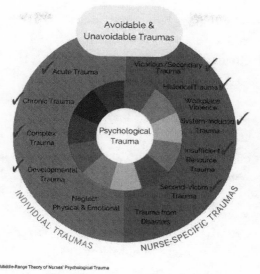

Adapted from Foli (2022). Middle-Range Theory of Nurses' Psychological Trauma

Jordan's Trauma History

various types of trauma, just as you did. For her homework, she reviewed the same information that you just read above regarding the circuits, hybrids, Threat Detector, and her Repository. She completed the Slow the Space Speed Bumps and — right along with you — is ever so gently becoming aware of her thoughts and the words she uses to signal safety to her Threat Detector. Before we sit in on Jordan's next session, take a peek at Jordan's graphic, which depicts her overall exposure to individual and nurse-specific traumas. Jordan noted four categories of individual trauma, including the pandemic, and five categories of nurse-specific traumas.

Lorre: [after welcoming Jordan to the session and giving her time to share her situation and symptoms] Thank you for being so open, willing, and courageous. I honor you and all that you're experiencing. [places both hands over heart]

Jordan: Honestly, I've been looking forward to this appointment. So much has happened!

Lorre: Yes, yes it has. Now that you've shared what you've experienced and are experiencing in detail, let's take a moment to explore how that sharing affected you in any aspect of your bodymindessence.

Jordan: OK, let's see. Well, I'm noticing that I'm tired, exhausted even. I mean, I just get utterly overwhelmed by my caseload. The charting system has so many redundancies that it takes me way longer to chart than it should. Like I'm saying the same thing twenty different times, it seems. My TMJ (temporomandibular disorder) is back. I clench my jaw, grind my teeth, and my shoulders are so tense that they feel like they're attached to my ear lobes. [laughs a little, then grows quiet, her energy collapsing]

Lorre: That's a lot to experience. Is there anything else you'd like to add?

Jordan: Um, how much time do you have? [chuckles] Cuz I can go on all day!

Lorre: There's an exercise I'd like to share with you in a moment that relates to this, so if you're comfortable with sharing a little more, that would be helpful.

Jordan: OK, so here it is. I can't sleep, I can't eat, I can't hydrate, I can't poop, I can't see my family, I can't spend quality time with my kids. I don't have time for exercise, rest, my spiritual practices, or any leisure activities. [The pitch of her voice raises as she speaks much faster.] I haven't gone on a hike since nursing school. I think I made a big mistake by getting into nursing . . . healthcare. I'm not able to care for people the way that I'm supposed to — the way they *should* be cared for [reaches for the box of tissues]. I mean, seriously, I made more money and worked about half the hours when I was a food server! I'm so over it! [She fights back the tears for a moment before she allows them to flow as she sobs quietly for a moment.]

Lorre: Thank you for sharing your deepest truths. I have experienced much of what you're experiencing, as have millions of nurses. I want you to know that you're not alone. There's nothing wrong with you. And there *is* a pathway from here to better life balance and a meaningful practice. I'll be with you every step of the way. [Jordan is visibly relieved.] Would you like to check out this exercise?

Jordan: I'll literally try anything. Whatever I need to do to get better, I'll do it.

Lorre: That's a great way to approach any challenge or healing opportunity. Do you remember the Healing-Centered Language & Reflection, where we explored the effect of the words *triggered* vs. *stimulus* and *unintegrated trauma* vs. *unhealed bits of wisdom*?

Jordan: I sure do! That was a powerful exercise. I'm really seeing how the words I use affect me and affect my Threat Detector.

Lorre: Absolutely, it is so helpful! Well, this exercise is very similar to that one. This time, we're exploring the thoughts and words you use surrounding your circumstances and how you are affected by them. [Passes Jordan the clipboard with the Expanded Healing-Centered Language & Reflection Activity] Shall we give it a whirl?

Jordan: [skims the worksheet] 100% yes, let's do it!

***

You may have noticed that I used "situation" to describe Jordan's trauma context and "symptoms" to describe how trauma was manifesting in all dimensions of her bodymindessence. I did this so as not to unnecessarily signal a potential threat to your (or Jordan's) Threat Detector. As you move through this book, you'll learn strategies to help you delve into your deeper layers of trauma and their specific manifestations. In these early chapters, you'll skim the surface in preparation for the deeper healing opportunities that come in later chapters while staying as stable and regulated in your NS as possible. The last thing you need is for me to overwhelm your system by doing too much, too fast, too soon. One step at a time, steady as you go . . .

In the session, I facilitated Jordan in reframing the narratives from Chapters 1 and 2 using this worksheet after ensuring she had clarity about what was happening in her current situation and symptoms. Now, it is your turn to do this activity. After you're done, we'll rejoin Jordan's session.

Expanded Healing-Centered Language & Reflection Activity

Let's take a moment to come together in awareness to reflect upon how the thoughts and words we use can influence the Threat Detector and which circuits and hybrids come online.

While it's very natural to need to talk about, write about, and otherwise express all the details of one traumatic experience or the symptoms that are manifesting, doing so repetitively may have negative unintended consequences, like engaging your or someone else's Threat Detector. This is how we can unknowingly perpetuate the trauma cycle. Once you have clarity about what is happening and how it is affecting you, use these words instead of retelling the entire narrative.

Situation(s): Use this word to globally describe whatever disturbing hardship, trauma, event, or circumstance you are experiencing.

Symptoms(s): Use this word to globally describe how the situation is manifesting in one or more dimensions of your bodymindessence.

Going forward, use the words "situation" and "symptoms" to describe your clear understanding of your existing situation and symptoms.

Note that there will be instances in the future where new layers to your situation and symptoms emerge. In those cases, you might say or write something like, "My situation has more layers to it. These new layers are —."

As the new layers become familiar to you and when no new information or insight is emerging as you think, write, talk, or express about them, it is then time to include them in the global statement of, "My situation . . ." or "The situation . . ." The same process applies when discovering additional symptoms.

Reflection, Journaling, or Creative Expression

As you reflect upon these terms, explore how they feel when you speak, write, or creatively express them. To contextualize this exercise, recall a situation or event that was very difficult for you. And by very difficult, on a scale from 0-10, go with something in the 1-5 range so as not to signal a potential danger to the Threat Detector. Then, ask yourself these questions and notice any sensations, thoughts, or feelings that emerge during the next 30-60 seconds, or longer.

1. **Situation Reflection:** Think, write, discuss, or creatively express to describe a trauma you've experienced, using the word "situation" in place of other descriptors.
2. **Symptom Reflection:** Think, write, discuss, or creatively express how a trauma you've experienced has affected one or more aspects of your bodymindessence. Use the word "symptom" or "symptoms" in place of other descriptors.
3. **Noticing:** You may or may not be detecting subtle differences in your perceptions, sensations, thoughts, feelings, or other bodymindessence experiences as you describe what is happening using the

healing-centered "situation" and "symptom" descriptors. This is a subtle yet powerful shift that signals safety to your Threat Detector. Well done!

Take home message: The Threat Detector is on duty 24/7, in service to your survival. Choose thoughts and words that signal safety to the Threat Detector. This will support the ventral vagal circuit to come online in its *I am and we are safe* mode. By doing so, you'll spend more time feeling calm, cool, collected, and connected.

Healing is happening.

The session with Jordan resumes.

Lorre: What did you notice as we moved through the activity?

Jordan: I didn't realize how many times each day I told the complete story about my situation and symptoms. I didn't know how deeply it was affecting me and how much I needed to talk about it.

Lorre: We all need to talk about our experiences, we're social beings who need to be seen, heard, understood, and accepted. It's perfectly natural to talk about your situation and symptoms. In fact, it's a hallmark characteristic of The Five Big Picture Phases of Haelan — do you remember enduring, uncertainty, suffering, hope, and The Three R's?

Jordan: I do, and now that you mention it, I feel like I'm in the . . . [flips through the pages on the clipboard to locate the handout] . . . I'm in the "motormouth" phase of enduring, right?

Lorre: Yes, that is where I see you, too. Now that you know where you are in the big picture, let's dial in and explore how to choose neutral thoughts and words to signal safety as you move through this and all of the phases.

Jordan: I totally get it. When I described what was happening and how I was feeling the first time, I guess I used it like a complete narrative, I could feel myself getting revved up stress-wise. My symptoms — which I won't elaborate upon [laughs heartily, with insight] — heightened, became exacerbated. But then, the second time, doing the activity, I stayed more centered . . . more calm . . . when I used the words "situation" and "symptoms." Wow, I had no idea, but it really does help!

Lorre: Ah, that warms my heart to share in this healing shift with you. I'm wondering how your coworkers and other nurse friends are experiencing their situations?

Jordan: Well, [laughs earnestly] they certainly are using *all the words*. Their narratives, just like mine was, are like the ticker tape that runs across the bottom of a newscast. It's non-stop, but that's because our situation is non-stop stress with a lot of trauma. [pauses to ponder] Is it OK that I used "non-stop stress" and "a lot of trauma"?

Lorre: You can use those and other neutral terms. Follow the wisdom of your NS. If you notice the thoughts or words you used signaling a potential danger to your Threat Detector, or if you experience an uptick or exacerbation of symptoms, then you'll know to use different words the next time. Everyone's Repository is different, so it's an exploratory process.

Jordan: Yes, and I definitely don't want to further disrupt my coworkers — we all have enough to deal with!

Lorre: You certainly do! And by virtue of your healing-centered language shift, you are starting a culture where nurses can heal and co-regulate with one another just by virtue of staying regulated in their nervous systems.

Jordan: I've heard those terms a lot in my newsfeed . . . like regulation, dysregulation, co-regulation . . . I sort of get it, but not really . . .

Lorre: There's a lot in the media on these topics right now. Let's walk through it together, shall we?

Jordan: Yes, I feel like it's really important to understand my situation and my symptoms — and what I can do to help myself.

Lorre: There's so much you can do to help yourself, and you're already in progress. You're doing great. But no one heals alone or in a vacuum. We need each other to heal, co-regulate, and thrive.

Jordan: Really? Because, honestly, I feel like I want to crawl into a dark cave, lick my wounds, and heal by myself.

Lorre: That's a natural response given where you are in your NS today. You'll learn more about how to navigate your circuits and hybrids as we go down the healing path together. For now, let's just think about how your NS is evolutionarily hardwired. No one gets through life alone. Mammals are social beings. Your survival depends upon your ability to connect, communicate, and collaborate with others.

Jordan: So, that's why we don't want to motormouth the big narratives of our situation and symptoms at work. So we can connect, communicate, and collaborate together? Just saying "situation" and "symptoms" and words like that . . . that makes it easier for us to connect with each other. Like, all the narratives are the static on the radio station before you tune in completely.

Lorre: Yes, great metaphor! And there's more. We also co-regulate in our NSs together. When one person is dysregulated — say one of your coworkers — their NS will innately start to harmonize with the other regulated NSs in the group. I'm wondering, is there someone at work that makes you feel calm, safe, relaxed, secure?

Jordan: OMG, yes, there's this one charge nurse on another unit. We literally call her the Buddha Incarnate! You just want to be in her world. She's so grounded and calm all the time. She's such a loving and caring person, no matter what.

Lorre: How wonderful to have that presence at work. When you interact with her, how do you feel?

Jordan: Oh, I think I know where you're going with this question! I feel calmer, with less symptoms. Like I'm more grounded, at more peace if only for a few moments. That's because I'm co-regulating with her NS, right?

Lorre: I strongly suspect that is the case! Excellent work today. Before our next session, I have some light reading for you to do about how your NS regulates, dysregulates, and can get hijacked. When we come back together, we can pick up from there and keep moving forward.

Jordan: [checks the time on her phone] Time sure does fly by here! That sounds great.

As our session drew to a close, Jordan took a few handouts with her that correspond with the next section, which you'll read below regarding how your nervous system can be affected by the conditions within which you work.

The Window of Tolerance

You've probably heard a lot about regulation and dysregulation in mainstream and social media. Let's refresh or build upon your knowledge base as it pertains to nurse traumatization and how it affects your NS at home and at work.

A Regulated Nervous System

Throughout each day and in response to lived experiences, you may feel times of mild stress and times of feeling open, receptive, calm, cool, collected, and connected (within and with others). A regulated nervous system can seamlessly fluctuate between ventral vagal tone with mild SNS engagement in responses to the stresses of daily life. It's a beautiful rhythm as you move into the *all-hands-on-deck* pathway so you can attend to the stress or threat. After the stress or threat has abated, a regulated NS can easily return to the ventral vagal tone of *I am and we are safe*. This natural process of moving from a SNS stimulated state to an open, relaxed, and socially engaged state is, as Dr. Dan Siegel describes it, the Window of Tolerance. But, for people who have been affected by trauma, the NS's ability to regulate — to move flexibly between the different circuits and hybrids in response to stressors — is compromised.

As we all learned in nursing school, the human body is always striving to move toward homeostasis in its physiological processes. The same can be said about responding to the cues from your inner and external environments. Your body, including your NS, is always working toward homeostasis — an optimal state of arousal or stimulation where we can optimally thrive in our daily functions. The Window of Tolerance describes how humans ideally function in an optimal arousal zone where the ventral vagal circuit and the SNS circuits are online, and the stressor is determined by the Threat Detector to be within the "I can" SNS response. Yes, it's a stressor, but it's one that the NS can address and then seamlessly return to ventral vagal tone. By contrast, an "I can't" SNS stimuli would be assessed by the Threat Detector as a potentially life-threatening one, which then signals for the dorsal vagal circuit to come online.

"When we are in our Window of Tolerance, we are in the sweet spot of our nervous systems."

Lorre Laws, PhD RN

When within your Window of Tolerance, you are able to optimally manage your emotions, and cope and adapt to ever-changing stimuli. You are calm, cool, collected, and connected within and with others. The Window of Tolerance is the "sweet spot" of your NS rhythms. However, prior and current trauma profoundly affects the degree to which your NS can thrive in the Window of Tolerance. Ideally, your Window is wide open. Then, you spend most of your time thriving in ventral vagal tone — grounded, centered, relaxed, connected, and effectively managing the ruptures, stressors, and disruptions of daily life.

As significant stressors or dangers emerge, you experience minimally hyper-aroused ("I can" SNS) or hypo-aroused ("I can't" SNS) temporary responses before returning to the Window of Tolerance. Should you experience extreme hyper- or hypoarousal or remain in these states for a prolonged period of time — such as a chronically under-staffed and under-resourced nursing role — then your Window of Tolerance closes or slams completely shut.

For those affected by trauma, the Window of Tolerance is smaller and/or more difficult to access depending upon your inner and external conditions. There are a lot of unhealed bits in Your Repository that are taken into account by the Threat Detector. You may not have had the people that you perceived that you needed before, during, or after the event. Your NS adapted to all that you've experienced and may be over-firing the "danger" response. This pushes us away from our NS's sweet spot, the Window of Tolerance, and into hyperarousal (overwhelmed, anxious, out of control, angry), or hypoarousal (freeze state, numb, disconnected, spacy, zoned out). Nurses who have experienced prolonged exposure to nurse-specific traumas report that their Window of Tolerance is either small or nonexistent most days. Perhaps you are among them. When I was healing through my traumatic experiences, it

Window of Tolerance

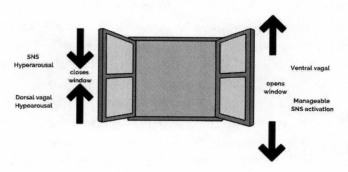

SNS
Hyperarousal

closes
window

Dorsal vagal
Hypoarousal

Ventral vagal

opens
window

Manageable
SNS activation

felt like a feather floating by would slam the Window shut. Simultaneously, my NS went from regulated to dysregulated in a nanosecond. It's a hard way to live. Throughout the rest of the book, you'll learn how to navigate and attend to your NS to ensure you're in your sweet spot, The Window of Tolerance, most of the time.

A Dysregulated Nervous System

When traumatic events occur, they may exceed your NS's capacity to self- or co-regulate with others. Factors that influence dysregulation include ancestral traumas that are transmitted from one generation to the next, individual traumas such as ACEs, disordered attachment experiences, other significant relationship disruptions, and the entirety of experiences in Your Repository and body. This is why two nurses working on the same unit on the same day can have two completely different NS responses. One nurses' Window slammed shut while the other was in their NS sweet spot with the Window wide open.

Dysregulation manifests in different ways for different people. Common dysregulation responses include an excess emotional response to a situation, difficulty calming down or ramping up, or avoiding difficult feelings, people, or situations. Persons experiencing dysregulation have difficulty coping or tend to ruminate over problems repeatedly. Dysregulation affects relationships secondary to externalizing, internalizing, or dissociating in response to stress. It is difficult to set or maintain boundaries, control impulses, or resist the urge to control anything or everything when dysregulation visits. From the overall quality of one's relationship with oneself to the quality of intimate partner relationships, dysregulation can make it very difficult to connect within and with others.

Being dysregulated can feel like your NS is stuck in the "on" or "off" position. When you feel stuck in the "on" position, the SNS circuit is online and driving you to respond, to do something, anything, NOW. You are hyperaroused. This creates additional and prolonged stress for all bodily systems. People who feel stuck in NS "on" position find it difficult to engage with mindful or stillness practices. Their NSs are screaming for them to move, react, respond. If you find yourself in this state, moving will be helpful — try tapping your foot while in a meeting, rubbing your thumb and forefinger together, rolling a pen or paper clip in your fingers, swaying, dancing, or engaging in any form of exercise.

Some people's dysregulated NS gets stuck in the "off" position, which results in hypoarousal manifesting as a freeze or shutdown. The stress or danger, combined with the unhealed bits in Your Repository, were assessed by the Threat Detector as potentially life-threatening. The dorsal vagal circuit comes online. It can feel like a punch to the gut that takes your breath away. That dorsal vagal tone can wreak havoc in the digestive system to the point that it can be difficult to eat, drink, or digest. It's also difficult to engage in normal daily activities when the dorsal vagal is online. Nurses report having to "drag" themselves into work and having no energy after work and on their days off. Laying on the couch or in bed is about all that seems manageable with the NS stuck in the "off" position. It affects every aspect of your life, and the people around you can't see or relate to how utterly exhausted and shut down you are internally. It's literally a *no-hands-on-deck* situation.

How Nurses' Nervous Systems Get Hijacked at Work
Ideally, nurses would practice from their wide-open Window of Tolerance. Absent the healthcare system inadequacies that frequently result in *avoidable* nurse traumatization (workplace violence, system-induced trauma, insufficient resource trauma, second-victim trauma), nurses are equipped to thrive and practice safely.

What Should Happen:
Nurses are Safe & Thriving

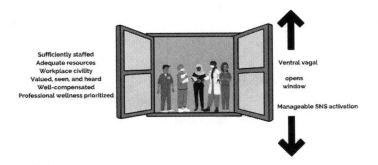

Sufficiently staffed
Adequate resources
Workplace civility
Valued, seen, and heard
Well-compensated
Professional wellness prioritized

Ventral vagal

opens
window

Manageable SNS activation

But nurses don't always feel safe because nurses aren't always safe. Your Threat Detector is scanning for safety, 24/7. If your working conditions are such that there is insufficient staffing, inadequate resources, workplace incivilities or violence, gaslighting, or other threats to nurse safety, your Threat Detector will pick up those cues. It will compare the current cues with Your Repository and signal accordingly to your NS, which will respond as it has adapted to respond. Remember, this is all occurring below the level of consciousness, so how you respond is not a choice, but rather an adaptation. Without an awareness of your NS adaptations, how to attend to and align them with your external world, the Window of Tolerance narrows, as does your ability to practice within it. You're at high risk for, or have already, dysregulated. It is not your fault if and when dysregulation occurs. This is your NS doing what it's supposed to do — keep you safe. The circuits and hybrids come online in service to your survival. Although we can't choose what circuits and hybrids come online and when, we can learn how to navigate our NS and partner with its wisdom to ensure we stay in the Window and regulated.

This is how nurses' NSs get hijacked at work. Our role requires us to be open, compassionate, connect with our

What Really Happens:
Nurses are Not Safe
& Pushed Out of the Window

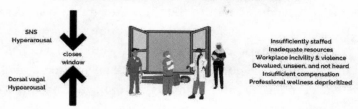

patients, and use therapeutic communication to deliver patient-centered, relationship-based care. In other words, our role requires us to be in the Window of Tolerance with our ventral vagal circuit online and stress levels that keep the SNS circuit in the "I can manage this stress" range of regulation instead of the "I can't manage this stress" as it starts to dysregulate.

Patient safety is the cornerstone of nursing care. Every nurse is well-versed in the importance of patient safety. We prioritize patient safety above all, and rightfully so. For, as WHO Director-General, Dr. Tedros Adhanom Ghebreyesus, has said, **"If it's not safe, it's not care."** Similarly, Joseph Q. Jarvis, MD, and Kindra Celani, DNP, remind us, **"When nurses are not safe, patients are not safe."**

When it comes to nurse safety — the pillar upon which safe patient care is delivered — healthcare systems fail. We have good people working in poorly designed healthcare systems that do not consider nurse safety and how threats to nurse safety contribute to nurse traumatization, dysregulation, and burnout. If nurses aren't safe and their patients aren't safe, it's no longer healthcare. It's risk management. It's the process of identifying, evaluating, and controlling threats and risks to an organization's capital holdings and earnings. It's also disease management, but that's a topic for another time.

Your Nervous System and Other People

Of paramount importance is the relational aspect of trauma, healing, and safety. We are hardwired and evolutionarily required to connect with others not only for physical safety, but for co-regulation. To highlight this point, imagine you are in a grocery store and you hear a loud sound, like a car's tire blowing out, or a gunshot. Your Threat Detector and limbic system respond to that stimulus before your upstairs brain can process what is happening. The first thing you'd do in that situation is scan the faces and body language of those around you in an attempt to locate the danger and identify those who represent safety. Our survival depends upon our ability to "read" people and position ourselves with those who represent safety. We don't live in a vacuum. We are inseparable from the contexts in which we live and work, including the people we encounter. To completely understand how to navigate your NS, it is important to understand how it works with other people.

Relationship Is Everything

Another key factor influencing whether or not you experience regulation or dysregulation in your NS has to do with how other people were and are able to be with you during hardship or trauma. Dr. Bonnie Badenoch reminds us that relationship is *everything*. It's not so much the nature of the trauma itself that influences its integration, as it is the people who were/ are with you at the time the event happened. Did you have the people you perceived that you needed before, during, or after the trauma? You may or may not have had who you needed. Or, if the people you needed were there, maybe they weren't equipped to help you in the way you needed — likely because they themselves were dysregulated or outside *their* Window. Not every person is fully equipped to meet the needs of another during times of extreme stress or trauma. To highlight the importance of co-regulation, community, and having who you need before, during, or after a trauma, let's turn to a case study of child soldiers in Nepal.

In Dr. Badenoch's work, she describes studies of child soldiers between ages 5-14 in which researchers examined how these child soldiers were reintegrated into two different communities after a horrific war experience. The researchers also analyzed whether the child soldiers developed PTSD and, if so, to what extent. In one village, the child soldiers returned to a community that embraced them with acceptance, compassion, and nurturance. As a whole, this community structure and dynamic also supported early childhood secure attachment development. After the war, the child soldiers were reintegrated into their village with supportive rituals and commune with elders, parents, families, and peers. The children showed few symptoms of trauma, and none of them were on the PTSD spectrum.

In contrast, another village had a reintegration process filled with rejection and judgment. This community, collectively, may have been less supportive of nurturing behaviors. The child soldiers were not embraced upon their return. Instead, they were harshly treated and shamed. The village community members who were with the children before and after the war weren't able to fully support the child's NS regulation, healing, and post-traumatic growth. There was evidence of PTSD across the village's community members, and the child soldiers also experienced PTSD symptoms.

"In general, those who are rejected continue to suffer in the most painful ongoing ways ... those who are accepted and nourished on their return thrive to the extent that there are very few signs of what they have experienced."

Bonnie Badenoch, PhD LMFT

Relationship Is Everything for Nurses, Too

How we, as nurses, perceive those who were/are with us before, during, and after exposure to nurse trauma affects our ability to integrate — or not integrate — the trauma throughout our embodied neural circuits and hemispheres. When it comes to trauma and our ability to integrate it through our embodied and relational brains, it matters immensely how we perceive those who are with us before, during, and after the event. There seem to be two camps regarding how nurses collectively respond to nurse trauma exposure. In the first camp, there is the "work family" response of unity, support, and inclusion. How many of us have, at one time or another, referred to our work bestie, work wife, work husband, or work family? Here, nurses are able to be who they need to be, with and for one another before, during, and after the event or prolonged situation.

The other camp is one where nurses tend to respond to the trauma exposure by rejecting one another with an "every nurse

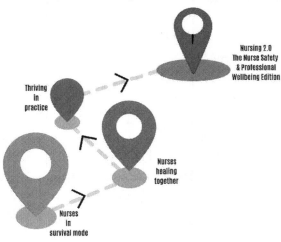

From Surviving to Thriving En Route to Nursing 2.0
The Nurse Safety & Professional Wellbeing Edition

Nursing 2.0
The Nurse Safety
& Professional
Wellbeing Edition

Thriving
in
practice

Nurses
healing
together

Nurses
in
survival mode

for themselves" response. In these instances, it is possible — if not likely — that the event or prolonged stress has exceeded the team's ability to manage. The collective Window of Tolerance is small, if it's open at all. The team has likely left-shifted, their upstairs brain has disconnected somewhat from the downstairs brain, the SNS circuit is on overdrive in the "I can't manage" zone, and the dorsal vagal circuit is online. Dysregulation is the norm, with the team in various NS adaptations of SNS hyperarousal by moving toward the threat with aggression, rage, or violence (physical, emotional, etc.) or away from the threat with fear, worry, or anxiety. The online dorsal vagal circuit brings with it behaviors that align with feeling trapped, shut down, hopeless, fawning, or freezing. Conditions are such that the Threat Detector cannot signal safety for their ventral vagal circuits to come online so they can more readily connect within themselves and with others. Instead, their Threat Detectors are signaling that conditions are not safe, and their NSs respond with survival mode behaviors.

This is why it is so important that we, individually and collectively, learn the language of our NSs and support one another in trauma healing. From a place of collective healed-ness, we can affect a "positive endemic" of mass change, as described by bestselling author and international journalist, Malcolm Gladwell, in his book *The Tipping Point*. As nurses, we are change agents and clinical champions, so we already live and embody the three tipping point "rules" to affect positive change for our patients. Now, it's time for us to do the same for ourselves and our profession. The three cleverly named rules that guide a tipping point of mass change for positive social endemics are *The Land of the Few*, *The Stickiness Factor*, and *The Power of Context*, each of which are described in the table below.

Within the current nursing crisis is tremendous opportunity and potential to affect sustainable change. It is my hope that you will join me in *The Land of the Few* as a like-hearted change

Gladwell's Rules That Guide Mass Change

1. The Land of the Few	It takes change agents and champions to deliver the message of hope and change. The author of this book is one of many change agents who are committed to ushering in Nursing 2.0: The Nurse Safety & Professional Wellbeing Edition.
2. The Stickiness Factor	How the positive change message "sticks" to the recipient or reader and resonates as truth with healing potential that ripples out to others as a positive contagion of professional and social change.
3. The Power of Context	The change message must survive, thrive, and spread throughout the contexts and systems within which nurses live and work, individually and collectively. Current workplace contexts are ripe for healing, change, and sustainable transformation as nurse safety and professional wellbeing are prioritized.

agent and champion. May nurses resonate with the healing truth and potential and use *The Stickiness Factor* to share this book and the healing opportunities with other nurses. May we all leverage *The Power of Our Contexts* as we heal and transcend the avoidable traumas we've experienced in deference to nurse safety and professional wellbeing.

By engaging with the teachings in this book, nurses can take the compassionate "What happened to you?" perspective, knowing that so many are doing their best given where they are in their NS adaptations, Window of Tolerance, and behaviors that

Tipping Point Rules for Mass Change
En Route to Nursing 2.0

- ① The Land of the Few
- ② The Stickiness Factor
- ③ The Power of Context

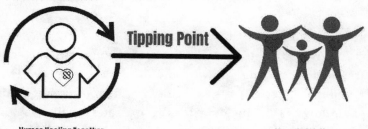

Nurses Healing Together

Tipping Point

Nurse Safety & Professional Wellbeing

Adapted from Gladwell (2006)

The Road to Nursing 2.0
The Nurse Safety & Professional Wellbeing Edition

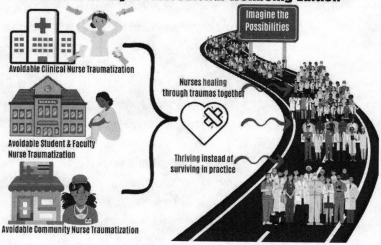

Avoidable Clinical Nurse Traumatization

Avoidable Student & Faculty Nurse Traumatization

Avoidable Community Nurse Traumatization

Imagine the Possibilities

Nurses healing through traumas together

Thriving instead of surviving in practice

manifest when someone is dysregulated. This is where Haelan Nurses embrace and support one another. We *are* the people we need to heal and co-heal, regulate and co-regulate, and thrive instead of just surviving in our practices. Whether at home, in practice, or returning from war . . . *relationship is everything.*

How to Start Navigating Your NS

You might be wondering where to start given all that you've learned about trauma, upstairs and downstairs brains, RH and LH collaboration, circuits, hybrids, regulation, dysregulation, the Window of Tolerance, and the ruptures and repairs that affect everyone. Rest assured that the rest of this book is dedicated to helping you navigate it all — with all of your beautiful layers. In the next chapter, you'll learn about your innate ability to heal and how to curate Your Innate Care Plan and practices. To prepare for the road ahead, the first step is to learn how your NS prefers that you partner with it. Navigating your NS isn't a "one and done" spa treatment. It's a lifestyle that will radically improve your health, wellness, and quality of life at home and at work. As it turns out, your NS wants you to take a MicroDoses Matter approach to partnering with its wisdom and navigating it so that you live regulated while thriving in your Window of Tolerance.

MicroDoses Matter

Given that your Threat Detector and NS are on duty 24/7, it is important to be aware of where you are in your NS and then tenderly attend to it using any number of practices in this book and elsewhere. Attending your NS with nurturing MicroDoses that signal safety to your Threat Detector is an important first step as you embark upon the journey from dysregulation to regulation, from surviving to thriving in your Window of Tolerance. Just like lifestyle choices can stave off many chronic conditions, attending your NS can do the same.

If you were discharging a patient who had a heart attack from the hospital, you would educate them on the importance of making incremental changes to diet, exercise, and other lifestyle choices and to sustain and grow them over time. You wouldn't tell the patient to just eat right, exercise, and cut down on the booze for just one day. That approach would not shift outcomes for the patient, just as taking this approach won't work for you. You know how this works. Small, incremental changes woven throughout each day as a sustainable lifestyle change is what we're going for here. Shifting from surviving to thriving in practice and in life.

This approach is exactly what your NS needs. It needs you to learn its language, harness its wisdom, and partner with it as you move toward wholeness — healthy, well, and thriving. The best approach to take is the MicroDoses Matter one, which is completely doable at home and at work. There are four

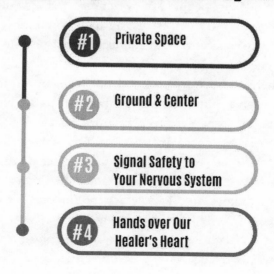

MicroDoses Matter™
Navigating your Nervous System

#1 Private Space

#2 Ground & Center

#3 Signal Safety to Your Nervous System

#4 Hands over Our Healer's Heart

MicroDose steps and the entire sequence can be done in under 30 seconds:

Step 1. Private Space: Your Threat Detector needs to detect safety, so step into the restroom, break room, supply room, a vacant patient room, or an unoccupied conference room. Less than 30 seconds is all that you need, and if more time is available, you can do several MicroDoses rounds or extend each step as desired.

Step 2. Ground & Center: Get into the habit of carrying a small pocket pal or nature artifact in your pocket. My go-to is a heart-shaped rose quartz crystal. Hold your pocket pal in your hand or rub it between your thumb and fingers. Do whatever feels soothing and natural to you. If time permits, do a lightning round of Bonnie's Body Scan. It goes like this, "Feet to earth, roots to the star at the center of the earth. I now sense my feet, my lower legs, my upper legs, my hips, my buttocks, my belly, my heart, and up to the sky." Adapt this however feels comfortable to you. Sometimes, I use my hands to lightly touch my feet, legs, torso, heart, and then raise them overhead stretched out to the sky.

Step 3. Signal Safety to Your Threat Detector & NS: The signal that works well for most people is to use their sense of smell or sight. Most people are overstimulated visually with all the technologies and devices. If you have a window or nature in your private space, you can connect with it visually to signal safety. My clients prefer to use their sense of smell and some form of aromatherapy, such as essential oil lip balm, aromatherapy patches, or even a cotton ball in a small plastic bag or container in your pocket. You're not concerned with efficacy or effectiveness here; you're signaling safety to your Threat Detector to help regulate or maintain NS regulation. Choose scents that evoke a sense of safety, comfort, love, and connection. I'm a fan of citrus and holiday baking scents. I also reach for lime and clove essential oils if I'm getting too much SNS engagement.

Play around with your five senses and explore what signals safety for *you*. Perhaps having a soft fabric, textile, or smooth button signals safety. Maybe it's putting in your earbuds to hear a quick excerpt from a favorite song. Or you might feel safe when tasting flower essence elixirs, your favorite dried fruit, or hard candy. Explore, have fun, and notice all the ways in which you can signal safety to your Threat Detector.

Step 4. Healer's Heart: To seal your MicroDoses Matter practice, place one or both hands over your heart to signal safety and nurturance. Being a human is hard. Being a nurse is even harder, especially in the current healthcare climate that is devastating to your healer's heart. Give yourself, your healer's heart, and your NS a moment of love, reverence, and compassion.

The second part of the Healer's Heart step is to position yourself to co-heal and co-regulate with other nurses. Remember, it matters immensely who is with us before, during, and after an event or situation. **We can be the people that we need to heal** as we usher in *Nursing 2.0: The Nurse Safety & Professional Wellbeing Edition*.

Minding Your Transition Gaps

Given where most nurses' NSs are during practice, it can be difficult to envision where to place those MicroDoses throughout a busy day. The easiest places are those transition moments — before brushing your teeth, while your coffee or tea is brewing, as you put on your shoes, as you buckle and unbuckle your seatbelt, and so forth. At work, look for those transition moments — before you enter a patient room or colleague's office, as you walk through doorways, while you wash your hands, when you enter the supply room, before you start to chart or return an email, and so on. I call this "minding your transition gaps." Throughout each day, we all move through seemingly endless transitions, each one of which contains a little gap where you can MicroDose. All that is required is a small perception shift and 10-30 seconds, a manageable goal for the extraordinarily busy nurse.

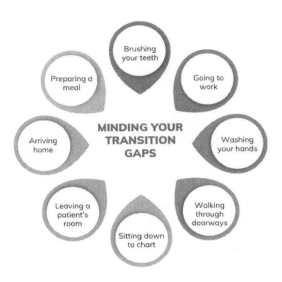

Super, Super Quick Solo MicroDose Practices

As you explore your MicroDoses Matter practice, you can draw from the Super, Super Quick MicroDoses Matter Menu shown in the table. Take creative liberties in adapting these however desired so you can expand your menu to regulate and co-regulate many, many times throughout the day.

Super, Super Quick *Solo* MicroDoses Menu

Super, Super Quick *Solo* Practices	Description
One Mindful Breath	One aware breath to separate yourself from the stressor. You are not the situation, you are the one nurturing your NS by attending to the situation. Haaaaa exhale, if possible, to signal safety and invite the ventral vagal circuit to come online. You're breathing anyway, so MicroDosing in this manner takes no additional time.

Pocket Pal 4x4	Keep a smooth object in your pocket. Rub the object between your thumb and fingers while doing one or more rounds of 4x4 breathing (each step to the count of four: inhale, hold, exhale —haaaaa if possible, hold, repeat).
Bear Hug Container	For NSs that feel like a live electrical wire without insulation. Put one hand under the opposite armpit. Put the other hand on its opposite shoulder. Do your choice of 4x4 or 4-7-8 breathing.
Elbow/Foot Doorway Tap	For when you're on the move. Every convenient time that you pass through a doorway, gently (or mentally) tap it with your foot or elbow while taking One Mindful Breath.
Hand Over Heart	Place or visualize your right hand over your heart. Left hand open. Visualize calming energy and support entering through the left hand while stress exits through the bottom of your feet into the earth.
Nurture with Nature	Use a screen saver, phone wallpaper, or actual artifact from nature that you can carry on your person. Use aware, relaxed breathing while connecting with the nurturing and restorative energies of Mother Earth.
Solo Notice, Name & Nurture	Pause briefly to notice bodily sensations, name your associated feelings, and nurture your NS using any super, super quick or preferred practice.

Super, Super Quick MicroDose Practices with Others
These practices offer the additional benefit of co-regulation with other Haelan Nurses or like-hearted colleagues and loved ones.

Super, Super Quick MicroDose Practices *with Others* Menu

Smize & Nod	As you pass or encounter another person, give them a soft smile with your eyes — a smize — and a gentle nod of the head. This simple act of connection facilitates co-regulation for you both, even if neither of you are aware of it at the time.
Bump it	For those comfortable with appropriate and therapeutic physical touch, offer a gentle and mutual elbow or foot bump as you pass by or engage in conversation or a shared task.
Heart Holding	Each person briefly places one or both hands over their own heart as a gesture of healing, co-regulation, and support.
Sidebar Debrief	If circumstances support a quick verbal exchange, take a moment for each person to express how their NS is being affected. Meet one another with nonjudgmental compassion and engage in a shared super, super quick or preferred practice.
Shall We Sway?	As the context allows, very gently and minimally sway your hand, arm, foot, or torso back and forth with a colleague to show mutual support, nurture your NS, and co-regulate together.

Healer's Heart Solidarity	Place one hand over your heart as you pass or engage with another Haelan Nurse or colleague. This signifies healing solidarity and co-regulation. My hands are over my heart many, many times throughout the day as I honor and facilitate healing for all.
Shared Notice, Name & Nurture	Each person holds co-regulation space for the other as each takes a brief pause to notice bodily sensations, name the corresponding emotion, and nurture your NS using any super, super quick or preferred practice.

Chapter Wrap-Up

In this chapter, you learned about your NS where trauma is concerned. The three circuits, the four hybrids, the Threat Detector, and Your Repository are all important and in service to your safety and survival. You learned about NS regulation and dysregulation, your Window of Tolerance, and the factors that help you to stay regulated and thriving within it. You also learned about some of the factors that cause SNS hyperarousal ("I can't" range) and the dorsal vagal circuit to come online, both of which shrink your Window of Tolerance to the point that you are partially in it, or not in it at all. Importantly, you learned how your NS gets hijacked at work, and how *relationship is everything* when it comes to trauma and healing. You practiced your first MicroDoses Matter round and learned that your NS needs many MicroDoses of nurturance throughout the day. All said, you learned the language of your NS and are beginning to navigate it — and you'll continue to do so in the chapters ahead. Before you move to the next chapter, please engage in the Haelan Nurse Activities below so you can get a little more MicroDoses Matter practice and integration.

Haelan Nurse Activities

Let's expand your MicroDosing repertoire as you continue to explore and practice. In the graphic, you'll find a list of the 14 Super, Super Quick MicroDosing practices that you can do solo or with others. Complete the table below, which I started for you, to create your unique MicroDoses Matter menu.

Recommended MicroDoses Matter dosing schedule: This is really up to you. The more you can MicroDose, the more stable and supported your NS will be. To start, try MicroDosing in the morning and evening before you brush your teeth. Then ramp up from there, adding before and after work and during any breaks you can take. Ideally, you'll ramp up to MicroDosing any time you notice a shift in your NS. It takes a little time and practice to discover the rhythm of your NS, and you'll be doing just that in the chapters ahead.

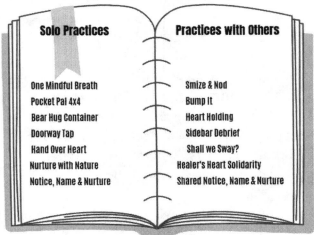

Super, Super Quick MicroDoses Matter Menu

Solo Practices	Practices with Others
One Mindful Breath	Smize & Nod
Pocket Pal 4x4	Bump It
Bear Hug Container	Heart Holding
Doorway Tap	Sidebar Debrief
Hand Over Heart	Shall we Sway?
Nurture with Nature	Healer's Heart Solidarity
Notice, Name & Nurture	Shared Notice, Name & Nurture

My MicroDoses Matter Menu

MicroDose Step	Ideas to Explore in my MicroDoses Matter Practice
1. Private Space	Brainstorm and list private spaces that you can access for 30 seconds or longer, at home and at work.
2. Ground & Center	Brainstorm and list small items that you can have on your person to help you ground and center. Then, add choices from the Super, Super Quick MicroDoses Matter Menu along with any other ideas that emerge.
3. Signal Safety to Your Threat Detector	Brainstorm and list ways in which you can signal safety to your Threat Detector. Start with the five senses, and then list your other ideas. • Smell: • Sight: • Hearing: • Taste: • Touch: Then, add choices from the Super, Super Quick MicroDoses Matter Menu along with any other ideas that emerge.
4. Healer's Heart	Brainstorm and list other ways in which you can honor yourself, your healer's heart, and the amazing that you and all nurses are at the core of their being. How I can honor myself and my healer's heart: How I can honor my colleagues and their healer's hearts:

Deeper Dive Resources

Badenoch, B. (2022). *Trauma & the embodied brain: A heart-based training in relational neuroscience for healing trauma.* Sounds True.

Maté, G. (2021). *The myth of normal: Illness and health in an insane culture.* Penguin Random House.

Porges, S. W. (2017). *The pocket guide to the polyvagal theory: The transformative power of feeling safe.* WW Norton & Co.

Van der Kolk, B. A. (2015). *The body keeps the score: Brain, mind, and body in the healing of trauma.* Penguin Books.

Section II

Healing Is Happening

Chapter 4

Your Innate Care Plan (YICP)

Now that you've brainstormed ideas for your MicroDoses Matter practice, it's time to put it into action. Think of MicroDosing your NS as staying hydrated throughout the day. You need that hydration to keep your cells and organs functioning just like your NS needs to be reassured that you are safe. By MicroDosing throughout the day, your Threat Detector can signal safety to your circuits and their hybrids. This, in turn, translates to more NS regulation and time within your Window of Tolerance. And, in its glorious positive feedback cycle, your upstairs and downstairs brains are connected, your RH and LH are collaborating effectively, and you are experiencing regulation. By being regulated and in your Window, you can now reap the benefits of neuroplasticity as you reshape your experiences from survival to thrive mode.

Button Jar Time Assessment

It can be challenging to notice when there is time for a MicroDose, especially when your SNS is online calling you into action — to do something, anything, NOW. Or, if your dorsal vagal circuit is online and requires you to stop or shut down NOW. When your upstairs and downstairs brain start to temporarily disconnect and your limbic system gets in the driver's seat, it will absolutely feel like you cannot take so much as one second to MicroDose. This is where your Button Jar Time Assessment tool comes into play. As shown in the image, visualize a jar of buttons with various shapes and sizes. Then, ask yourself, "How much time do I have for a MicroDose right now?" If you're at work, you may feel like you don't have any time at all. That would represent the smallest button in the jar,

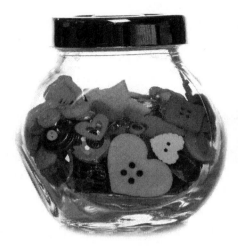

Button Jar Check-In

for you always have time for one deep, mindful breath. You're breathing anyway, so it's not taking any more time. You're just shifting your perspective to MicroDose when bandwidth is extremely narrow.

But let's say you have somewhere between 10-30 seconds. Those can be easily embedded throughout your day. You can MicroDose before you brush your teeth, before you put on your seat belt, or before you enter public transportation. Many nurses MicroDose as they're punching in on the time clock, before sitting down at the computer, before entering a patient room, before withdrawing medication to administer, while washing their hands, etc. These short MicroDoses would correspond to some of the smaller — but not the smallest — buttons in your jar.

The medium-size buttons could represent 1-3 minutes, the medium-large buttons 5-10 minutes, and so forth. It's your button jar, so play around with how much time each button represents and MicroDose commensurately. The goal is to not let a dysregulated NS make the decisions. There is always time to MicroDose because you're already breathing. And, unless you're in the middle of a code or rapid response, you probably have 10 seconds to MicroDose. Becoming aware of what your NS is signaling and then accurately assessing with your button jar will help to keep you, and not your limbic system, in the driver's seat.

Rx for MicroDoses Matter

As you start this mission critical practice, do so first in the mornings and evenings so you can get comfortable in the four steps (private space, ground & center, signal safety, healer's heart) and what strategies work best for you. Then build up to every four hours until a habit begins to form. From there, titrate up to MicroDosing at least once throughout every waking hour of the day to optimize your Window of Tolerance. Then, add PRN MicroDoses whenever you sense stress or dysregulation coming online.

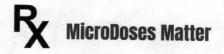

R̪x MicroDoses Matter

✓ Morning and night until comfortable

✓ Every four hours until a habit forms

✓ Every waking hour throughout the day to optimize Window of Tolerance

✓ Add PRN MicroDoses whenever you sense stress or dysregulation

Dr. Lorre
Signature

Continue to engage in your MicroDoses Matter practice throughout our time together in this book and beyond. It is an integral foundation to Your Innate Care Plan (YICP).

Your Innate Care Plan (YICP): The Basics

Given what you've learned thus far regarding your unique journey through hardship and trauma, you can now see that your lived experiences and unhealed bits of wisdom that are stored in Your Repository are unique unto you and you alone. Accordingly, Your Innate Care Plan (YICP) is also unique unto you. YICP is grounded in integrative nursing philosophy and science, one of the principles that speaks to every person's innate capacity to heal. Its design and practices will help you leverage your innate capacity for regulation, health, and wellness. YICP is the "how" you will move from survival to thriving mode, which can be distilled into this one actionable formula: $3A + B \rightarrow 3R$. The 3As are Awareness, Attending, and Alignment. This is how you nurture your NS. The B stands for Balance, which is conceptually similar to the "self-care" concept but with a more well-rounded approach. The 3Rs represent where we're going as individuals and a nursing community — Regulation, Reconnection, and Restoration. Let's explore each component separately below and then more fully develop YICP formula in the next chapters.

Awareness describes how you shift your perception as you gently and compassionately view yourself through the lens of "What happened to me?" instead of "What's wrong with me?" Awareness involves mindfully responding to your inner and outer lived experiences instead of habitually knee-jerk responding to them. Through your field of awareness, you see yourself as the person who is experiencing or has experienced hardships and traumas instead of *being* the trauma or its NS adaptations.

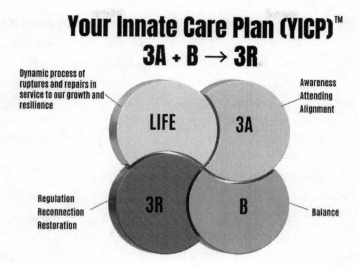

Your Innate Care Plan (YICP)™
3A + B → 3R

Dynamic process of ruptures and repairs in service to our growth and resilience

LIFE

3A

Awareness
Attending
Alignment

Regulation
Reconnection
Restoration

3R

B

Balance

Attending means honoring your NS and all that it has experienced, stored, and adapted to in service to your survival. You attend, nurture, and nourish your NS through practices that align with where your NS is at any given moment. Attending is the overall term for how you partner with your NS's evolutionary wisdom and navigate it in response to internal and external stimuli and as unhealed bits arise. By attending and nurturing your NS, you create a warm and welcoming environment for your unhealed bits — and their corresponding energetic activations — to emerge and be healed.

Alignment, in its simplest sense, is congruence or correspondence between your inner realities and outer lived experiences. This includes reconciling the inner impact of past or current traumas and how your NS adapted then with what is happening in your outer world now. It is very common for your NS adaptations to become patterns. While those adaptations or patterns served you well in the past, they may be maladaptive in the current context. Alignment is a process that starts on the inside after you've attended and nurtured your NS, like threading a needle from the inside and then pulling it to the outside. Examine if your NS adaptation is serving you well in the current context. If so, you are aligned and can crack on as you are. In most cases, you'll see an adaptation that could benefit from some tweaking or a full remodel. Then, you gently transform that adaptation and translate it into your current external reality. The alignment process is very subtle and so very powerful.

Being aligned can feel like being in a flow state or in oneness with life because you are aligning with your truest nature. For those whose beliefs include spirituality or religious connections, alignment includes your connection to whatever you know as a higher, omnipotent power that is greater than your human experience. It is also the process of honoring your deepest truths, and perceived life purpose, which changes as you do. Factors that favorably influence alignment include awareness, NS attending, gestures of inclusion for emerging unhealed bits, and being regulated in the Window of Tolerance. As we become more aligned, we internally expand so that life-force energy (chi, prana, unitary beingness, or however you identify with the grander context of life) can flow more fully within and throughout your external world. When aligned, your deepest inner truths are reflected in your external life. This is when you begin to live your highest and most authentic life, however you define it at the time.

Sometimes it's helpful to think of the 3As (Awareness, Attending, Alignment) as part of a spiral staircase. The lower three stairs are the 3As, which are where you connect with your inner world. From our inner world 3As, we can see how our outer world is affected in the Balance component, which includes the externals of daily living. By aligning our inner truths with our external world, we can move toward being more balanced and healthier in daily living.

YICP Making the Alignment-Balance Connection
Inner Wellbeing → Outer Wellbeing

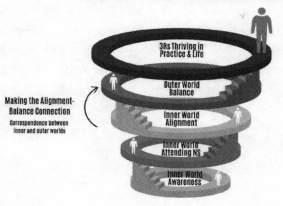

YICP Connection

Balance is reported to be the easiest part of YICP. It's all about the tangible externals in life and what you would typically view as self-care. Balance involves showing up for yourself with personal responsibility for and a commitment to healing and thriving, with others. It includes these components: body and mind wellness; connections and relationships; beliefs, values, and purpose; personal and professional contexts; financial wellness; and the all-important yet frequently sacrificed domain of regulating, relaxing, and recharging. I like to visualize the balance concept as a bicycle wheel, with the balance components making up the wheel. When you are balanced in your external living, it's like riding a bike with a fully functional wheel and inflated tire. But when you're imbalanced, so is your bicycle wheel. The ride becomes bumpy. The wheel rim is bent, the spokes are broken, and the tire isn't holding air. But still, you must ride it through the day, pushing against all the barriers that result from being out of balance. I much prefer a balanced external life, riding through each day on a fully inflated wheel, with ease and grace.

The 3Rs describe how you move toward healing and wholeness. The healing process *is* the destination given the inherent rupture-repair rhythm of life. The 3Rs include **R**egulation in your nervous system, **R**econnection within and with others, and **R**estoration of your healer's heart. When you are fully realizing the 3Rs, you are also fully thriving in your Window of Tolerance. The 3Rs reflect haelan, or healing, as a transformative process through which you reinterpret your life and sense of wholeness in bodymindessence. Being regulated, reconnected, and restored brings a much higher level of quality to your life.

How to Approach YICP

Partnering with YICP for healing is more of a "low and slow is the way to go" process than a "IV push" one. Positioning yourself in right relationship, with others, to facilitate healing is a gentle process of self-discovery. You can go as fast as your NS can go. Trust me on this one and know it to be true. Most nurses, including me, try the IV push method, only to find themselves knocked right out of the Window of Tolerance, dysregulated, overwhelmed, and usually in a freeze or shutdown.

What NOT to do: Don't be like me. Before I was a trauma-informed nurse and educator, I tried the IV push, *bring-it-on* approach. I literally set a goal to get my healing all done right now. STAT. I just wanted my suffering to end, to be done with it all. I longed for the land of rainbows and unicorns, where I would be at peace forever more. But that's a story for another time. In a very left-shifted way, I thought I could make a list of all the traumas and aspects that I needed to work on and chart them on a calendar. I believed that I could tackle them all and complete the healing process in a matter of days or weeks. I took a left-brained, Type A personality, bring-it-on mechanistic approach to a very complex, nuanced, and layered healing process.

This was a recipe for disaster. It was as though my unhealed bits, seemingly all of them at once, flooded into my field of awareness, longing to be attended and healed. It was *a lot* of energy to receive in one macro IV push dose. It was way too much for my NS. My dorsal vagal came online and *shut me down*. By taking the IV push approach, I actually added another trauma layer and experienced a setback. Although my intentions were earnest, my process was the exact opposite of what was needed. My NS was utterly overwhelmed. I didn't have all the right people that I needed for co-regulation, co-healing, and trauma healing-integration. Given the enormity of unhealed bits stored in my Repository, which I summoned to emerge all at once, my Threat Detector perceived and signaled extreme danger. My dorsal vagal came online, the dimmer switch almost fully on. I was in the deep freeze part of the freeze hybrid spectrum. I needed several days for the freeze to start thawing and about a week before I returned to my Window of Tolerance. Life was definitely living me. And, despite my best intentions to heal, I brought on a NS freeze adaptation instead.

So, don't be like Lorre. Don't bring it on. No IV pushes. No trying to race to the finish line (there isn't one) to get it over with. Your unhealed bits, like mine, could emerge en masse and overwhelm you instead of emerging in a healthy, titrated manner corresponding to YICP and NS. Doing too much, too fast, too soon, will assuredly overwhelm your NS and start to nudge you out of your Window of Tolerance and into a dysregulated state. Or, as it was for me, push you out of the Window altogether.

What to do: Move with compassionate, noble tenderness and gently respond to the wisdom of YICP. Know that your healing process will emerge in its own perfect time. YICP doesn't respond well to left-shifted dominance and rigid lists, tasks, checklists, timelines, and expectations. YICP cannot be forced, coerced, or mandated, for it is your sacred healing roadmap. Its timing is highly attuned to your healing layers, lived experiences, and unhealed bits. YICP is assuredly not bound by the LH constructs of time, clocks, and calendars. This is a RH-LH-RH process of softening, opening, trusting, allowing, adapting, supporting, and being supported — by yourself, your trusted loved ones, Haelan Nurse Communities, and your trauma-informed healthcare team.

YICP is far more accessible through your Window of Tolerance. When you're disrupted, dysregulated, or the Threat Detector is signaling a red alert, it's like putting a dark, damp, gray blanket over YICP. Yes, it's still there, but it is so much harder to get to if you're in a freeze or shutdown adaptive state. Or, if your SNS circuit is hyperaroused and in the "I can't" zone, you won't be able to see the big picture of your healing process. So, **the first goal is to live within the Window of Tolerance** by MicroDosing regularly and in frequent intervals. Even if it's one deep, conscious breath, that counts and matters immensely.

The second goal is to understand that YICP access increases every time you MicroDose and engage with YICP practices. Throughout this book, you'll create a unique YICP Menu filled with your favorite and most effective strategies and practices. YICP is a synergistic practice that works if you work it. The more you put into practice, the more healing gains you'll realize. Approach YICP with heartfelt self-compassion, love, and unconditional acceptance of yourself — in all the ways, throughout all the times, and in all your beautifully NS adaptations and unhealed bits. Be gentle. In the chapters ahead, you'll learn how to titrate YICP doses just as you would medication rites of administration, with the right dose at the right time using the right route for the right reason. In all things healing and in life, move gently, with ease and grace. **Healing is happening.**

Your Innate Care Plan (YICP): Practice Preferences

The first step in curating YICP is to explore your practice preferences where self-nurturing is concerned. Depending upon which circuits and hybrids are online when you engage with YICP, you'll align your practices with where your NS is at that moment. It makes good sense to partner with the 300–500 million years of evolutionary NS wisdom. It usually doesn't bode well to fight against your NS. For example, if your SNS circuit is online with the dimmer switch setting in the "I need to move or do something" range, then forcing yourself to sit down and be still could result in frustration and further aggravation to your NS. Similarly, there will be times when you want to be still, playful, alone, or with others. The key is to follow your NS's lead as to what it needs and then partner with it through your favorite YICP practices.

To ensure you have the resources and practices that you need for your NS at any given time, we'll explore practices from The Tree of Contemplative Practices. Many nurses are familiar with this free resource, and if you're not, then visit the website at: https://www.contemplativemind.org/practices/tree. I offer my heartfelt gratitude to The Center for Contemplative Mind in Society, Maia Duerr, and Carrie Bergman for their offering to humanity and our nursing community.

The Tree of Contemplative Practices is intended to help you develop your practices while cultivating awareness and building stronger connections within, with others, and to your spiritual or religious ways of being or not being. The tree is organized by different groupings of practices, whose definitions are fluid and overlapping. It's not so much about how the tree is organized as it is how you connect your practice preferences to it. You'll explore your tree and then populate your preferred practices into a YICP Menu in the Haelan Nurse Activities at the end of this chapter. For now, the Contemplative Practices Table may get your brainstorming juices flowing.

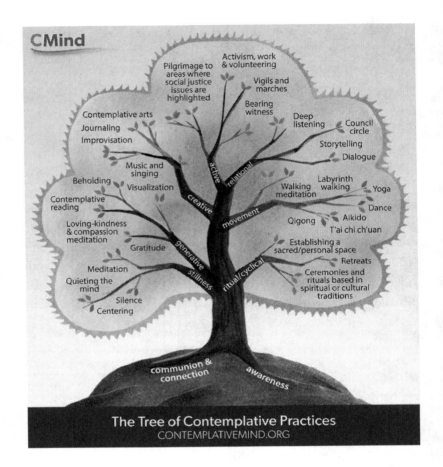

The Tree of Contemplative Practices
CONTEMPLATIVEMIND.ORG

Practicing Solo and with Others

The healing process is both a solo and relational pursuit. There are aspects of healing that involve inner work, such as the Awareness and Alignment components of YICP (3As + B → 3Rs). Other healing aspects — such as Attending or some of the Balance components — can be done individually or with others, as aligns with your NS and context. As you begin to conceptualize YICP, be sure to consider both the solo and relational aspects of healing in mind, for both are mission critical to thriving with Regulation, Reconnection, and Restoration in your Window of Tolerance.

Contemplative Practices Table

Contemplative Practice Category	Examples of Practices (partial list, categories may overlap)
Stillness	Meditation, silence, centering, quieting the mind, mindfulness practices, body scanning, breathing practices (4x4, 4-7-8, etc.), mindfulness apps and videos, welcoming your thoughts, feelings, and sensations.
Generative	Gratitude, visualization, beholding, contemplative reading, loving-kindness and compassion meditation, embracing preferred wisdom, indigenous, cultural and spiritual traditions, opening to interconnectedness with all other living beings, cultures, and societies.
Creative	Music, singing, improvisation, contemplative arts, journaling, any form of creative expression through any medium (drawing, painting, sketching, sculpting, arts and crafts, building, modeling, etc.).
Active	Engaging with, supporting, or bearing witness to social justice issues (vigils and marches, activism work and volunteering, pilgrimages, etc.).
Relational	Deep listening, dialogue, council circle, storytelling, poetry reading, acting, playing, authentic sharing with trusted loved ones.

Movement	Walking meditation, labyrinth walking, yoga, dance, aikido, qigong, t'ai chi ch'uan, shaking, jumping, swaying, any form of exercise that you enjoy, including hiking, climbing, biking, lifting, etc.
Ritual/Cyclical	Retreats, establishing a sacred or personal space, ceremonies based in spiritual or cultural traditions, celebrations, practices, etc.

To prepare you for YICP development, let's start thinking about how you'll map your preferred preferences to common NS circuits and hybrids. In the Practices to Nurture My Nervous System Alone & With Others table, you'll see how to sort your preferred practices. Just skim it for now, for you'll be completing the table at the end of the chapter as part of your Haelan Nurse Activities. This is a launching off exercise — let your instincts guide you. As you become more comfortable with navigating your NS, you'll update this table and use it to inform YICP. Everything here, like in life, is a work in progress. There's no right or wrong, just you exploring your preferences where your NS is concerned. Resist the temptation to overthink on this one! These practices can and should be incorporated into your MicroDoses Matter routine however possible.

Practices to Nurture My Nervous System
Alone & with Others

Below, brainstorm and think about how you'll complete this table with your preferred practices as it aligns with where your NS might be at different times. You can use or reuse any practice that feels right for any NS circuit or hybrid. This is an exploration activity and one that you'll refer to and update as

NS Practices

Practice Choices	Play Hybrid (feeling safe, relaxed, energized)	Stillness Hybrid (feeling safe, grounded, centered, present)	SNS Hyperaroused Circuit (feeling unsafe, fight or flight response)	Fawn Hybrid (feeling unsafe, fight or flight isn't available; must please and appease)	Freeze Hybrid (feeling very unsafe, stuck, shutdown, hopeless, lethargic, no energy)
	Indicate both solo and practices you you can do with others.	Indicate both solo and practices you can do with others.	Indicate both solo and practices you can do with others.	Indicate both solo and practices you can do with others.	Indicate both solo and practices you can do with others.
Stillness					
Generative					
Creative					
Active					
Relational					
Movement					
Ritual/Cyclical					

you get better acquainted with your NS, how it responds, and what it needs. These practices can and should be incorporated into your MicroDoses Matter routine, as desired.

Riley's Case Story

Let's explore how Riley, one of Jordan's charge nurses, approached using her innate care plan. Recall the very challenging, short-staffed, under-resourced unit in which Jordan's team worked. Compounding these challenges were the signs of traumatization that overwhelmed each nurse's NS. Being regulated and in one's Window of Tolerance was a rare luxury for the nurses working on this unit. Jordan's team members described their unit as "beyond toxic." Riley, one of two charge nurses, was often in the heart-wrenching position of being availed of limited personnel and resources from upper management from which to effectively lead the unit. She described this frustration as needing to pay rent at the first of the month with only half of a paycheck. It was never enough.

As a charge nurse, Riley was an engaged, compassionate, and effective leader who was well-liked and respected by all. In our early conversations, Riley described how her healer's heart felt like it was put through the paper shredder every day at work. Being deprived of the resources and personnel needed to deliver safe, high-quality care weighed heavily on Riley and resulted in nurse-specific traumatization and moral injury as the near misses, adverse and sentinel events became more frequent. As a charge nurse, Riley was a staunch advocate for improving staff ratios and resource allocation. The team enthusiastically supported Riley's efforts and often expressed gratitude verbally and through random acts of kindness. Over time, as upper management offered little more than platitudes and rare quick-fix resources, Riley and the team experienced all forms of nurse-specific traumatization.

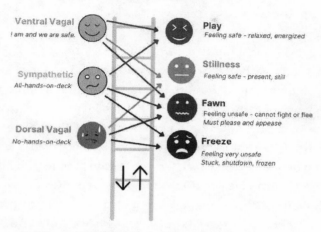

Riley's Team: Online Circuits & Hybrids

As you can imagine, every team member's Threat Detector was signaling danger as the external circumstances grew increasingly dire. Each nurse responded differently in their NS adaptations because each had unique inner unhealed bits in their Repository that were being concurrently assessed by their Threat Detector. No one's Threat Detector was signaling safety. Riley and her team had every circuit online, from the SNS "I can't" hyperarousal, to all three circuits' engagement in the fawning hybrid, to the dorsal vagal circuit's "I can't" hypoarousal and freeze hybrid. No one was practicing within

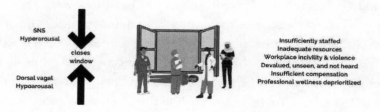

Avoidable Nurse Trauma Pushing Riley's Team out of Their Window

their Window of Tolerance given the vast amount of *avoidable* nurse trauma they were exposed to every day and over a prolonged period.

Riley's Innate Care Plan

During our early sessions, Riley described what once was a joyful, compassionate, and meaningful nursing practice. She was answering the call of her healer's heart and fulfilling her dream of caring for people in their greatest time of need. Over time, Riley started to feel less content and fulfilled and became more worried and anxious. On some days, the fear of avoidable system-induced adverse events hung over Riley like a dark, black cloud. Other days felt like a steady stream of frustration and agitation in the wake of staffing shortfalls and resource deprivations. Several years before our time together, Riley worked hard to prepare herself to serve in a leadership role by earning her master's degree in clinical systems leadership. She longed to be a part of the solution instead of being constrained by the problems.

Riley was quickly promoted to charge nurse and, following a brief and transitional honeymoon phase, learned that the charge nurse role was fraught with even more challenges. Riley felt helpless to properly staff and resource the nurses who were so devoted to the care of their patients. She often took patients for team members in addition to her charge nurse duties. Riley described how a sense of shame and hopelessness grew over the hope that once resided within. Empty promises were replaced by even more patients, many of whom had complex needs that exceeded the unit's resources and personnel expertise. Riley anguished when she had to decline team member requests for much needed paid-time-off requests. The team desperately needed their earned time off, but there were no other nurses available to cover their shifts. In a noble act of solidarity, Riley vowed to work overtime and not request any earned time off, opting instead to avail that time to the team.

I'm betting that you have experienced shades of what Riley experienced in your role. Every nurse knows that working beyond one's capacity for prolonged periods of time simply isn't sustainable in any bodymindessence aspect. Yet, we either volunteer or are required to work beyond reasonable and safe expectations in service to our patients and one another, at the expense of our health and wellbeing. In our early encounters, Riley arrived in my office depleted, exhausted, and burned out, opting to lay down on the sofa rather than sit on a chair for our informal yet professional sessions. To Riley's credit, she came with an earnest desire to heal and a willingness to do whatever was required to regulate, reconnect, and restore herself. This open willingness is everything. Riley was ready to position herself in right relationship for healing, with others. This openness is literally the gateway to her healing and to yours.

Slow the Pace Speed Bump: Ventral Vagal Breathing Practice

Riley's story may feel like . . . a lot. You've probably lived parts of this case story yourself. Let's take a moment to step back, lean in, and do some noticing and naming with tender gestures of welcoming inclusion. You, like Riley, have seen, felt, and experienced so much.

Drop down from the LH into the body circuits and just notice. Feet to floor, floor to earth, earth to feet. Notice the skin and muscles in your lower then upper legs. Become aware of belly and chest sensations. Place your hands over your heart and then, in one big inclusive gesture, do a big self-bear hug and embrace all the parts of your bodymindessence with loving kindness.

Stay in this space as long as desired. Should you long for connection, reach out to a trusted loved one or Haelan Nurse. Breathe, notice, and nurture whatever emerges for you.

When you're ready, let's gently engage the ventral vagal circuit by doing a Ventral Vagal Breathing practice. As you know, the vagus nerve moves through the diaphragm, so various diaphragmatic breathing exercises help to engage this circuit.

- Sit or recline in a comfortable position.
- Observe your natural breath, allowing your lower belly to rise outward and fall inward as you inhale and exhale. Do a few rounds until it feels natural . . . because it is when we're in ventral vagal tone.
- Begin to inhale through the nose and draw the breath back toward the sinuses.
- Exhale through the mouth with a soft "haaa" sound, like you are misting a pair of sunglasses before cleaning them. If you're in a public space, you can "haaa" very softly to honor your privacy. It's not about the sound as much as it is about the diaphragmatic ventral vagal stimulation.
- Resist the temptation to not use or observe your voice as it makes the soft "haaa" sound. The act of making and listening to this sound is music to the ventral vagal nerve, which, in turn, will engage so you can expand your Window of Tolerance.
- Repeat the inhales and expand the length of the soft "haaa" exhales to further attune ventral vagal stimulation. Do as many rounds as desired.

Use the above steps at any time while doing other activities. Even while working and especially while charting. Continue with these next steps to reset the ventral vagal system.

- Use the above steps to engage the ventral vagal system.
- Now, at the top of your gentle inhale, pause for the count of three to further stimulate the vagal system.
- Gently "haaa" exhale to the bottom of your expiration valley or for as long as comfortable. Repeat for a few rounds.
- To support you in maintaining the ventral vagal tone after this exercise, use "soft eyes" by opening them ever so slightly while gently looking at a point below you. Strive to keep your eyes soft and stationary.
- Continue with the breathing cycles, taking the breath inward to the top of the inspiration hill and "haaa" exhaling to the bottom of the valley.
- Repeat for a few rounds.
- Gently close your eyes and allow your natural breathing pattern to resume.
- With eyes still closed, compassionately observe your internal and external sensations.
- When you are ready, gently open your eyes and observe the effect of your engaged ventral vagal system. You may observe a subtle or profound effect, or perhaps an imperceptible one given your current context. Whatever you observe is perfect for this moment. Keep leaning into this practice and observe as you realize healing gains.

Healing is happening.

Chapter Wrap-Up

We'll continue with Riley's case story and see how she puts her YICP into action in the next chapter. In this chapter, you learned how to use the Button Jar Time Assessment to guide which MicroDose practices to use, ranging from when there is seemingly no time to when there is plenty of time. You learned the basic formula for YICP: 3A + B → 3R. You are brainstorming how to align your preferred practices with your MicroDoses Matter routine and thinking about how you can nurture your NS with individual and group practices. All of this will inform YICP Menu, which you'll continue to explore and develop throughout the book. **Healing is happening.**

Haelan Nurse Activities

Button Jar Time Assessment: Complete the table below to make the connections between your button jar and the approximate amount of time each button represents. You're creating a visual map to reference when your SNS circuit is trying to convince you that there isn't time for you to MicroDose or nurture your NS. I started the first row for you. The rest are yours to complete with whatever makes sense for your MicroDoses Matter routine.

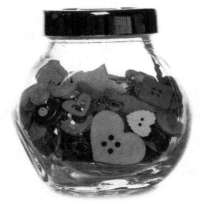

Button Jar

Button Jar Time Assessment Table

Button Size	Time (seconds, minutes, hours, days)	Corresponding Practices for MicroDosing
There isn't a small enough button for me right now	There is literally no time to MicroDose.	You're breathing anyway, so this practice doesn't take any additional time. Shift your perspective and do one deep inhale and slow exhale. If you can make a soft haaaaaaa exhale sound to encourage your ventral vagal circuit to come online, please do so.
Teeny tiny button		
Small button		
Medium button		
Large button		
The biggest button that will fit in your jar		

Practices to Nurture My NS: It's time to start conceptualizing YICP by first completing the Practices to Nurture My Nervous System Alone & With Others table. Then, write an "M" by those practices that you can incorporate into your MicroDoses Matter routine.

Once you've completed the table below, it's time to share in this healing process with other Haelan Nurses and your trusted

NS Practices

Practice Choices	Play Hybrid (feeling safe, relaxed, energized)	Stillness Hybrid (feeling safe, grounded, centered, present)	SNS Hyperaroused Circuit (feeling unsafe, fight or flight response)	Fawn Hybrid (feeling unsafe, fight or flight isn't available; must please and appease)	Freeze Hybrid (feeling very unsafe, stuck, shutdown, hopeless, lethargic, no energy)
	Indicate both solo and practices you can do with others.	Indicate both solo and practices you can do with others.	Indicate both solo and practices you can do with others.	Indicate both solo and practices you can do with others.	Indicate both solo and practices you can do with others.
Stillness					
Generative					
Creative					
Active					
Relational					
Movement					
Ritual/ Cyclical					

loved ones. Have some fun brainstorming and aligning nurturing practices with the NS circuits and hybrids. **Healing is happening.**

Deeper Dive Resources

CMind. (2021), *The tree of contemplative practices.* The Center for Contemplative Mind in Society. https://www. contemplativemind.org/practices/tree.

Dana, D. (2018), *The Polyvagal theory in therapy: Engaging the rhythm of regulation* (Norton series on interpersonal neurobiology). WW Norton & Company.

Kreitzer, M. J. (2015), *Integrative nursing: Application of principles across clinical settings.* Rambam Maimonides Medical Journal, 6(2), e0016-e0016. https://doi.org/10.5041/RMMJ.10200.

Kohrt, B. A., Ottman, K., Panter-Brick, C., Konner, M., & Patel, V. (2020), "Why we heal: The evolution of psychological healing and implications for global mental health" in *Clinical Psychology Review,* 82, 101920. https://doi.org/10.1016/j.cpr.2020.101920.

Chapter 5

Putting YICP into Action

In this chapter, you'll build upon what you learned in the last chapter by taking your preferred practices and populating them into a YICP Menu. Recall that your MicroDoses Matter routine and YICP practice are lifestyle choices to help stabilize and nourish your NS so you can move towards thriving in your Window of Tolerance. By consistently engaging in your MicroDoses Matter and YICP routines, you'll discover that they provide fuller, richer healing in your deeper layers. Both are necessary for you to consistently thrive in your Window of Tolerance while living your highest and best life, however you define it (and that definition changes and grows as you do). Here's a quick refresher of YICP components:

> ### YICP: 3A + B → 3R
> Awareness-Attending-Alignment + Balance → Regulation-Reconnection-Restoration

Before we resume Riley's case story, recall your MicroDoses Matter Menu from an earlier chapter. Those solo and shared practices can also be included in YICP Menu, just as Riley did in hers. Follow your intuition and partner with your NS's wisdom as you explore the various practices.

With that refresher in mind, let's now preview the YICP Menu that you'll be developing at the end of the chapter in the Haelan Nurse Activities. Here's what a YICP Menu template looks like:

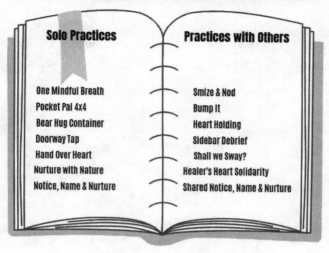

Super, Super Quick MicroDoses Matter Menu

Solo Practices	Practices with Others
One Mindful Breath	Smize & Nod
Pocket Pal 4x4	Bump It
Bear Hug Container	Heart Holding
Doorway Tap	Sidebar Debrief
Hand Over Heart	Shall we Sway?
Nurture with Nature	Healer's Heart Solidarity
Notice, Name & Nurture	Shared Notice, Name & Nurture

YICP Menu of Preferred Practices
(Ongoing: Add your preferred practices to
the ones listed below)

Stillness Practices
Meditation, silence, centering, quieting the mind, mindfulness practices, body scanning, breathing practices (4x4, 4-7-8, etc.), mindfulness apps and videos, welcoming your thoughts, feelings, and sensations.

Generative Practices
Gratitude, visualization, beholding, contemplative reading, loving-kindness and compassion meditation, embracing preferred wisdom, indigenous, cultural and

spiritual traditions, opening to interconnectedness with all other living beings, cultures, and societies.

Creative Practices
Music, singing, improvisation, contemplative arts, journaling, any form of creative expression through any medium (drawing, painting, sketching, sculpting, arts and crafts, building, modeling, etc.).

Active Practices
Engaging with, supporting, or bearing witness to social justice issues (vigils and marches, activism work and volunteering, pilgrimages, etc.).

Relational Practices
Deep listening, dialogue, council circle, storytelling, poetry reading, acting, playing, authentic sharing with trusted loved ones.

Movement Practices
Walking meditation, labyrinth walking, yoga, dance, aikido, qigong, t'ai chi ch'uan, shaking, jumping, swaying, any form of exercise that you enjoy, including hiking, climbing, biking, lifting, etc.

Ritual/Cyclical Practices
Retreats, establishing a sacred or personal space, ceremonies based in spiritual or cultural traditions, celebrations, practices, etc.

YICP Menu of Preferred Practices Table

	YICP Awareness Both Solo & With Others	YICP Attending Both Solo & With Others	YICP Alignment Both Solo & With Others
Your Circuits & Hybrids			
Play Hybrid *I am safe and feel like being active.*			
Stillness Hybrid *I am safe and feel like being still.*			
SNS Hyperaroused Circuit *I feel uneasy, threatened, or unsafe - I need to do something to move towards or away from the stimulus.*			
Fawn Hybrid *I feel uneasy, threatened, or unsafe - I can't fight or flee, so I must please and appease.*			
Freeze Hybrid *I feel uneasy, threatened, or unsafe. I have little or no energy. I just can't.*			
Suitable for all circuits and hybrids (Solo practices that can be adapted to do with others.)			

Our House of Haelan

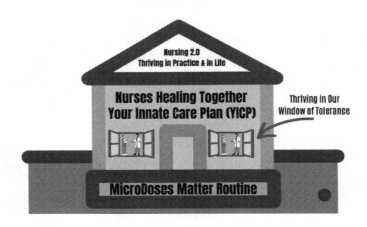

It may be helpful to think of your MicroDoses Matter routine as the foundation and YICP as the structure that sits atop the foundation. Together, they form Our House of Haelan. As you continue to engage in your MicroDoses Matter and YICP practices, you'll weave your own unique and beautiful tapestry of healing, regulation, and thriving as you regulate, reconnect within and with others, and restore your healer's heart and bodymindessence health and wellness. This is a personalized process that leverages *your innate capacity to heal*. With that in mind, let's return to Riley's case story and see how she is starting to develop her YICP Menu.

The First A: Awareness

In our early sessions, Riley's field of awareness was severely compromised. She shared her stories through the lens of "something is wrong with me" as if the circumstances, clearly beyond her control, were due to her own shortcomings or failures. Riley placed everything on her shoulders and then made herself feel wrong, incompetent, and like an utter failure. Life was living Riley — hard. Instead of perceiving herself as an incredible human who was experiencing a natural, adaptive response to a dire situational problem, Riley perceived herself *as the problem.* Riley and I talked about how her responses of fawning, fighting, fleeing, freezing, shutting down, and breaking down were NS adaptive responses and not conscious choices. Instead of welcoming how she was feeling, Riley was unknowingly pushing her perceptions, sensations, unhealed bits, thoughts, and feelings away. This ultimately led to further disconnection within her and contributed to the disconnection with others. Oftentimes, this "pushing away" adaptation is connected with a left-shifted hemisphere. Riley was unaware of how her left-shiftedness was affecting her. To help her become aware of all aspects of herself, we added the **Welcoming Yourself Home** practice to Riley's YICP. This awareness practice can be used for any circuit or hybrid that is online for you. I've added this practice to YICP Menu in the Haelan Nurse Activities at the end of the chapter so you can continue to use it throughout our time together and beyond. Until then, please join Riley and I in her session below.

Welcoming Yourself Home

Riley arrived at our appointment feeling overwhelmed. She shuddered at the thought of welcoming in her discomfort, pain, and unpleasant bodily sensations.

Riley: Why should I welcome the bad things that are happening to me . . . or have happened to me?

Lorre: That's a great question. I'm not suggesting that you welcome the bad things that you've experienced. Instead, I'd like for you to welcome *your complete self* home, including all those NS adaptations, unhealed bits, perceptions, feelings, or sensations that may feel uncomfortable, awkward, painful, or any other kind of way. When you or anyone else is dysregulated or out of your Window of

Tolerance, there's a sense of disconnection within and with others.

Riley: So, I don't want to disconnect further by pushing parts of myself away, is that what you mean?

Lorre: That's exactly what I mean! Remember when we talked about how it matters immensely that we have who we perceive we need before, during, and after a hardship or traumatic experience?

Riley: Yes, I do. That really makes so much sense.

Lorre: Well, in the Welcoming Yourself Home exercise, you are learning to be just that person for yourself. You are the first person that you need on your healing team. You are one of the people that you need before, during, and after your trauma exposure.

Riley: [nodding affirmatively] OMG, yes. I so get that! That must be what you mean when you talk about showing up for yourself.

Lorre: Yes, in part. There are so many ways in which we can and should show up for ourselves. For now, we'll focus on Welcoming Yourself Home.

***

I asked Riley to close her eyes if she was comfortable doing so, which she was. Together, we did a few rounds of 4-7-8 breathing (inhale to the count of four, hold to the count of seven, "haaaa" exhale to the count of eight). Riley started to relax. Her hands went from clenched to relaxed, as did her jaw. She looked and verbalized feeling comfortable and ready to do the Welcoming Yourself Home practice.

I asked Riley to open her heart and mind to a time when she felt very, very comfortable and welcomed. A time when it felt good to be Riley, surrounded by trusted loved ones who were always 100% Team Riley. The corners of Riley's mouth turned up in a gentle, partial smile. I asked Riley to notice the weather and how the air felt on her face and skin. I asked a gentle series of questions to guide Riley in connecting to a felt sense of being safe, supported, and welcomed. What types of clothes were you wearing? What smells and sounds are you observing? Who is with you? Do you have warm hugs? Conversations? Are there foods, flowers, or other treasures from nature with you? Riley's soft smile expanded and she gently opened her eyes and sat upright. I asked Riley if she would like to share what that smile was about. With a chuckle, she nodded yes.

***

Riley: I remember how wonderful our Sunday picnics were when I was a child. That was when my Nana was still alive. She had this beautiful home just outside the city, on a large parcel of land. There were rolling hills and grass as far as the eye could see. Most Sundays, we would drive to Nana's house for an afternoon picnic. [Her energy level rises, as does the color in her cheeks and the lift in her voice.]

Lorre: How wonderful, I can see this beautiful setting in my mind's eye.

Riley: We didn't have to do chores on Sunday and got to wear our best clothes to Nana's house. She always made us good food. She could cook! There was always a homemade dessert. Oh, I remember her peach pie with vanilla ice cream. We'd eat it on the back porch as we talked the afternoon away or played cards while her staticky radio played in the background. Then, as it started to get dark, we would gather the lawn chairs and sit around the fire pit . . . [Her voice trails off as she recalls this welcoming memory.]

***

Riley and my eyes meet softly, in a knowing gaze of shared understanding. Riley shared how she felt so safe, seen, understood, and welcomed by her Nana. I asked Riley to close her eyes if she'd like to spend more time in this safe, welcoming inner space that she curated with the unconditional love of her Nana. Riley closed her eyes and I asked her to place one or both hands over her heart, so she could feel this deep connection and sense of being welcome, exactly as she was then and is now. I guided her to notice her bodily sensations, starting with the feet, lower then upper legs, including her skin and muscles. Riley started noticing her belly, her heart, her arms, and then the air and atmosphere around her. She looked as peaceful as a napping kitten. Riley rested within this inner welcoming field of love and support for several minutes.

When I sensed that she was ready, I asked if she was open to inviting present-day Riley into the scene, as a Welcoming Yourself Home gesture of inclusion. We talked about how she could return to this inner sanctuary, her inner home, anytime. All these Sunday afternoons with her Nana were also embodied and stored in her Repository. Creating a safe and welcoming inner home is an essential awareness practice that also signals safety to the Threat Detector and nourishes the NS.

***

Riley: [contemplates with her eyes looking upward for a moment before resuming eye contact]

Won't my hot mess of a life ruin my inner home, my sanctuary?

Lorre: Your Welcoming Yourself Home practice is one where you can always feel safe, seen, heard, and supported, just as you were with your Nana during those lovely weekend picnics and bonfires. No matter what is happening in your life or what unhealed bits are emerging, no harm or disruption can come to your inner sanctuary, your home within yourself.

Riley: I can already feel my NS quieting down. I'm not nearly as stressed and contracted as I was before. Such a simple yet powerful awareness practice!

***

After we completed this Welcoming Yourself Home practice, we talked about how this inner sanctuary is always available,

24/7. Most people, over time, develop a number of Welcoming Yourself Home inner spaces using visual cues from indoors, outdoors, in this world or beyond, with or without other people or animals. Riley and I talked about how she could, as present stressors or prior unhealed bits emerge, use her Welcoming Yourself Home awareness practice to welcome all parts of herself to this safe inner space as a radical gesture of self-inclusion, self-acceptance, and self-love. Spontaneously, Riley placed her hands over her heart as she welcomed the parts of herself that would have otherwise been ignored or pushed aside, down, or away. Now it's your turn to do your first awareness practice by Welcoming Yourself Home.

Slow the Pace Speed Bump: Welcoming Yourself Home

Using Riley's case story as a guide, it's your turn to explore your inner sanctuary, which may be based on a real-life experience as Riley's was, or it may be based on favorite passages from books, movies, music, or nature. Anything goes! Allow your imagination to lead the way — no left-hemispheric forcing here.

Start with a few rounds of 4-7-8 breathing. Gesture inclusion while noticing and naming sensations or perceptions as they emerge. If it feels comforting, place your hand over your heart and/or belly or gently rock or sway.

Should you begin to feel overwhelmed or start to shut down, it's OK to step away from this practice. Take time to connect with a trusted loved one, Haelan Nurse, or health professional. Your NS will signal when it's ready for you to move forward and when to take a break or connect with others. Your job is to be aware of these sensations and honor them with self-love and self-compassion.

After your 4-7-8 breathing rounds, allow your inner sanctuary to emerge. Notice the images, colors, sensations, smells, tastes, etc. Notice if others are with you, from the physical or other dimensions. Welcome yourself home . . . all your parts and unhealed bits. Bask in the glorious inner sanctuary of safety, peace, and tranquility.

When you're ready to return to the external present moment, do a gentle wiggling of feet, legs, hips, torso, shoulders, arms, neck, and head to welcome yourself back here in the present moment, too.

In the space below jot, sketch, or reflect on your inner Welcoming Yourself Home sanctuary using any creative medium of your choosing. You can add to this sanctuary or create new ones at any time. Set a goal to visit your inner sanctuary several times each day — if only for one aware breath — so you can deepen your awareness as the first A in YICP: 3A + B → 3R.

***

My Inner Welcome Home Sanctuary:
Jot, sketch, draw, write, or creatively depict your inner sanctuary. You may have more than one sanctuary, and they can change as you do. Aside from being an unconditionally safe place, there are no limits or restrictions in your inner sanctuary.

***

***

***

Healing is happening.

Movie Theater or Bird on Shoulder Awareness Practices

Riley continued with her Welcoming Yourself Home awareness practice. She created several inner sanctuaries into which she could retreat for a few breaths or up to a half-hour, sometimes longer. Riley was eager to expand her YICP Awareness repertoire and wanted to explore other awareness practices. In this session, Riley added the Movie Theater and Bird on Shoulder awareness practices to her YICP. I added them to YICP Menu below, so you can explore them further at the end of this chapter and beyond. Let's join Riley's session, where she opened by expressing her frustration with trying a meditation practice.

*****

Riley: I can't meditate. Every time I try, I just do it wrong!

Lorre: In which ways do you feel that you're doing it wrong?

Riley: Well, I just can't get my mind to stop. Why can't I turn my mind off so I can meditate?

Lorre: Honestly, I hear this a lot from clients and colleagues. There's a lot of misinformation out there, in general, where mediation, awareness, and mindfulness practices are concerned. Let me ask you a few questions so we can explore this together.

Riley: Sure!

Lorre: When you are doing some of your MicroDoses Matter and preferred practices, like breathing exercises, gesturing inclusion to your whole self, or Welcoming Yourself Home, are you expecting your heart to stop beating while you're doing them?

Riley: [appearing puzzled] Um, no . . .

Lorre: [with a tender, curious voice] Do you expect your lungs to stop breathing?

Riley: [chuckling] Definitely no! [nods her head in expectation of the next question]

Lorre: Then why would you expect your brain to stop producing thoughts?

Riley: [laughing now] I never thought about it that way! No, I wouldn't ask my brain, heart, or lungs to stop doing their job while I'm MicroDosing at work or at home.

Lorre: Exactly!

Riley: So, why would I expect my brain, heart, and lungs to stop while I'm trying to meditate?

Lorre: Precisely. And I'm glad you used the phrase "trying to meditate." Awareness practices, including meditation, are more about *allowing* and *being* than they are about *trying* and *doing*.

Riley: How so?

Lorre: Do you remember our earlier conversation about how the RH and LH collaborate?

Riley: I do! It's like how we go back and forth between the hemispheres, like lacing our shoes.

Lorre: That's right. Many people take a LH approach to awareness or meditation practices. Their LH wants a plan, a roadmap, or an instruction manual. While it's helpful to have a general LH sense of what an awareness practice is, as we've talked about before, we also need for there to be inner space for the RH and its neural nets to weigh in.

Riley: That makes sense. I'm starting to see how left-shifted I am! [chuckles]

Lorre: Most of us are left-shifted. There's evidence of it everywhere, especially in healthcare. But it hasn't always been so. Think back to times before the industrial and technological revolutions. We were far more hemispherically balanced in those days.

Riley: I know. Even from the time I was a child until now! [gestures head exploding]

Lorre: If meditation isn't your thing, or if your SNS circuit is in the upper portion of the dimmer switch range, then I have other awareness practices for you to explore.

Riley: [exhales, appearing relieved] Yes! I'm over trying to meditate right now!

Lorre: Many of my clients enjoy YICP-Awareness using the Movie Theater or Bird Watching approaches. Do you have a preference?

Riley: Can I learn about both?

Lorre: Absolutely! Let's learn by doing and start with the Movie Theater exercise. Go ahead and get comfortable and close your eyes. Choose whatever breathing technique feels good to you and I'll guide you through it.

Riley: Let's do that ventral vagal breathing exercise. [Lorre facilitates as described in an earlier Slow the Pace Speed Bump.]

Lorre: Good, let's start with the Movie Theater practice. Imagine that you have before you the biggest movie theater screen you can imagine. You could be at an indoor venue, with those long, deep colored curtains, stairs, and reclining chairs. Or, you could be outdoors, at an amphitheater or drive-in theater. Your movie theater screen can go anywhere, so with your mind's eye, play around with different venues and see what feels good for today.

Riley: [after several moments] OK, I'm in my movie theater. Now what?

Lorre: With soft inner eyes, keep your movie theater screen in view while placing your attention on the natural rhythm of your breath. If any sensations emerge, just welcome them in. You can stop this exercise at any time should uncomfortable thoughts or sensations arise.

Riley: OK. What do I do with these thoughts that are whirling around?

Lorre: Perfect timing for that question! Whatever thoughts, emotions, scenes, conversations, or memories that emerge, allow them to drift away from your mind and onto the screen. As they do, you stay in your comfy theater chair and just observe, watch the show. Notice but don't cling to or otherwise attach yourself to those thoughts. Let's be together in this space, in noble silence, for a few minutes so you can *observe* your thoughts instead of *being* those thoughts.

Riley: [several minutes later] What do I do with the thoughts that are stuck in my head? Some of them won't go onto the screen.

Lorre: Just notice them and allow them to be as they are. Return to your breath while your inner eyes softly view the theater screen. Meanwhile, gently focus on your natural breath and inner movie screen.

Riley: That's amazing! As soon as I stopped worrying about those thoughts, they moved through . . . like . . . [pauses, searching for the words]

Lorre: Like clouds passing in the sky?

Riley: Yes, just like that!

Lorre: Good work. Stay in your field of awareness and just observe. Lovingly detach from the thoughts and feelings and allow them to be as they are. Meet any resistance or reluctance with gentle gestures of inclusion to welcome all parts of yourself home. Stay with your breath and your inner movie theater with open curiosity and self-compassion. When you're ready to leave this inner space, gently wiggle your arms, legs, torso, and head before opening your eyes and joining me in the room.

Riley: [after several minutes, wiggles and opens her eyes] Wow. That was amazing. I've never experienced anything like it. Before, when I tried to meditate, it was like I was in battle with my thoughts, trying to make them all go away or disappear. But when I allow them to be, like you say, as they are, they sort of dissolve or disappear by themselves.

Lorre: Yes, they sure do! Sometimes, if thoughts are particularly sticky or persistent, I lovingly detach from them . . . or I visualize cutting the energetic cord. I tell myself that if I want to call that pesky thought back at any point, I can do so. I've never had anyone call back a sticky thought though.

Riley: I think I get it. So, is this what you meant by "human as being"? Just being with my thoughts instead of trying to do something with them?

Lorre: Yes, precisely. We are all so conditioned to be "doing" all the time, many of us from the first moment we awaken to the last moment before we drift off to sleep. Through your field of awareness, you can balance your inner human-as-doing and human-as-being scales.

Riley: I totally get it. This is super helpful. So, how do I do the other awareness practice, the bird one?

Lorre: The Bird on Shoulder practice is exactly the same — except for the perspective. Instead of being in a movie theater and observing what appears on the screen, you take your favorite bird and place it on your shoulder.

Riley: What kind of bird?

Lorre: Any bird that feels safe and comfortable for you. I've had clients choose all sorts of birds, from hummingbirds to finches, sparrows to owls, ravens to eagles. The type of bird doesn't matter so much as your level of comfort. I've also had clients use mythical, spiritual, or religious deities in place of the bird. Anything goes!

Riley: [closes her eyes for a moment] OK, I have my bird. It's on my shoulder. Now what?

Lorre: As before, ground and center with any breathing exercise that feels good. When you feel settled, shift your perspective so that you are observing your life, thoughts, feelings, sensations, and emotions through the bird's point of view.

Riley: That's kind of weird . . .

Lorre: It may take a few moments to adjust to . . .

Riley: Oh, I get it now. OK, so the bird is like a scribe. It's like I'm using the bird's eyes to see myself and everything. This is so cool. It's like being a stargazer, but I'm looking at my life.

Lorre: Wonderful. As before, just notice, observe, gesture, and welcome all parts of yourself.

***

After Riley's bird watching practice, we debriefed, Riley set her goals for our next appointment, and we ended the session. Her energy field was noticeably lighter. Her eyes were bright, she had a lift in her step, and there was a softness to her facial expressions. Healing was happening. Now it's your turn to explore these awareness practices, along with any others that you may already have in your repertoire.

Your Turn: Movie Theater or Bird on Shoulder Awareness Practices

Using Riley's case story as a guide, engage in one or both awareness practices. You can do these practices anywhere, so long as you aren't driving or operating anything with wheels. It's helpful to be very comfortable — in stillness, while moving, whatever feels right for you. You can be indoors or outdoors. Some people enjoy using noise canceling technologies to minimize background noise and distractions, while others prefer to listen to instrumental music.

Jot, sketch, draw, write, or creatively depict your reflections and experiences here or elsewhere.

***
***
***

Healing is happening.

The Second A: Attending (and Nurturing) Your NS

Before we take a deeper dive into how you can attend and nurture your NS, it is important to disclose that there are pharmacological, psychological, psychotherapy, psychosocial, and other traditional and integrative strategies to clinically manage trauma or post-traumatic stress disorder. While these approaches and strategies are beyond the scope of this book, I have linked a number of resources for you at the end of the chapter in the Deeper Dive Resources. It's also prudent to disclose that while this book is grounded in many scientific disciplines, it is not intended to be used as a diagnostic tool or a substitute for professional health or mental health care. I recommend that you, like me, personally engage in proactive mental health wellness and care. Please consider working with a trauma-informed provider as needed or desired. This book is an educational resource with self-nurturing practices. Healing is always possible and available in all of your layers. That said, let's explore how you can attend your NS as the foundation of a self-nurturing practice.

You've already been attending and nurturing your NS by engaging in your MicroDoses Matter and YICP practices. In the graphic, you'll find a summary of the practices you've learned about thus far.

MicroDoses Matter & YICP Menus

MicroDoses Matter Practices		YICP Practices	
Solo		**Your Preferred Practices**	
One Mindful Breath	Pocket Pat 4x4	Stillness	Relational
Bear Hug Container	Doorway Tap	Generative	Movement
Hand Over Heart	Nurture with Nature	Creative	Ritual/Cyclical
Notice, Name & Nurture	Bonnie's Body Scan	Active	Others
With Others		**Awareness Practices**	
Smize & Nod	Bump It	Welcoming Yourself Home	
Heart Holding	Sidebar Debrief	Movie Theater	
Shall we Sway?	Healer's Heart Solidarity	Bird on Shoulder	
Shared Notice, Name & Nurture			

To these Attending & Nurturing practices, we'll add Speed Dating Your NS, Group NS Dating, and Haelan Community Group Dating.

Speed Dating Your Nervous System

You can't always fully attend to your NS in the moment, especially on those days where it feels like you're getting slammed from the moment you arrive to the moment you leave. MicroDoses, while incredibly helpful, don't always fully address our NS's needs. MicroDoses are intended to be administered along with MacroDoses of NS attending and nurturing. Please resist the temptation or habit of turning YICP into a chore or task. They aren't tasks to be hurriedly completed for the sake of crossing them off your mental list. Your healing requires all of you to show up for yourself, with your whole healer's heart filled with self-love and compassion.

Instead, attending and nurturing your NS is intended to be a rich, juicy, and felt experience that is savored just as a small child leisurely cherishes their favorite soft blanket, stuffed animal, doll, or other toy. Attending and nurturing your NS satisfies natural and primal needs that, once you're comfortable with them, can be playful and enjoyable. Let's learn how you can date your NS as an attending and nurturing NS practice.

Speed Dating Your NS Practice

At the end of each workday, integrate a quick speed date with your NS to attend to any lingering stress, sense of overwhelm, or dysregulation. Sometimes, it is necessary to temporarily *suspend but not reject* emerging sensations, thoughts, and feelings. While at work, you strive to attend to and regulate your NS through your MicroDoses Matter routine. As soon as your workday is done, a speed date with your NS is a wonderful self-nurturing act.

Speed Dating Your NS doesn't have to take a lot of time. It doesn't matter so much how long you show up for yourself. It matters immensely *that* you consistently show up for yourself. Some of the Haelan Nurses I work with speed date their NS in the parking lot after work by taking time to breathe, release, and restore. Others like to drive to a nearby park or use headphones or earbuds while using public transportation. Many nurses like to enjoy their speed date during or after a shower or bath. Your speed dating practice is ideally a consistent and sustainable one that you enjoy as soon as comfortably possible after work.

Explore what works well and what doesn't. Partner with the wisdom of your NS and let it lead. What does it need? Do you want to be indoors or outdoors? Do you need to move? Play? Be still? Be alone or with others? Many nurses enjoy listening to music or using mindfulness or self-care apps on their phones, while others enjoy noise canceling headphones. What feels warm, nurturing, soft, tranquil? Or, if you feel like you need to move, what kind of movement feels good? On one speed date, you might feel like being still. On other dates, you might crave movement. Sometimes you may want to both move and be still. Or play. By consistently speed dating your NS, you'll develop your speed dating rhythm. **Healing is happening.**

Group NS Dating Practice

Recall that *relationship is everything.* We need one another for co-regulation, co-healing, and survival. It can be easy to slip into the mindset of wanting to heal alone like a wounded animal, alone in a cozy cave, in times of dysregulation. And while there are times when solo speed dates are the best fit, there will be just as many times when Group Nervous System Dating is beneficial. You can weave MicroDoses Matter With Others practices throughout the day as a launching point. As time and bandwidth avails, you can expand your speed dates into whatever feels right for you — both during and outside of work. The goal is to weave a web of co-regulating and compassionate support throughout the day.

Some nurses use a move or still Group NS Dating approach. For the move approach (when conditions in their setting permit), they climb a few flights of stairs together or do a quick lap around the building. Others like to have a swaying or shaking minute in a private space. Anything goes as long as it's suitable for your work environment.

By far the most popular stillness-based Group NS Date activity is the *Team Zen Sand Tray*. Start by placing a sand tray in the break room or another shared space. Everyone is invited to bring in nature artifacts or meaningful relics from home and contribute to that day's zen tray. Throughout the day, team members mindfully attend to the zen garden by adding, removing, or rearranging materials, miniature stones, flowers, or other items. As you and your colleagues embark upon your Group NS Dating process, lean into one another and draw from your creative and playful nature. Be boldly inspired. Explore and have fun. Nurses who co-regulate together, heal together . . . and that makes everything better! Let's see how Riley's unit approached their Group NS Dates.

The First Haelan Nurse Community

Continuing with Riley's case story, she learned how to attend to her NS using the same strategies that you are. Riley wanted to help her nursing friends and colleagues with their healing process and decided to take a leadership role for their Group NS Dates. To start, Riley's team brainstormed and came up with a list of NS attending-nurturing activities that they enjoyed and tailored it with activities they could do together as a group. They grew excited about all the ways that they could be there for one another. This group started with 5 members and morphed into more than 15 members over time, though not every member attended every event.

Riley volunteered to get them started with fun and relaxing social activities. This group's goal was to deepen their healing process while having lighthearted fun and laughter, with each member taking turns to lead them through various attending activities. They met once or twice a month using a drop-in-when-you-can approach, meeting in one another's homes, parks, coffee shops, yoga studios, and arts and crafts venues. Riley's group varied their activities — sometimes just the nurses would attend, other times spouses, significant others, and children would join the fun. Here's a quick list of some of the activities they enjoyed, with room for you to add ideas for your trusted loved ones and Haelan Nurse Community.

Over time, Riley's group of diverse nurse collaborations morphed into the first Haelan Community. Along the way, they encountered some obstacles. Everyone had full lives and a scarcity of discretionary time. Riley's group expressed frustration — they wanted to carve out time for themselves and for their healing with one another — but it felt like a logistical nightmare. They scheduled a session with me to discover a pathway through the left-shifted time scarcity perspective.

During that meeting, we opened with grounding, centering, and attending practices. Then they discussed and decided upon a goal for that session, which was how to overcome the time and logistics barrier. The conversation that followed yielded rich information: (a) given their dynamic schedules and limited paid-time-off approvals, there wasn't going to be a perfect time that worked for everyone all the time; (b) if they shared planning and hosting responsibilities by rotating a Haelan Host each month (or twice-monthly, when possible), no one would be unduly burdened; (c) the Haelan Host would be responsible for scheduling, planning the activities, and communicating with the group; and (d) at the end of each event, they would reflect, discuss, and make recommendations for the next Haelan Host.

Working within those parameters, we did a white board reflection where the group members listed all the reasons why they didn't have time for healing and self-caring activities. I

Haelan Community Group Dating

Mindful tasting parties — savor beverages and foods together	Arts and crafts: fiber arts, painting, ceramics, jewelry making, macrame
Chair massages	Walking, hiking, jogging
Yoga, Tai Chi, Qigong, movement-mindfulness	5-4-3-2-1 exercise
Dance or exercise class	Spa day
Shinrin-yoku forest or nature bathing	Manicure-pedicure party at home or at a salon
Labyrinth walking meditation	Explore one another's spiritual, religious, cultural, or familial traditions
Aromatherapy	Hot pot or fondue party
Sound or music therapy	Field trips to local attractions
Singing, humming, chanting	Staycation getaway
Coloring book party	Music appreciation, with or without swaying, shaking, or dancing
Shared self-compassion session	Gentle stretching or yin yoga
Meditations: loving kindness, sitting with difficult emotions	Gardening — at a community garden or at home, in containers — anything goes!
Leaves on the Stream visualization (put each thought on a leaf and watch the stream carry it away)	Board games, charades, mystery parties
Guided imagery and visualization exercises	Cooking classes, progressive dinner parties

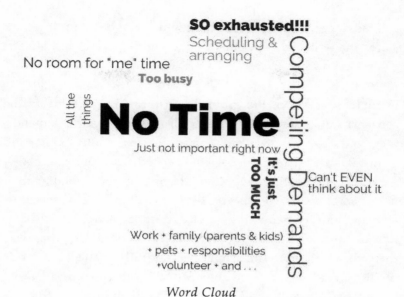

Word Cloud

hastily constructed a word cloud of their list. I invited the group to drop down from their LH and into their body while they sat with their word cloud — to just be with it in gentle compassion, while gesturing inclusion for any sensations, thoughts, or emotions. The energy in the room grew heavy with reverent contemplation. After a few moments, I encouraged the group to look at the white board as though it were a mirror. I asked each group member to share what the word cloud meant to each of them.

Jordan: That there's no time for me in my life . . .
Chin-Mae: Some of this stuff isn't really that important to me.
Taylor: I need to edit my life.
Gabi: Wow, that's . . . concerning . . .
Riley: How can it be that my life isn't even about me?!
Lorre: It's a lot to take in. If you feel ready, let's take a deeper dive by answering the question of "Where does my discretionary time go?" Be sure to reflect screen time — TV, streaming,

media, social media — all of it, which can be a big time sink for many of us. Especially in the era of hi-tech, left-shifted societal norms.

***

In rapid succession, the group brainstormed and came to the consensus that, despite busy schedules and competing demands, they could carve out a couple of hours each month to heal and grow together. All of the usual left-shifted distractions emerged — media binging, online shopping, internet and social media rabbit holes, scrolling ourselves to sleep, etc. Numbing, distracting, and disconnecting are all evidence of unhealedness that is ripe for our time, attention, and engagement. Now seeing a pathway through which more time could be mindfully availed, the group easily agreed upon a flexible SMART (specific, measurable, achievable, relevant, time-bound) goal and self-reported that this goal seemed attainable. Their SMART goal was:

Riley's Haelan Community SMART Goal

Within the next month, schedule our first five gatherings where each member hosts and facilitates a fun activity that supports our regulation, reconnection, and restoration.

We kept in communication as the group explored their preferences and gathering dynamics. I met with the group again, after each member served as a Haelan Host. They were thriving in the group through fun, rich, and meaningful activities that also helped them to co-regulate and live within their Windows of Tolerance. Being a small part of their process filled my healer's heart with joy and purpose. Healing was happening, and their transformations were palpable and infectious in the best sense of the word. Central to the healing shifts that they were making — within and with one another — was their commitment to change and willingness to do whatever was necessary to keep moving forward. They transcended their collective left-shifted mindset of "There's no time for me" to "There's always time for me."

"Some changes look negative on the surface, but you will soon realize that space is being created in your life for something new to emerge."

Eckhart Tolle

The Third A: Alignment

Alignment is the personal, intimate relationship between your inner truths and outer lived experiences in all aspects of bodymindessence. This includes reconciling the impact of unhealed bits that emerge from Your Repository with how they are manifesting now in your outer world. If the inner impact is lived maladaptively in your outer world, that signals that realignment is needed. Similarly, if you observe your once highly adaptive NS responses aren't serving you well in the current context, then realignment is needed. It's a subtle but oh so powerful process of reconciliation, from the inside out.

Many people are so left-shifted and disconnected that they're out of touch with their deepest, most vulnerable truths. Being out of alignment reflects the adaptations to your NS over time that likely resulted in left-shiftedness. There is no blame or shame where misalignment is concerned, for NS adaptations are not choices we get to make. They are adaptations in response to trauma and hardship. So, strive to take that tender, compassionate "What happened to me/us/they/them?" perspective. We all are where we are because of the brilliance of our Threat Detector and NS that kept us safe. Honor these adaptations, for you wouldn't be where you are today without them. Just as we honor the unhealed bits of wisdom that emerge when conditions are ripe for healing. All in service to your growth, strength, and resilience.

185

The goal of alignment is to heal those misalignments so you may connect with your ever-evolving deepest truths, dreams, aspirations, and life purpose. It's like tuning into a radio station in your car. At first, there's nothing but static and noise. But as you keep aligning that tuner to the music, the static fades away and the beautiful music can be heard clearly. Similarly, when you are aligned internally and externally, you are in a flow state of oneness within yourself and with the grander context of life — however you perceive it. You are living your highest, best, most authentic life. And it feels *good*. When you are misaligned, there is incongruence and disconnection between your deepest truths and outer realities. It feels like something's missing or that you're just going through the motions. You aren't fulfilled in the ways that matter to you most.

Reconnecting your inner sensations and feelings with your outer reality can feel, at first, a little overwhelming, ambiguous, or unattainable. Let's sit in on one of my sessions with Gabi, who is on the same team with Riley, Taylor, Chin-Mae, and Jordan (before she changed employers). Gabi and his family were displaced from a war-ravaged country to the United States. Gabi was a nurse in his native country, but his credentials weren't recognized in the US. So, he had to start over in a new country, a new culture, and a new (hot mess of a) healthcare system. He had to re-do nursing prerequisites and attend nursing school again. Life required Gabi to embody an "I'll do whatever I need to do" attitude, and he responded in kind. He was a valued and wonderful nurse who supported his team wholeheartedly. In our group sessions, he was comfortable with the awareness and attending practices, but the concept of alignment was a perplexing one. Here's what we discussed:

***

Gabi: I'm feeling good about my awareness and attending practices. They're so helpful. I use them a lot [chuckles], like . . . really a lot! But when practicing alignment, it's so . . .

confusing. It's like it's all garbled together . . . like a ball of . . . chaos. I don't know what to do with it.

Lorre: I hear the word *chaos* a lot in my practice. So much has happened to you. Your NS adaptations and perseverance are brilliant. As a result of all that's happened, much of it is stored in the body and neural nets that . . .

Gabi: ... [recalling our prior sessions] They hang out as unhealed bits of wisdom, right?

Lorre: Exactly.

Gabi: So why does this make alignment practice so hard for me?

Lorre: Tell me some of the ways in which alignment is hard for you.

Gabi: Well, I get centered and grounded. It's hard sometimes. I love Bonnie's Body Scan. Somehow, being anchored to the star at the center of the earth helps me to stay in my body.

Lorre: That's wonderful. Then what happens?

Gabi: So, [long pause] I do the welcome home thing and . . . it feels like I don't have a home. I mean, yes, I have a home that we live in, but I don't have a home within myself. Everything is go here, do this, do that. It's exhausting.

Lorre: Have you discovered any sense of an inner home?

Gabi: Yeah, but it's not much of a home. [chuckles] It's more like a deserted island.

Lorre: Tell me about this deserted island, using all of your senses. Let's try closing your eyes for a few minutes, if that feels comfortable. [Gabi nods affirmatively and we do Bonnie's Body Scan.] Now, let's go to your island. Let me know when you get there.

Gabi: [after a few moments of silence] I'm there. [audibly exhales]

Lorre: Good. Tell me what you see and hear.

Gabi: It's like this island in the middle of the sea. There's like a small mountain, lots of trees, and brownish-gray sand.

Lorre: Do you feel comfortable exploring this island? I'll be right here with you.

Gabi: Yeah.

Lorre: Wonderful — tell me everything! Whatever you see, hear, smell, taste, touch, or feel. Let's explore your island!

Gabi: Well, it's windy. The sea is choppy and there are gray clouds in the sky. It looks like it might rain later. I can smell the sea. [nods his head] I can taste the saltiness of the air on my tongue. And I can feel the sea air on my skin. It's hot, but the wind is cool.

Lorre: Oh, I am so feeling what you are describing! Let's walk around a little. What's it like behind you? Around you?

Gabi: There's a lot of jungle bushes and tall trees. I don't know what they are, but they're amazing. Wait, hold on. I think I see a path or a trail or something . . .

Lorre: Would you like to see where this trail goes?

Gabi: Way ahead of you — it goes through this thick ground covering towards the butte or mountain, or whatever that hill thing is. I'm kinda jogging right now. [laughs] Does this count as exercise for today?!

Lorre: [also laughing] It definitely counts as inner exercise! Keep going. I'm right here with you.

Gabi: The trail is narrowing and getting rocky as I climb. Now it's turning to the right. I'm about half-way up this mountain and I can see the other side of the island. Wow . . .

Lorre: Go on . . .

Gabi: This other side is completely different. The sea is calm, there's a blue sky with some white clouds. There's a gentle breeze. The water is more . . . blue . . . I guess.

Lorre: Do you want to go to this other beachy area?

Gabi: Already there! The sand is a lot softer and whiter here. I'm barefoot and I can feel the sand between my toes. [exhales, relaxingly]

Lorre: Sounds glorious. Would you like to take a few moments here?

Gabi: Yes, [laughs] and I may never leave! [He takes several moments and appears calm — tranquil, even — with jaw unclenched, hands softly open, and a relaxed breathing rhythm.]

Lorre: Do you feel at home on this side of your island?

Gabi: Totally.

Lorre: If it feels right, we could move into your attending and nurturing practice.

Gabi: I'm in.

Lorre: So, let's start the alignment practice from the calmest spot in your Welcome Home space. Today, it's this calm side of the island. Tomorrow, it could be the same or different places. We just go with whatever emerges. Alignment is a process of allowing. There's no doing in this practice. It's about holding this inner sacred, safe space and seeing what emerges, if anything. Sometimes nothing emerges, and that's OK. That just signals that inner trust is being reestablished or is growing.

Gabi: But what if I just start thinking about everything and get overwhelmed again?

Lorre: That happens sometimes. It's just the left-shifted hemisphere making sense of what it's getting from the right. Can you let those thoughts be as they are? Let them pass you by, like clouds in the sky?

Gabi: I'll try . . .

Lorre: [chuckles] Trying is such a complex word, isn't it? Let's put "trying" into perspective using Eckhart Tolle's work. Trying is a *human-as-doing* thing. See if you can shift from doing into *human-as-being*. Just be. Allow the energy of these thoughts to dissipate in their own perfect time. Just be. Notice your breath . . . this calm side of the island. [Gabi's jaw relaxes again.] Good. Let me know when you're ready for more.

Gabi: Yeah, I'm good. And you're right. I just allowed the thoughts to be. They hung around for a bit and now they're gone. They just sort of dissipated!

Lorre: Your awareness practices are paying dividends — wonderful! Now, to help you reconnect with your deeper self from this calm, peaceful, and safe inner island, let's draw from your imagination. On your island, or whatever inner safe space you are inhabiting, is a magic wand or other artifact familiar to you. Take a look around and see what you find.

Gabi: [looks puzzled] Really? Okay . . . [laughs excitedly] I found something!

Lorre: Do tell!

Gabi: There was this Aladdin's lamp thing under a bush. [grunts softly as he gestures that he's looking inside the lamp] No genie though.

Lorre: Whatever your imagination produces, or doesn't, is just fine. Let's say that with this Aladdin's lamp, all things are possible. Some clients find magic wands. Or pixie dust. You get the idea. You can use either or anything else that appears. There are no limits or restrictions, no sense of time or money.

Gabi: Ooooh, I like where this is going!

Lorre: Now, if this Aladdin's lamp could bring, change, or do something for you, what one thing would it be?

Gabi: Just one thing?! There are so many. [laughs]

Lorre: Just one — for now. That will help you navigate any inner static as you move into your deeper layers, from the bottom of your heart, as they say. What is the one change, one shift that you would like to be realized in your life?

Gabi: I'm going to need a minute . . . [rubs his eyes with perhaps the beginning of a tear emerging]

Lorre: There's no time in this inner Aladdin's lamp sanctuary. If that one wish, that one deep truth, emerges, you can keep it private or share it with me, whatever feels comfortable.

Gabi: There's this one thing . . . well it's not really a thing . . . it's a *big situation*. [grows verklempt, rubs both eyes]

Lorre: Just be with that *big situation*. Allow whatever message your deeper self has to emerge. You are safe on your island, and with me.

[Note to reader: Insert any *big situation* you have or are now experiencing as you read through Gabi's transcript.]

Gabi: I know I need to change this *big situation*. I just don't *want* to . . .

Lorre: The head and the heart don't always arrive at the same place at the same time. Stay with your breath, gesture inclusion. Allow your deeper self to be heard.

Gabi: OK, but I don't *want* to change it. But I really, really *need* to change it.

Lorre: Good, stay with it, you're brushing up against your resistance. Allow your resistance to be as it is — just like those clingy thoughts from a few moments ago. Just observe and allow. Time doesn't exist on our inner island sanctuary.

Gabi: OK.

Lorre: When the discomfort of the resistance abates, forecast what your outer world would look and feel like *after* you moved through the change process. Your *big situation* is in the rearview mirror now.

Gabi: [jaw softens, the corners of his mouth turn upward ever so slightly] It looks . . . good. Really good. It feels amazing, actually. It's like I can see my life without . . . chaos . . . that chaotic static in the way. After I make the alignment, I can see that everything will flow better in my life . . . especially this one really difficult part . . .

Lorre: Stay with this feeling for as long as you'd like. When you're ready, you can follow your breath, start to gently move your feet and hands, and open your eyes.

Gabi: [eyes open, body relaxed] Do your other clients have experiences like this? Wow. That was incredible.

Lorre: Most do — it's the best part of my job! You just laid down the very first neurons to change the *big situation* as you weave a new tapestry using the threads of new synaptic connections and neuroplasticity. Wonderful! Let's talk a little bit about your experience. At the beginning of this alignment exercise, how did you feel?

Gabi: I felt . . . overwhelmed. Like I didn't know where to start.

Lorre: And then your LH jumped in to make sense of how you were feeling before you were done feeling it. The sensations you were experiencing, the feelings that were emerging — would you say they were more comfortable or uncomfortable?

Gabi: Definitely uncomfortable!

Lorre: Coming into our deeper truths is often accompanied by the discomfort of resistance. Those subjective, juicy feelings from the body's neural streams and RH. Most of us are adaptively left-shifted, so it makes sense that the LH would step in and take over, so we can be spared our temporary discomfort.

Gabi: I never would have thought of it that way . . . but . . . that's exactly what happened.

Lorre: Would you like to take another alignment step? [Gabi nods yes.] Let's use your Inner Straw as a connector between your inner and outer worlds. In your mind's eye, can you envision such a straw?

Gabi: Yes, I got it.

Lorre: Great. Think about the early part of this alignment practice. When all the perceptions, emotions, and sensations were being felt, the discomfort of it. And then all those LH thoughts came rushing in.

Gabi: Those thoughts were vicious, man. Like a tsunami on my island.

Lorre: [chuckles] That's a great way to put it. Now, going back to that Inner Straw that connects your inner and outer worlds. What did it look like? Feel like?

Gabi: [laughing] Honestly, it looked like one of my son's bendy straws, what do they call those things?

Lorre: I think they were originally called crazy straws, but bendy straw works! What if your spirit, life energy, life force, chi, prana, or however you relate to it . . . was flowing through that straw, back and forth between your inner and outer worlds? Would that energy, containing your inner, deepest, and most vulnerable truths . . . would it flow with ease and grace, to be readily realized in your outer lived experiences?

Gabi: Um, that's a no. I couldn't even find my inner truth, let alone have it flow. Have you ever tried drinking out of one of those bendy straws? They are so much work!

Lorre: They *are* a lot of work — and you don't get much to drink when it has to travel through all the twists, turns, and bends. The same is true for our life energy. It gets all stuck and stagnant in the bendy straw.

Gabi: Or it's just too much work. So you don't bother with it. That's what I do with my son's bendy straws. I just don't use them. [laughs]

Lorre: And that's what happens to your alignment over time. Because of all that has happened to you, your brilliant NS adapted so you could be safe. You had to store that which you couldn't process during those times. The right people, those who could aid you in fully processing before, during, or after the trauma, weren't there or weren't able. So, without knowing how to navigate everything, it's natural to left-shift. But when we do so, there's a sense of inner disconnection from the juicy, subjective part of ourselves from which our deepest truths can emerge. In other words, your Inner Straw morphed into a bendy straw.

Gabi: I totally see how that happened. So that's why I did the Welcome Home exercise before the attending practice? To get me more balanced in my hemispheres? So I could more deeply feel and then understand what I need to do about the situation?

Lorre: Our thoughts can feel chaotic or tangled up sometimes. Especially when our inner and outer worlds are in that bendy straw flow state. Now, remember what it felt like after you allowed the thoughts, and then the resistance, to be as they were. You allowed them to pass, like clouds in the sky.

Gabi: That's exactly what happened.

Lorre: Tell me how that invisible straw looked and felt during that part of your alignment practice.

Gabi: Wow. OK, I see it now. It's like this clear, no wait . . . like, how do you say it . . . like soft rainbow colors?

Lorre: Iridescent?

Gabi: Yes, iridescent! It's like there's this steady ebb and flow going through this iridescent straw.

Lorre: That's right. Through your alignment practice, you allowed a subjective, juicy, deep truth to emerge, to be heard by you. As you projected this truth into your external world, albeit in the future, you made an alignment gain. And you forged a new neuroplastic trail of synapse that can wire and fire together as you continue aligning.

Gabi: It's one thing to make an alignment gain here [taps his facial temple], but nothing has changed out there [points outward].

Lorre: It hasn't changed *yet*. Whether or not you use your alignment gains to affect change depends upon you, your free will, and your decision-making process. How you respond to your inner truths, if at all, is your choice to make.

Gabi: Oh, that makes sense. But if I understand correctly, it's hard to change when I'm in bendy straw mode. Dysregulated, if you will.

Lorre: Fantastic insight. The more you nurture your NS, the more you will thrive in your Window of Tolerance, and the more opportunities there will be for alignment gains. You get to decide if you will live your life through the chaotic, kinked, bendy straw or if you will live it through the Inner Straw of iridescent ease and grace.

Gabi: [shoulders slightly slump forward] It's not going to be easy making this *big situation* change that I need to make . . .

Lorre: Change can be difficult. And a little scary while you're in the midst of it. It can also be amazing, wonderful, liberating, and glorious. Remember how it was difficult to sit with your thoughts and resistance earlier?

Gabi: Very uncomfortable.

Lorre: But you did it. You created inner space and allowed the resistance to pass while you connected to your deeper truth. The inner tends to reflect the outer. If you decide to make this *big situation* change, do so in the most compassionate manner for all. People, generally speaking, don't like change — often because it's uncomfortable. Once you get more familiar and comfortable with your subjective, juicy inner world while navigating the left-shifting and resistance, you'll find it easier to do so in your outer world.

Gabi: That's why you call it an alignment practice, right? Because I'm feeling a little wobbly about it, if I'm to be honest.

Lorre: It's natural to feel a little wobbly when learning anything new. It's like learning how to ride a bike — we have someone helping us, then training wheels, then the training wheels come off, and before long, you're riding that bike everywhere.

Gabi: [laughing] That's exactly what we're doing at home. Teaching my son how to ride a bike! That makes perfect sense. This whole alignment thing reminds me of that quote from Hermes Trismegistus, "As within, so without. As above, so below."

Lorre: Brilliant!

***

After our session, I reflected upon Gabi's use of the word "chaotic," as so many nurses before him had similarly remarked. At the risk of geeking out too much here, I pondered this sense of inner chaos in the context of complexity science and complex adaptive systems. We live in our inner systems, our outer systems, and in the spaces in between. Ideally, we would thrive in alignment — with connectedness, congruence, and correspondence between these inner and outer systems, through which we are influenced and inextricably linked. This innate alignment gets disconnected or misaligned in the aftermath of trauma.

To the left-shifted hemisphere, absent the full story as would otherwise be conveyed from the now wounded right hemisphere, these yet-to-be-deciphered patterns appear and feel disordered, chaotic. We long for this sense of connectedness, being in alignment. In response to what happened to us, we adaptively disconnected and became misaligned for the sake of survival. As we heal through our past and present wounds, together, we can support one another in this inner-outer unification process of alignment. As a result, our many truths of past and present begin to align, harmonize, and heal as we move toward wholeness. The chaotic nature of our misalignment begins to self-organize and move toward healed wholeness. Disrupted, chaotic patterns of misalignment return to the innate, ordered, and aligned patterns that were prevalent in the pre-trauma life chapter(s).

"What we call chaos is just patterns we haven't recognized. What we call random is just patterns we can't [yet] decipher."

Chuck Palahniuk

Preparing for Alignment Practices

Taking a left-shifted approach to alignment is a recipe for overwhelm and frustration. We need to get the whole story from our bodily neural nets, circuits, and RH. Looking back at my early alignment practices, I have to chuckle at the degree to which my substantial left-shifted worldview tried to rule this process. Here's the list of what NOT to do tips to consider as you approach your alignment practice:

Alignment: What NOT to Do

- **Don't do this practice when you're dysregulated or outside your Window of Tolerance.** There's too much static and energy interference. If that's the case, do a Micro- or MacroDose and start the YICP cycle. Do an awareness practice. Then attend and nurture your NS. When you feel grounded, centered, and within your Window, then proceed with the alignment practice.
- **Don't come in hot, sharp, or impatient.** This isn't an interrogation or interview process. Coming in with "What is my purpose?" or "What is my deep inner truth?" while you impatiently tap your foot, check the time, and expect an immediate, clear, and direct answer is like adding another brick to your inner wall of resistance.
- **Don't expect your deeper truths to emerge in any particular order, or in any specific time frame.** You've probably felt threatened, unsafe, or dysregulated for some time — maybe decades. You're like a rosebud before it blooms. No matter how much you want it to bloom, it

does so in its own perfect time and manner. As is the case for your healing and blooming process.

- **Don't deflect, dismiss, disregard, minimize, marginalize, ignore, or argue with your deepest truths when they emerge.** Your Threat Detector is on duty 24/7, even during YICP practices. Honor what emerges instead of pushing back or resisting it, lest you signal potential danger to your Threat Detector and add another layer of bricks to your inner wall of resistance.

- **Don't think of your alignment process as a board game.** You can't push, steer, maneuver, or direct your alignment process. There are no shortcuts or secret passages.

Alignment: What TO Do

- **Start with MicroDose and YICP Awareness & Attending practices.** These practices help you ease into your alignment practices. With ease, grace, and tender nonjudgmental curiosity, create loving inner space to welcome any sensations, awareness, insights, epiphanies, symbols, messages, images, or direct knowing to emerge. Alignment is a practice of *allowing* from our human-as-being-ness. Resist temptations to take a human-as-doing approach to alignment. Without an agenda or timeline, just notice what — if anything — emerges.

- **Bypass your Wall of Inner Resistance** by using the Aladdin's Magic Lamp or a magic wand approach. Ask "If I could change, be, or do one thing, what would it be?" The answers you seek often emerge in their own time and format, often through abstract symbols or a clear sense of inner knowing. Sometimes a few key words come through. Sometimes nothing appears while you are creating and sustaining this safe inner sanctuary in preparation for the answers you seek.

- **Welcome whatever appears** as you do with your gestures of inclusion practice. The safer and more welcoming you are in your response to the fragments of inner truth that emerge, the more you will receive. You'll begin to see patterns amid what feels like inner chaos. Should you feel that your Window of Tolerance is getting smaller or that you have engagement in your NS circuits, flow into awareness-attending practices before resuming your alignment practice in this or a future session.

- **Approach alignment practices like a beautiful jigsaw puzzle**. As the clues and pieces of your deep inner truths emerge, welcome and accept them for now. The preliminary goal is to experience your inner reality more clearly. Then, from your deepest and most vulnerable truths, you can later decide if and when to take action to reflect these truths externally, if at all.

Your Turn: 3A's Inner Flow Practice

Your alignment practice is one of allowing, as human-as-being. It flows from the awareness and attending practices. Use this guide as a launching point and trust the inner wisdom of YICP and NS as you instinctively modify this guide to best support your inner flow practice.

- This practice may feel like a vulnerable one for your NS. You may have ACEs or other traumatic experiences where you didn't feel safe to be seen, heard, or understood. Start by creating a safe, nurturing, and private environment. Surround yourself in sights, sounds, smells, textiles, and flavors that signal warmth, safety, and comfort.

- Ease into an awareness or Welcoming Yourself Home practice that feels most supportive and comfortable. Be in this compassionate and nonjudgmental inner space for several moments, or longer.

- Move into your favorite NS attending and nurturing practice. Welcome any sensations, perceptions, or unhealed bits that may emerge. Continue attending until you sense you are close to or within your Window of Tolerance. If you feel dysregulated or mostly outside your Window, continue with attending practices. Take as much time as you need to reconnect with your Window of Tolerance.

- From your Window and reasonably regulated NS, proceed with your alignment practice. You may find it helpful to visit your inner sanctuary and use the Aladdin's Magic Lamp or magic wand approaches to gently inquire about what your deepest, truest self would like for you to know at this time.

- Your LH may try and swoop in to make sense of this subjective, creative inner space. If that happens, thank your LH for doing its job, but it's not time yet. Notice if you are holding onto the need for control, order, or an immediate answer. If that's the case, see yourself opening and allowing while creating safe inner space for your bodily neural circuits and RH to receive that which wants to emerge. Allow the LH dominance to float by as a cloud in the sky for now.

- It's possible that you may feel inner resistance as your deeper truths emerge. For many people, our inner truths were adaptively forsaken or sacrificed in deference to our survival needs at that time. It's natural to feel mild resistance or discomfort as we now safely and lovingly allow ourselves to be seen, heard, valued, appreciated, and understood.

- If you experience inner resistance, signal signs of safety inwardly and connect to your environmental comforts using your five senses. If it feels comfortable, you can retreat to your inner sanctuary.
- When you feel ready to conclude this inner flow session, honor and thank your deepest, truest self for being willing to be safely seen and heard, with welcoming, nonjudgmental compassion. Send signals of safety, support, reassurance, and gratitude. Make a mental note of the sensations and perceptions you experienced, so you can better hear and feel your deepest self in the future.
- Close your inner flow practice by gently moving your limbs, jaw, neck, head, and torso. Give yourself a big bear hug. You took — and will continue to take — monumental steps toward healed wholeness in bodymindessence.

Healing is happening.

B Is for Balance

Congratulations on moving through the 3A's of YICP formula. Next up is the B for Balance component.

YICP: 3A + B → 3R

Awareness-Attending-Alignment + Balance → Regulation-Reconnection-Restoration

You probably noticed that the 3A's were inner practices. The inner flow practices of awareness-attending-alignment really support your deeper self, bodily neural circuits, unhealed bits,

Balance Components

Balance Component	Description
Personal Responsibility	Speaks to getting into the driver's seat of your adult life and lovingly caring for all dimensions of self in bodymindessence, including your NS and unhealed bits of wisdom. Facilitating your healing, with others.
Body & Mind Wellness	Describes supporting your physical and mental health and wellness by engaging in health-promoting ways of being and doing in your daily life while addressing health disruptions, illness, or disease that emerges over time.
Connections & Relationships	Considers your healthy connections and relationships with your loved ones, friends, family, communities, groups, and teams while addressing any unhealed-ness, codependency, power imbalances, or disease within your social relationships.
Personal and Professional Environments & Contexts	Includes the environments and contexts within which you live and work and are influenced by (physical, emotional, intellectual, social, spiritual, environmental, relational, occupational, ergonomic, etc.), which are ideally safe, supportive, creative, and healthy, as well as the need to address disruptions or dynamics that interfere with bodymindessence wellbeing.

Financial Wellness	Speaks to your relationship with resources, money, and money management, including the ability to meet current and future financial needs in support of your optimal safety, security, health, and wellness in bodymindessence.
Regulate, Relax & Recharge	Describes how we take care of our NS and regulation as foundational to relaxing and recharging our bodymindessence. This includes YICP practices, healthy sleep and screen time, relaxing alone, with trusted loved ones, and Haelan Nurse Communities, and leveraging the health and wellness properties to regulate, relax, and recharge.
Beliefs, Values & Purpose	Includes living in alignment with your perceived core values, beliefs, and life purpose, which change and evolve as you do. Showing up with and for yourself and your deepest truths while lovingly and compassionately making changes in your outer world to align with living your highest and best life, as defined by you.

and RH information to be safely expressed. You are or will start noticing your deeper truths, which may or may not be reflected in your external lived experiences. That's where the balance practice comes in — to give an external framework so you can explore, maintain, adjust, pivot, or discard that which is misaligned. As you become more comfortable with the alignment and balance aspects of YICP, you'll begin to see where there is alignment (or misalignment) between your inner truths and outer experiences. Most nurses find the balance aspect of YICP the easiest one to address, for you can see, feel, touch, and experience the balance components that are described in this table:

Returning to our bicycle tire example from the preceding chapter, we ideally glide through life in aligned balance, on a fully inflated tire. Let's drill down a little further into this metaphor and look at the bicycle wheel as a visual representation of YICP. At the center of every bicycle wheel is a hub — that metal piece that resembles an empty spool of thread, to which all the spokes connect. Where balance is concerned, personal responsibility is the hub. This is the point of self-empowerment. Within the hub are the unseen but critical inner infrastructure of the 3A's (awareness-attending-alignment). Now, envision your inner, deepest alignment truths as the spokes on the wheel. Your deepest dreams, hopes, and ever-changing life purpose emerge from the depths within to be realized in your outer world. These truths, the spokes, emerge to connect to your outer balance components (body and mind wellness, connections and relationships, environments and contexts, financial wellness, regulate, relax and recharge, and beliefs, values and purpose).

YICP: Balance

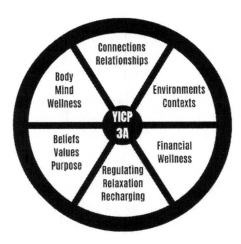

Notice that there are overlapping characteristics within and across the alignment and balance components, which reflect the complexity of our being-ness in bodymindessence. From the 3A's embedded in the hub, and through the spokes supporting the wheel, attaches the tire itself, represented by the balance components.

It's natural to think of these components as individual parts that comprise our whole lived experience, but that isn't so. Instead, envision the synergistic relationships between the balance components as the air we put into our tire before we ride into each day. Are your body and mind health and wellness needs fully met? Give your tire a big infusion of air. If these needs aren't fully met, make note and give a small infusion of air.

How are your connections and relationships faring? Are you engaged in healthy, balanced, and meaningful relationships that are free of codependency, addiction, and sticky attachments? If so, infuse a good amount of air into your balance bicycle wheel. If not, make note, and infuse a small amount of air. Similarly, evaluate the remaining balance components of environments and contexts, financial wellness, regulate, relax and recharge, and finally your beliefs, values and purpose. Commensurately inflate your tire relative to the degree you are fully or partially addressing each component. Once the air is in your tire, does it feel full and firm, ready to easily ride the road ahead? Or is half-way inflated? If so, you may make it through the day, but it will be a bumpy and uphill ride for most of it. Perhaps your balance tire is flat and you'll have to put a ton of effort into just getting through the day, riding on the rims when you can, and pushing the bike when you can't.

You get the idea. YICP has your back. Everything you need is already within you. Living YICP is a practice, a lifestyle. It all begins with and is about you. Notice how much you have learned and are learning as you partner with the wisdom of YICP and NS. You are the healing that you seek, solo and with others. You are the change agent of your life, your nursing practice, and — with other Haelan Nurses — the change agent for our profession. And you are not alone. You are so fully and richly supported by me, your trusted loved ones, your personal and professional communities, and our Haelan Academy & Communities. Lean in. **Healing is happening.**

The 3 R's: Regulation, Reconnection, and Restoration

The ways in which you grow by partnering with YICP are unique unto you in the broadest sense of your bodymindessence. Your growth will always include NS regulation gains, an improved sense of inner and outer reconnection, and restoration, to varying degrees, in all aspects of bodymindessence, including your healer's heart. It's important to note that YICP is not a one-and-done equation where you emerge completely healed in all-the-ways. Our left-shifted, drive-through, instantaneous results culture would have you believe that this is the case, but it simply isn't so. We know that life is a process of hardship and healing, rupture and repair — with no end destination. We iteratively move *toward* healed wholeness, but never arrive, for we do not live in silos or vacuums where we can control every aspect of our lived experiences. Healing is a spiral-like process and destination unto itself. It provides a pathway toward living a richer, more fulfilling, purposeful, meaningful, high-quality life. One where life's hardships and ruptures are readily addressed, with relative ease and grace, by the incredible tools and practices that you developed by honoring and partnering with YICP and NS.

For your learning purposes, I initially used the equation in the box below to describe YICP. Our LH likes to construct order, systems, and formulas out of the juicy and subjective information it receives. Since most of us are left-shifted, it made sense to initially present a very LH approachable formula:

Your Innate Care Plan (YICP)™
3A + B → 3R

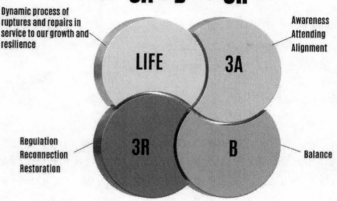

Dynamic process of ruptures and repairs in service to our growth and resilience

Awareness
Attending
Alignment

LIFE

3A

Regulation
Reconnection
Restoration

3R

B

Balance

YICP: 3A + B → 3R

Awareness-Attending-Alignment + Balance → Regulation-Reconnection-Restoration

---

Now that you've made your first pass through the framework of YICP, let's keep the same formula. Now visualize YICP as a dynamic, iterative, and circular process, as shown here.

There will be times in which you will more readily or fully engage than others, but YICP is always there. Just as your NS is. It's a matter of shifting your field of awareness and engaging with them. You can't separate yourself from YICP or NS, but you certainly can choose to put your head in the sand, like an ostrich, and refuse to participate in your healing process. That's always an option. Healing requires tremendous courage and unwavering commitment. Not everyone is ready or willing to engage. Wherever you are on this path is where you are — there is no expectation, judgment, comparison, or shame. Your healing journey is yours to take, in your perfect time and manner.

"There's a version of yourself you haven't met yet. Keep showing up until you're introduced."

Jim Kwik

Haelan Nurse Activities

Now that you're better acquainted with YICP components, it's time to do some exploration and sorting as to where you think they might best support your NS in its various circuits and hybrids. In the graphic, you'll find the MicroDoses Matter and YICP practices you've learned about this far. You can always refer to the earlier chapters and Haelan Nurse Activities if you need a refresher.

In the table below, add practices to YICP so you will have the tools you need for every circuit and hybrid. For now, you'll focus on the 3As. You may use the same practice multiple times, in different ways. Even if you're not super comfortable with every

MicroDoses Matter & YICP Menus

MicroDoses Matter Practices
Solo

One Mindful Breath — Pocket Pal 4x4
Bear Hug Container — Doorway Tap
Hand Over Heart — Nurture with Nature
Notice, Name & Nurture — Bonnie's Body Scan

With Others

Smize & Nod — Bump It
Heart Holding — Sidebar Debrief
Shall we Sway? — Healer's Heart Solidarity
Shared Notice, Name & Nurture

YICP Practices
Your Preferred Practices

Stillness — Relational
Generative — Movement
Creative — Ritual/Cyclical
Active — Others

YICP Practices
Awareness Practices

Welcoming Yourself Home — Movie Theater
Bird on Shoulder

Additional Attending Practices

Speed Dating Your NS — Group NS Dating
Haelan Community Group NS Dating

Alignment Visualization Practices

Aladdin's Magic Lamp — Magic Wand
Inner Straw

Balance Bicycle Wheel Sections

Personal Responsibility — Connections
Environments & Contexts — Finances
Regulate, Relax & Recharge — Body Mind Wellness
Beliefs, Values & Purpose

MicroDoses Matter & YICP Menus Expanded

YICP Menu of Preferred Practices PLUS

	YICP Awareness Both Solo & With Others	YICP Attending Both Solo & With Others	YICP Alignment Both Solo & With Others
Your Circuits & Hybrids			
Play Hybrid *I am safe and feel like being active.*			
Stillness Hybrid *I am safe and feel like being still.*			
SNS Hyperaroused Circuit *I feel uneasy, threatened, or unsafe - I need to do something to move towards or away from the stimulus.*			
Fawn Hybrid *I feel uneasy, threatened, or unsafe - I can't fight or flee, so I must please and appease.*			

Freeze Hybrid

I feel uneasy, threatened, or unsafe.
I have little or no energy. I just
can't.

Suitable for all circuits and hybrids (Solo practices that can be adapted to do with others.)		Visualizations:
• Welcoming Yourself Home	• Speed Dating Your NS	• Aladdin's Magic Lamp
• Movie Theater practice	• Group NS Dating	• Magic Wand
• Bird on Shoulder practice	• Haelan Community Group Dating	• Inner Straw

Exploring YICP Flow Practice

Time Available	When I can do a YICP Flow Practice (busiest days)	When I can do a YICP Flow Practice (busy days)	When I can do a YICP Flow Practice (not as busy days)
15 minutes			
30 minutes			
45+ minutes			

practice yet, just tentatively note them in the table knowing that you can and will be moving things around as you grow in YICP practices and begin thriving in your Window of Tolerance.

The next step is to start YICP Flow Practice, on a daily basis for now, or more frequently if that feels right for you. You'll make the most gains if you dose YICP Flow Practice to gently challenge but not overwhelm yourself. Use this table to explore the dose and frequency of YICP Flow Practice.

Deeper Dive Resources

Brown, B. (2012). *The power of vulnerability: Teachings of authenticity, connection, and courage.* Sounds True.

Complex Trauma Resources. (n.d.). *Core topics, treatment, and resources.* https://www.complextrauma.org/.

Kabat-Zinn, J. (2018). *The healing power of mindfulness: A new way of being.* Hachette UK.

Tolle, E. (2004). *The power of now.* New World Library.

Chapter 6

Leaning Into Our Layers

In the last chapter, you learned how to put YICP into action. Your House of Haelan now has a strong MicroDoses Matter foundation and a YICP Menu to guide YICP Flow Practice. In this chapter, you'll learn how to lean into some of your deeper layers while being well supported by the tools and practices in YICP. Your House of Haelan is growing ever stronger, your NS is being nurtured, and you are able to spend increasingly more time in your Window of Tolerance. Healing is happening as you move towards wholeness and thriving in practice and in life.

Before we lean into those deeper layers, let's review how you can approach self-exploration and your awareness practices. As nurses, we do assessments all the time as the first step of our ADPIE nursing process (assess, diagnose, plan, implement, evaluate). So, it's easy to take this approach as we lean into the deeper layers of YICP. You'll be doing some gentle

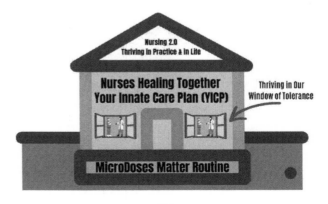

self-exploration in this chapter. While doing so, strive to stay balanced in your RH-LH-RH collaboration. It would be easy to slip into a more empiric, left-shifted approach, which is not quite what we're doing here. We need to create a safe, receptive space within, so the emerging unhealed bits and subjective, juicy RH information can be seen and fully reflected to the LH, then the RH, back to the LH, etc., for optimal hemispheric collaboration. This approach will gently harmonize YICP and NS to synergistically work on your behalf. YICP is unique unto you and comprises the totality of your lived experiences and innate capacities for health and wellness, so please give yourself the time and space that you need to explore in the fullest sense of the word.

Leaning into the layers of YICP, Your Repository and NS is like doing a holistic, full assessment versus a quick, focused assessment. Lean into those layers while maintaining a sense of gentle self-inquiry within your nonjudgmental, compassionate, welcoming, inclusive, and self-loving field of awareness. It's also important to relate to YICP and NS through the lens of your personal and professional wellness, and not through the disease management lens that is the focus of most healthcare systems. Trust that you are exactly where and how you need to be in this moment, for, as Eckhart Tolle reminds us, it could not be otherwise. The totality of your lived experiences and that of your ancestral lineage are being reflected and lived through you. You are doing a brilliant job of adapting and managing it all. It may *feel* like you are broken, fractured, drowning, stuck, disconnected, or utterly overwhelmed. Know that you are not broken. You are adaptive.

Through the lens of celebration and self-acceptance, look at you now! Here you are, in your glorious magnificence. Safe and so richly and earnestly supported by me and our Haelan Nurse Community. Your highly evolved and wise NS adapted and kept you safe. It stored that which couldn't be processed at the time because, among other factors, you didn't have who you needed before, during, and after the traumatic event(s). It may feel like life has been living you, but you are healing and pivoting toward living your highest and best life, as you define it, with ease and grace. Sure, there will always be disruptions, ruptures, repairs, and healing as you continually move toward homeostasis and wholeness. Again, please know this to be true: You are not broken. You are adaptive. By leaning into your deeper layers, you will continue to adapt by positioning yourself in *right relationship* for healing, regulation, reconnection, and restoration. Healing is happening and will continue to happen as we move forward together. Let's gently move into your deeper layers together.

"You are not broken. You are adaptive."

Lorre Laws, PhD RN

Leaning Into Our Awareness Layer

Terminology Refresher: Awareness

Awareness describes how you shift your perception as you gently view yourself through the compassionate lens of "What happened to me?" instead of a judgmental lens of "What's wrong with me?" Awareness is a practice that facilitates healing through the purposeful, non-judgmental attention to that which arises within you during any given present moment — all in service to your growth, development, self-understanding, and wisdom.

To start leaning into the awareness layer, let's sit in on a session with Nathifa from Taylor, Riley, Chin-Mae, Gabi, and Jordan's unit. Nathifa is an excellent nurse and self-proclaimed introvert who struggles with burnout and presenteeism at work. She is a single mother of two young children who doesn't receive much support from the father. Her family lives several hours away, but they stay connected through frequent video calls. Nathifa's financial situation is a stable paycheck-to-paycheck one that leaves little room for discretionary spending. She feels stuck in her life. When describing her work life, Nathifa says, "I love, love, love my team and my patients, but everything else at work is a sh*t show." Throughout our sessions, she describes feeling frustrated and hopeless about working conditions improving. She dreads going to work. Even on her days off, the thought of having to return to work hangs over her like a dark, black cloud. You may recognize some of the individual and nurse-specific traumas in her story.

Here's an excerpt of our conversation:

Nathifa: Everything in my life feels like a mess. Work is a freaking nightmare. I'm exhausted when I get home. My kids need me, as they should. I try to spend quality time

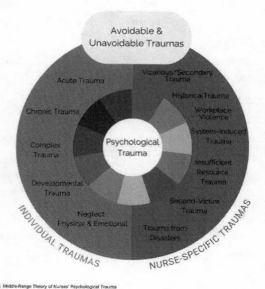

Adapted from Foli (2022) Middle-Range Theory of Nurses' Psychological Trauma

Avoidable & Unavoidable Traumas

with them on my days off, but I can't get off the couch. Like, making a cup of coffee is a major chore. Forget about taking a bath or going to the park. Then work is blowing up my phone, asking me to cover shifts, come in early, or go to meetings — on my day off! I feel like such a failure. [eyes turn downward, torso slumps]

Lorre: It's understandable why you're feeling this way. Sometimes, what we perceive as a failure is really evidence of growth and healing.

Nathifa: [laughs and takes a big sip of coffee] So, laying on the couch all day is growth?!

Lorre: It can signal both an adaptive response and a positive sign of healing. Let's take a moment to ground, center, and explore. Do you have a practice preference?

Nathifa: I like them all, but I can't remember them by name . . .

Lorre: We've used 4-7-8 breathing, ventral vagal breathing, and . . .

Nathifa: Oh, let's do that ventral vagal one. It's gooooood!

Lorre: That is a good one. [facilitates the ventral vagal breathing exercise from Chapter 4]

Nathifa: [after completing the exercise] It's amazing how effective that is. I feel better . . . a little . . . regulated . . . I guess you would say.

Lorre: Wonderful! Let's lean into your awareness layer and explore how your NS feels today. Do you remember this sheet from last time? [passes the How My Nervous System Feels Today and ANS Spectrum Circuits and Hybrids survey to Nathifa]

Nathifa: I sure do! Circle whatever I'm feeling, right?

Lorre: You got it! [chuckles] Explore how you're feeling, and then we'll see where you feel you're at in your ANS Spectrum today.

***

Worksheet #1: How My Nervous System Feels Today (circle all that apply)

***

Circuit 1: I feel . . .
Circuit 1

Calm	Safe	Social
Connected	Relaxed	Lighthearted
Grounded	Empathetic	Settled
Rested	Relaxed digestion	Open
Capable	Breathing easy	Curious
Healthy	Engaged	Compassionate
Vital	Relatively low stress	Mindful
Present	Seeing the big picture	Relatable and relating

Number of Circuit 1 Circles: _____

***

Circuit 2: I feel . . .
Circuit 2

Frustration	Difficulty sleeping	Vigilant
Irritation	Activated	Constipated
Rage	Overly energized	Fidgety
Concern	Increased HR, BP, RR	Alert
Anger	Sweating/not sweating	Concentration challenges

Restless	Enlarged pupils	Emotionally constricted
Worry	Dry mouth	Panic
Swallowing challenges	Annoyed	Anxiety
Moderate-high stress	Appetite increase/ decrease	Not seeing the big picture

Number of Circuit 2 Circles: _____

***

Circuit 3: I feel . . .

Circuit 3

Numb	Trapped	Decreased sexual desire
Collapsed	Stuck	Depressed
Immobile	Fearful	Emotionally detached
Helpless	Decreased HR, BP, RR	Flat
Depressed	Shallow respirations	Brain fog
Disconnected	Lightheadedness	Overwhelming stress
Dissociated	Increased pain threshold	Withdrawn
Shame	Fatigue – general	Fatigue – muscle
Apathetic	Shutdown	Socially disinterested
Hopeless	Limited social interest	Can't big-picture think

Number of Circuit 3 Circles: _____

***

For sensations or perceptions not described above: I feel . . .
(Use the space below to name any other feelings or sensations
that were not identified above. If what you're feeling corresponds
to one of the three circuits above, add it to that list, circle it, and
then adjust the tally below accordingly.)

***

***

***

Worksheet #2: Spectrum of Circuits & Hybrids
Step 1. Using the "How My Nervous System Feels Today"
exploration exercise, record the number of circles for each
circuit in the table below.

Circuit Categories

Safety Circuit	Danger Circuit	Extreme Danger Circuit
Online circuit: Ventral vagal *I am and we are safe*	Online circuit: SNS *All hands on deck*	Online circuit: Dorsal vagal *No hands on deck*
# of Circuit 1 Circles from How My Nervous System Feels Today (above) _____.	# of Circuit 2 Circles from How My Nervous System Feels Today (above) _____.	# of Circuit 3 Circles from How My Nervous System Feels Today (above) _____.

Note any sensations, feelings, and perceptions here:

***

***

***

Refer to YICP Menu and list which practices feel right for where you are in your NS right now:

***

***

***

Step 2. Using the number of circles for each circuit in Table 1 above, explore if your NS is in one of the hybrid states now. Recall that the circuits and hybrids are like dimmer switches that can come online in varying degrees. It is possible for one or more circuits or hybrids to be online at a time.

Hybrid Categories

Play Hybrid	Stillness Hybrid	Freeze Hybrid	Fawn Hybrid
Online circuits: Ventral vagal SNS *I am safe, engaged, and joyful.*	Online circuits: Ventral vagal Dorsal vagal *I am safe, open, curious, and still.*	Online circuits: SNS Dorsal vagal *I can't. I just can't.*	Online circuits: SNS Dorsal & ventral vagal *I can't escape, so I'll please and appease.*
# of Circuit 1 ___ & Circuit 2 ___ Circles.	# of Circuit 1 ___ & Circuit 3 ___ Circles.	# of Circuit 2 ___ & Circuit 3 ___ Circles.	# of Circuit 2 ___ & Circuit 3 ___ Circles.

Note any sensations, feelings, and perceptions here:

***

***

***

Refer to YICP Menu and list which practices feel right for where you are in your NS right now:

***
***
***

Nathifa completed both worksheets. She had a lot of circles in Circuits 2 and 3, with a few from Circuit 1. Nathifa noted these circles in her "ANS Spectrum of Circuits & Hybrids worksheet," after which our conversation continued.

***

Nathifa: So, I'm feeling like I'm in a freeze. Some days it feels like a deep freeze. [laughs heartily]

Lorre: Terrific. Walk me through your worksheet process.

Nathifa: Well, when I did the Circuits circles, I was kinda all over the place circuit-wise. I'm over it at work, but I feel powerless to do anything because I have no time, money, or energy.

Lorre: That's a wonderful insight and one that we absolutely can work with. Building on this awareness, with which circuit or hybrid do you feel most resonance?

Nathifa: [ponders a moment, scanning the paper] Well, I guess since I can't be a frozen ice cube at work [laughs], then I'd say I'm in the fawn hybrid. But at home, I'm in the freeze or deep freeze.

Lorre: [laughing with Nathifa] I suspect that's the case. One of the side effects of the fawn, or please-and-appease response, is that it makes it difficult for us to hear our own truth, to access our inner wisdom. I'm wondering if leaning into this fawning response would be helpful.

Nathifa: Probably. How do I lean in?

Lorre: Well, in addition to the exercises you've learned so far, you could add a reflective journaling practice. How do you feel about journaling?

Nathifa: It's like "meh" for me. That blank page is a little intimidating . . .

Lorre: [chuckles] I'm so familiar with how that blank page feels sometimes! Would writing down some journaling prompts first help with getting started?

Nathifa: Oh, yes — I have used other journals with writing prompts in them and it was much easier for me to write.

Lorre: Let's move in that direction by doing this Inner Truth Awareness exercise. You can use these prompts to reflect, journal, or converse with your Haelan Nurses and trusted loved ones. It goes like this:

Slow the Pace Speed Bump: Inner Truth Awareness
Adapted from Schwartz (2021).

Take a moment to do the 3As of YICP Flow Practice.

Before you respond to the journaling and conversation prompts below, do a quick body scan. Then, as you move through this exercise, monitor for signs of discomfort or overwhelm. Should that occur, pause this exercise. You can return to it any time. You can also do it with others. It's important to honor the sensations and titrate the stimuli (these prompts) to engage Your Repository, but not overwhelm the NS. Low and slow is the way to go!

Reflect upon what you are experiencing now — at work, at home, and in your relationships. Then respond to the prompts below.

Journaling and Conversation Prompts
It hurt me when _____.

The worst thing about this pain is that you said or did
_____.

The thing that makes me most afraid is _____.

What I wanted to say or do, but couldn't then, is
_____.

You can never take _____ away from me.

I know I am strong because _____.

I need for you to know this about me now _____.

My truth in this situation is _____.

I choose to _____.

Healing is happening.

We moved through the rest of Nathifa's session, where she set a SMART goal to gently lean into her awareness layer — for 10-20 minutes, once daily when she was on duty and twice daily when she was not. Nathifa verbalized being concerned about how much time she could actually devote to her YICP Flow Practice. She mistakenly thought she had to do ALL of the menu options for ALL of the steps, for 10-20 minutes. She was greatly relieved to learn that the YICP Flow Practice is dynamic and that she could lean into one of the 3As more than the others. For example, she could lean into her awareness layer for 10 minutes while flowing through her attending and alignment layers in 2-3 minutes. The bottom line is for Nathifa and you to follow your intuition and the wisdom of your NS. There's no right or wrong way to lean in or do a YICP Flow Practice. Explore, notice, and allow your innate capacity to heal and its rhythm to emerge.

You might be curious about how to lean into your awareness layer, as Nathifa did. As you likely anticipated already . . . you'll have an opportunity to lean in at the end of the chapter while doing your Haelan Nurse Activities. You're welcome to take a reading pause and do the Inner Truth Awareness activity now, or you can do it after you read this chapter, or anytime in the future. Honor your inner wisdom and NS and then do what feels most comfortable and manageable.

Leaning Into Our Attending Layer

Terminology Refresher: Attending

Attending the NS is honoring, nurturing and nourishing your NS and all that it has experienced, stored, and adapted to in service to your survival. We attend to our own and other's NS through the compassionate lens of what happened to me/we/us/you/they/them. Attending practices complement the wisdom of your NS and help it to regulate so you can thrive in your Window of Tolerance.

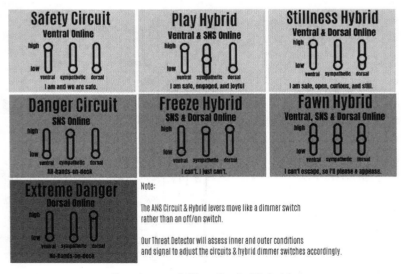

Spectrum of Circuits & Hybrids

Nathifa and I texted back and forth in between her last session and this next one. She was consistently doing her inner flow practice while leaning into her awareness layer. She began to see how her toxic workplace was affecting her NS and other body systems, mood, ability to sleep, and exercise intolerance. I passed Nathifa a clipboard with the Spectrum of Circuits & Hybrids worksheet on it and reminded her that the dimmer switches go online and offline, in varying degrees, as inner and out conditions fluctuate.

After refreshing her memory and exploring where she was in her NS that day, Nathifa was ready to share what she was feeling and experiencing. Let's sit in on part of Nathifa's next session where she describes her current challenge.

***

Nathifa: I am beyond exhausted. It is all I can do to get through the day. I just want to crawl into the bottom of my bed and stay in the fetal position all day. Even on my days off, I don't have the energy to even turn on Netflix, it seems. I take good care of my kids — know that — but *I just can't* with everything else . . . [drops head, sighs deeply]

Lorre: I am feeling your energy and am here with you. You're not alone, and there's much we can do to support you in this low-energy state. I'm wondering if you recall a related comment that you made at the end of our last session.

Nathifa: Hmmm, let me think [eyes look upward] . . . honestly, I don't remember.

Lorre: No worries. A lot has happened since then. It's perfectly natural not to remember a passing comment from two weeks ago. [chuckles, as does Nathifa] I jotted it down, just in case you wanted to refer back to it.

Nathifa: I'm bursting with curiosity! What did I say?!

Lorre: As you were moving toward the door, you said, "Sometimes, there's just nothing in the tank."

Nathifa: OMG! I *do* remember saying that. And that's exactly how I've felt. My mind wants to do the things that I'm supposed to do, but my body is like, "I can't, I just can't." Every day is like an inner tug of war. It's exhausting. I'm exhausted.

Lorre: I've been there. Many times. I totally get it. Would you like to lean into this exhaustion and see what's going on?

Nathifa: Absolutely — I know the drill! Start with a safe and comfy space, like your Zen Den office here. Ground and center is next, right?

Lorre: Impressive! [facilitates Nathifa's choice of 4-7-8 breathing practice using the haaaa exhale to stimulate the ventral vagal circuit] Does the first step in YICP Flow Practice come to mind?

Nathifa: Oh, yes, hold on, wait a minute. It's the . . . the . . . Awareness!

Lorre: Yes, it is! So far, YICP has five awareness menu options: Welcoming Yourself Home, Movie Theater, How My NS Feels Today, Spectrum of Circuits & Hybrids, and Inner Truth Reflection.

Nathifa: Snap! Look how much I've learned, y'all!

Lorre: Brilliant work! Which of these YICP menu options would you like to use for your awareness practice?

Nathifa: [leans forward and reaches toward the small coffee table between us] Girl, I'm all about these! [grabs a pen and completes both worksheets - How My NS Feels Today and Spectrum of Circuits & Hybrids]

Lorre: [after she completes the worksheets] So, tell me. How are you feeling in your NS today?

Nathifa: Well, surprising no one in *this* room [laughs], I'm all up in Circuits 2 and 3 (SNS and dorsal vagal). I got a lot more Circuit 3 circles than I did last time. That dorsal ventral circuit is back online. I can feel it.

Lorre: Such an astute insight. You're really getting acquainted with your NS, which is wonderful. You go, you!

Nathifa: [chuckles] I try!

Lorre: Were there any circuits with which you felt resonance?

Nathifa: Well, do I have to pick just one?

Lorre: No — your NS is shifting and adapting all the time, every moment of the day. Depending upon the stimuli you are experiencing internally and externally, you can move through many circuits and hybrids throughout the day.

Nathifa: I figured that was the case. I just wanted to double check . . .

Lorre: Like any nurse would! [We both laugh.]

Nathifa: Well, at home I feel like the dorsal vagal is online a lot more. It feels like I'm walking in quicksand, underwater. Like there's this heavy energy around me. Every time I try to do something, it's like my body is saying, "I just can't."

Lorre: Beautifully stated. Tell me about how you're feeling when you're on duty, at work.

Nathifa: [chuckles] Have you ever heard the term "dead man walking"? I feel like a "dead nurse walking" or like a zombie a lot of the time. I'm doing my very best [eyes tear up, voice thickens] . . . but my brain gets foggy, and I get so . . . [sobs] . . . overwhelmed . . .

Lorre: Let's take a minute for your deeper truth to emerge and be welcomed, heard, and included. I'm here with you. Anything that is said stays right in this room.

Nathifa: [reaches for a tissue, dabs eyes] Well, it's like I'm doing my very best, and I *am* taking good care of my patients, but I feel dead inside. Hollow. I'm not my usual bubbly self. It's all I can do to just get through the shift. Then we're always so short staffed. I don't have time or energy to be with my patients the way I'm supposed to — and want to. This isn't what I signed up for. This isn't the kind of nurse I want to be . . . [She drops her head into both hands and sobs quietly while I extend my hand for her to hold, which she does while giving my hand a squeeze in a beautiful gesture of co-regulation.]

Lorre: You have a lot going on and you are so brave, so courageous. [I squeeze her hand back and we both put our hands back in our laps.]

Nathifa: I feel like a failure. I can't do anything the way I normally would.

Lorre: It's natural to feel that way. It's hard to live life underwater while walking through quicksand. But it's important to know that how you're feeling and what you're experiencing is not a choice. It's not a reflection of your character, strength, or anything else.

Nathifa: [lifts head, her eyes looking into mine] Really? Because that's not how it *feels*.

Lorre: You are experiencing an involuntary response to past or present trauma — your brilliant NS has and will always adapt to keep you safe. What you are experiencing is an adaptation, not a character flaw or other weakness.

Nathifa: I suppose so . . .

Lorre: How do you feel about me dimming the lights and getting you a cozy blanket to snuggle?

Nathifa: Sounds divine. I may never leave this room. [chuckles while I dim lights and get her favorite blanket]

Lorre: Let's light a candle together, to symbolize our NSs coming together, in a co-regulating splendor of light, love, and healing. [She nods affirmatively.] Which candle is calling you?

Nathifa: That vanilla scented one, it's my fav. [We each light one long matchstick and light the candle together. Nathifa relaxes back into the corner of the sofa and exhales deeply.] This is what I need . . .

Lorre: Sometimes, we need to just "not." Your inner wisdom is serving you well. How do you feel about doing a breathing exercise or a body scan so we can ever-so-gently explore and attend?

Nathifa: I'm down for a body scan. [I facilitate Bonnie's Body Scan practice, after which I ask Nathifa to share what she experienced.] Wow. I'm really tense. My jaw hurts, all my muscles are tight. I feel like I need a long massage! [chuckles]

Lorre: Good work noticing this — your body has stored the past/present trauma activation energy in those body parts, especially the muscles. Let's do a visualization exercise to explore this stored energy. [Nathifa closes her eyes and relaxes back into the sofa, with the soft blanket wrapping her shoulders like a warm hug.] Breathe however feels comfortable and use your mind's eye to explore the energy in your body. Where does it feel tight or constricted?

Nathifa: [after she explores for a moment] Well, all the usual suspects I noticed a few minutes ago were tight, but what is really, *really* tight are my hips. I need a yoga class. [chuckles]

Lorre: A yoga class sounds wonderful! Let's do the Dorsal Defrost Practice. Staying with your visualization, let's use your mind's eye to go to a yoga class. See yourself arriving at your favorite yoga studio. It's warm there, with a lot of natural light, wood floors, gentle water fountain sounds, potted plants, and a big bouquet of your favorite flowers just outside the classroom door. Pause by these flowers and take in their beauty. If you enjoy the scent of these flowers, lean in and take a few deep inhales through your nose.

Nathifa: [takes three long inhales through her nose and exhales out her mouth using the "haaaa" sound] These lilies are stunning and they smell so good! It's like a lily aromatherapy session up in here. [chuckles]

Lorre: Exactly. Stay with your inner aromatherapy experience for as long as you like. When you're ready, find your space in the yoga studio, set up your mats and any props.

Nathifa: You know me so well! I'm all about those props for this stiff body! [laughs heartily]

Lorre: I use a lot of props myself — if I can't get to the floor, I bring the floor up to me. [laughs with Nathifa] Are you all set up in your inner yoga studio?

Nathifa: I am . . . and those lilies . . . they're everything . . .

Lorre: Wonderful. I'll be your inner yoga instructor, so you can relax and mentally enjoy whatever practices or poses feel good for you, OK?

Nathifa: OK, I'm ready.

Lorre: As I guide you through the practice, just nod your head when you're finished with each section, and then flow into the next.

Nathifa: Will do. I'm loving this inner yoga practice. It feels like I'm really there!

Lorre: That's fantastic. This inner yoga practice is available to you any time. And if yoga doesn't sound good, you can swap it for any other activity that feels right. You can choose anything from YICP Preferred Practices Menu, at any time. For now, we'll continue this inner yoga session and start with you visualizing a grounding moment in your favorite seated position. Nod your head whenever you're done grounding. [Nathifa nods after a moment.]

Lorre: Great. Now, in your mind's eye, do some gentle lower body and then upper body stretches to warm up your body. [Nods after a few moments.] Are you familiar with sun or moon salutations? [Nathifa nods affirmatively.]

Lorre: Great, when you're ready, visualize flowing into your choice of sun or moon salutations. [Nods after a few moments.]

Lorre: If it feels comfortable, go ahead and stand up in your mind's eye. If it doesn't feel good to visualize standing, then move into child's pose or savasana.

Nathifa: I didn't think I'd want to stand in my visualization, but I am. So, what now?

Lorre: Now, you can use your mind's eye to flow into your favorite balance pose. Tree pose, mountain pose, chair pose — whatever resonates.

Nathifa: Oh, that tree pose is too much! [chuckles] I'm going with a mountain pose.

Lorre: Good work honoring your inner wisdom. Mountain pose is an excellent choice. Feel the gentle, nurturing energy of the earth entering through your feet, up through your legs, torso, arms, neck, and then through and out the top of your head to whatever higher power, planet, or star to which you feel a connection.

Nathifa: Oh, Mother Earth — she feels so good! It's like reiki or tai chi energy. I love it!

Lorre: You're so right, and you're doing brilliant healing work here. Stay in this energy as long as you'd like. [After a few moments, Nathifa nods.]

Lorre: If seated or supine postures feel good, try visualizing a gentle restorative twist of any kind. Perhaps a revolved belly pose feels good? [Nathifa nods.] Laying on your back, bring your knees to your belly and then gently bring them toward the floor on one side — using a block to bring the floor to you whenever needed. Turn your head in the other direction if that feels good. Visualize that stored energy that was making you feel tight. See yourself gently squeezing it out of your body, as you would with a wet, soggy sponge. All that old energy is gently moving, no longer stuck or stagnant. It is leaving you as Mother Earth life force energy takes its place.

Nathifa: [sighs heavily] This is amazing. I have no words . . .

Lorre: Beautiful, no words are needed. When you're ready, use your mind's eye to gently twist to the other side and do the same. Nod when the other side is finished. [She nods after a few moments.]

Lorre: Now, we'll move into our last visualization pose — your choice of savasana, legs up the wall, child's pose, or any other deeply relaxing pose. Stay there as long as you'd like, and when you're ready to join me here back in my Zen Den, gently wiggle your hands and feet, and then open your eyes.

Nathifa: [after completing the inner yoga practice] Oh my. That was wonderful. I feel like some of that tension — that tightness — is better. And I didn't so much as lift a finger!

Lorre: You did great, truly. When our dorsal vagal circuit is online, we need to discharge the stuck energy and bring in present moment energy — one drop at a time. If we do too much, too fast, too soon, then we overwhelm our system and keep the dorsal vagal circuit online. So, we take a "low and slow is the way to go" approach. We titrate the first energy dose by *visualizing* the energy and movement.

Nathifa: This is so powerful. I can definitely feel a shift. A good shift.

Lorre: That's what we're looking for — small energetic gains first, followed by small physical movement when it feels comfortable and manageable. Would you like to physically release some of that stored energy? Or does that feel like it might be too much right now?

Nathifa: Well, I'm not looking to run a marathon or anything, but yes, getting rid of some more of this tightness would feel good.

Lorre: Excellent point. We definitely don't want to overwhelm your NS further by doing too much movement too fast or too soon. A lot of my clients try to take that "let's run a marathon" approach and it never ends well. Your inner wisdom, YICP, is guiding you to the "low and slow is the way to go" approach to releasing this energy. Brilliant! Let's bring this tightness into the present moment. How does it feel?

Nathifa: It feels like I want to stand up, move a little.

Lorre: Let's stand up and gently move, walk, stretch — whatever feels right. Let that tightness and your inner wisdom lead the way. Would you like to play some music? [I point to the tablet and music app. Nathifa scrolls for a moment and makes her selection.]

Nathifa: Can I keep this on? [wraps soft throw blanket around her shoulders, like a shawl]

Lorre: Absolutely! As you're moving — and anything goes — you can describe what you're feeling or experiencing, whenever you feel moved to do so.

Nathifa: [laughs] That will be easy. I externally process *everything*! [She laughs, and then we both get up and start moving, swaying, and stretching organically.] I feel like my jaw is in a vice. [She opens and closes her jaw several times.] There it goes. It's loosening up. My neck feels stiff. [She gently moves her head up and down, side to side.] My shoulders, my upper back — yikes. Are they ever locked up. [She does a spontaneous swan dive breath, which she practiced in a prior session.] My legs . . . they're like . . . [shakes one leg, then the other] overloaded with electricity or something [shakes both legs again]. Wow, that felt good. [shakes legs again]

Lorre: Look at you! [Nathifa sits down, as do I.] You did good work today. Healing is happening. [I gesture a heart mudra.]

Nathifa: [smiles, looking pleased] Why do I feel a little . . . a lot, actually . . . better?

Lorre: Much has happened. And it was all you. You arrived at this session so open, so willing to do whatever was required to shift from that feeling of dorsal ventral stuckness. I observed how receptive and engaged you were throughout our session. It was remarkable — as are you!

Nathifa: As the saying goes, "I'm so sick and tired of being sick and tired" that I'll try anything, [laughs with animation], well, *almost* anything!

Lorre: Good for you! By taking this approach, you are literally positioning yourself in *right relationship* for healing in all bodymindessence dimensions. You're engaged with repatterning, regulating and co-regulating your NS. That is key. You're leaning into your layers, with the love and support of your friends, family, and our Haelan Nurse Community.

Nathifa: I can't wait to do this with our Haelan Nurse group. It's my turn to host and facilitate next month — do you have any resources to help me do what we just did?

Lorre: Absolutely! I call the exercise we just completed The Dorsal Defrost Practice. It's a great attending practice to use whenever that dorsal ventral circuit is online. Remember earlier when you said you weren't looking to run a marathon?

Nathifa: [chuckles while nodding] Yes, ma'am, I do!

Lorre: That was the wisdom of YICP signaling that your system wasn't ready for a lot of energy or sympathetic activation.

Nathifa: Well, I'll be . . . [pauses in epiphany] . . . I had no idea. But you're so right. There it is. I see it now. My innate care plan, in action. So, is that why we did a yoga visualization before we got up and moved?

Lorre: Precisely! I like to think of the three ANS circuits like a treadmill. If the dorsal vagal circuit is online, it's like the treadmill is turned off or on a crawl-pace setting. We have to warm up the dorsal vagal. First, we gently and slowly release stored energy. Then, and only then, can we increase the speed setting on our treadmill to slowly walk, moving a little more energy while signaling to the SNS that there is now inner bandwidth for it to gently come online, followed by the ventral vagal circuit. But not too fast, lest we overwhelm the NS and bring the dorsal ventral back online.

Nathifa: So *that's* what just happened. I drug myself in here, like a frozen snowman. Like, I felt like . . . [looks upward, searching for the right word] I was stuck. Left to my own devices, I would have put my frozen a** in the microwave and blasted it on high to thaw as quickly as possible.

Lorre: [chuckles along with Nathifa] But that's not what happened — you honored YICP and declared that there would be no marathon running today. That's wonderful. Now you know what you can do next time that dorsal vagal is online.

Nathifa: Yep. Instead, I'll cozy up by the fire and do a gentle defrost. No microwave for me!

Lorre: [chuckles] Good point. Going back to that treadmill example, as you can tolerate more energy and movement, then you can slowly turn the treadmill on to go a little bit faster — say a slow walk, a gentle stretch, or a restorative hike.

Nathifa: Let me guess. We're moving up the ladder to the SNS circuit, right?

Lorre: Nailed it! [gestures mic drop] And then what would you do, assuming you felt comfortable doing the slow-to-medium SNS treadmill walk?

Your Repository
Threat Detector & Circuits

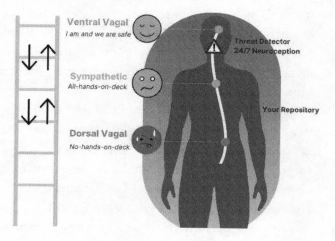

Nathifa: Well, two things come to mind. The first is that I could slowly increase the treadmill speed to get the ventral vagal more online . . . [pauses, questioningly so]

Lorre: Good — keep going!

Nathifa: But really, I'm getting that Window of Tolerance opened up, with me in it!

Lorre: Yes! When you're in your Window, you're calm, cool, collected, and connected.

Nathifa: I just want to stay in that Window all the time. It seems like every time I'm in it, I just get knocked out of it again. It's so frustrating . . .

Lorre: You are learning how to navigate your NS so you can stay in your Window, and you're making such good progress. When we're in the Window, we're vacillating through the online circuits — the ventral vagal is online with splashes of SNS in response to inner and outer conditions.

Nathifa: I get it — but [laughs loudly] I feel like my kid. "I want it now!"

Lorre: You are making such good progress! Partnering with YICP, your NS, and engaging in these healing practices — independently and with others — is establishing your psychological flexibility and your ability to regulate. The mindful awareness practices, the attending practices, they are helping you to stay in the Window. By virtue of doing your awareness-attending-alignment practices, you become aware of limiting beliefs and misalignments between your inner and outer worlds.

Nathifa: So, I'm already helping to keep that Window open?

Lorre: You are! YICP is a fantastic place to start. Some clients like to complement these practices with support from trauma-informed professionals. There are many therapeutic options available — somatic experiencing, eye movement and desensitization and reprocessing (EMDR), limbic system retraining, primal trust, and the list goes on from there. These and other options are always available for you to explore if and when it feels right to do so.

Nathifa: Well, that's good to know. It's like I'm already making progress and I didn't know it!

Lorre: Exactly. As you know, I'm a big mental wellness advocate. I think everyone, myself included, should routinely benefit from the support of mental health professionals.

Nathifa: I agree. It's so important to take care of your mental health. I mean, if we get our lady parts checked every year, our teeth checked twice a year, then [laughs] the least we can do is get a mental health check-in every few months or so!

Lorre: Absolutely! [chuckles] I couldn't have said it better myself!

As we closed our session, Nathifa set her goals for the upcoming weeks. She described feeling ready to work on her attainable goals. Before she left, Nathifa asked for the Dorsal Defrost Practice so she could use it with her Haelan Nurse group. Here's the exercise, which you can explore now or refer back to any time:

Slow the Pace Speed Bump: The Dorsal Defrost Practice

Start with finding a safe and comfy space. Take a moment to ground and center. Then, from YICP Menu, select and do an awareness practice. You're now ready to attend and nurture your NS with the Dorsal Defrost Practice.

Move into a visualization exercise where you can use your mind's eye to do any form of gentle movement activity like a stroll on a sunny day, a gentle hike in nature, stretching, yoga, tai chi, qigong, or any sport that you enjoy. You can refer back to YICP and Your Preferred Practices for inspiration.

Notice how your body responds to the visualization. If it starts to feel a little overwhelming or uncomfortable, pause and return to an awareness practice. Just notice and welcome whatever perceptions, feelings, or sensations that are emerging. Do a couple of rounds of 4-7-8 breathing.

When you're ready, continue with the Dorsal Defrost Practice of visualizing a gentle movement-based practice. In your mind's eye, move with great care and tenderness. Low and slow is the way to go. Pause to rest as often as you'd like.

After your Dorsal Defrost visualization, explore to see if your body feels ready to do some gentle physical movement. If a lot of movement doesn't sound good, then just do a little — like changing positions, doing a gentle stretch, or slowly do some range of moment in whatever joints are calling.

If a little physical movement sounds good, start slow, with gentle stretches, swaying, strolling and observe how your body responds.

Should you start to feel stiff, tense, or overwhelmed, consider dialing down the level of activity.

If you tolerate the movement and would like to keep moving, then slowly titrate up the activity level while being mindful not to overwhelm your system. Low and slow is the way to go.

Healing is happening.

Leaning Into Our Alignment Layer

Over the weeks that followed, Nathifa periodically updated me on her progress. Like most people, Nathifa's healing process was a spiral one. Some days she felt like she made quantum leaps, while on others it felt like a "two steps forward and one step back" process. She was moving forward and meeting her goals while occasionally expressing frustration or angst when she didn't progress in a linear fashion. I reassured her that what she was experiencing was part of the healing process — which is anything but linear. After reflecting further, Nathifa agreed that she *was* progressing and that she wanted to learn more about leaning into her deeper layers in her solo and Haelan Nurse community.

Terminology Refresher: Alignment

Alignment is congruence, correspondence, or connectedness between our inner realities and outer lived experiences. Being aligned is like being in a flow state or in oneness with life. It is the process of honoring our deepest truths, life purpose, and emerging unhealed bits in bodymindessence.

Nathifa arrived at her next appointment with a lot of angst and energy. Since we last spoke, her landlord informed her that they were selling the property that was home to her and her children. They would not be renewing the lease, and she would need to move within the next 45 days. Nathifa verbalized feeling overwhelmed, anxious, worried, and "downright pissed off because this isn't the first time this has happened to me." She described how her family relocated every year or two throughout her childhood as employment conditions changed. Here's how our session went that day:

Nathifa: I don't effing believe this! There's no way I can move in 45 days. I don't even know if I can scrape together the money for first, last, and deposit — let alone all the other expenses ... [Her voice trails off as her eyes grow misty.]

Lorre: That's a lot of change to navigate in a short amount of time. It's understandable that you're feeling all the feels as you process this unexpected news.

Nathifa: It's like I just can't catch a break. It's one thing to have work be a hot freaking mess. But now my home life is going to be a mess. Isn't there one place on this planet where I can just be . . . [sniffles] . . . left alone for a minute?

Lorre: It's understandable to feel unsafe, especially when you've felt that way before, when you experienced abrupt housing changes. Your Threat Detector is signaling a threat or danger, from this situation, which is touching upon your prior experiences. Would you like to explore how this is affecting you now so we can work toward your next steps?

Nathifa: Girl, I thought you'd never ask. Let me assume the position. [She laughs and grabs her favorite soft throw blanket and candle, which we light together before she relaxes into the corner of the sofa.]

Lorre: Beautiful. Are you feeling safe and comfortable? [Nathifa nods affirmatively.] Great, let's move into a grounding and centering practice.

Nathifa: Honestly, I don't think I can ground and center myself. Like, I can't even sit still. [She points to her fidgeting leg as she shakes it up and down slightly.]

Lorre: I totally get it. That's your NS signaling that some physical movement may be helpful. How does that sound?

Nathifa: That sounds better than being still. Let's try it.

Lorre: OK ... [passing Nathifa a Physical Grounding Activities handout], do any of these sound like a good fit?

Physical Grounding Activities

☐ Slowly open and close your jaw several times.
☐ Rub your palms together as fast as you can, feel the heat.

☐ Sway, swan dive, or dance.

☐ Stomp or jump up and down.

☐ Tear pages out of a phone book, newspaper, or magazine.

☐ Yell or scream into a pillow.

☐ Do some stretching exercises.

☐ Get some exercise — even 10 jumping jacks or pushups will do!

☐ Mindfully make a hot or cold beverage and feel every sensation as you drink it.

☐ Any other physical movement that feels safe and supportive.

Nathifa: I'm all about tearing some pages!

Lorre: [handing her a short stack of newspapers and magazines] Tear away — and don't worry about cleaning up afterwards. Your job is to tear those pages to your heart's content. You can tear, crumple, toss, drop, or anything you'd like with those torn out pages. Don't hold back and don't worry about cleaning everything up. That will be my job, later.

Nathifa: Sounds good. [She tears the magazines tentatively at first, then more robustly for the next few moments.] Can you come to my house and clean up after my kids, too? [laughs] This is great! [heartily tears more pages, crumples some of them and throws them towards the trash bin] What a release!

Lorre: [chuckles] Yes, yes, it is! Crack on for however long you'd like. [Nathifa tears several more pages and then settles back into the sofa.]

Nathifa: Whew! That was . . . liberating. I'll have to remember this for when my kids get a little squirrely.

Lorre: Kids love physical grounding activities. They're a lot of fun and very effective. Let's take a moment so you can do a quick scan to see if you're feeling a little more grounded and centered.

Nathifa: [closes her eyes for a few moments] I never would have thought that moving around, tearing pages, would be grounding . . . but I do feel more grounded . . . like . . . more connected to my body. I was a big ball of energy before.

Lorre: Keen observation — and yes — I could feel your energy today, too. Do you feel ready to see which NS circuits and hybrids are online today?

Nathifa: Let's do it! [She chuckles as I hand her the How My NS Feels Today and Spectrum of Circuits & Hybrids worksheets, which she enthusiastically completes.]

Lorre: How are you experiencing your NS today?

Nathifa: Well, today most of the circles are in Circuit 2, with some in Circuits 1 and 3. I can feel that the SNS circuit is online. [laughs] If I were a bartender, I'd say I have a shot of SNS with a splash of dorsal with a ventral floater in the glass!

Lorre: Sounds like you know your NS . . . and your cocktails! [chuckles] So, just to keep us on track, where are we in YICP Flow Practice now?

Nathifa: Well, let's see. We're working on the 3As. We did Awareness and we're doing the Attending part now. After, we'll do the third A of Alignment. Right?

Lorre: Exactly! Good work. Now that we know your SNS is online more than the others, let's see if a stillness or movement attending practice feels best for you. Thinking about YICP Flow Practices, which of the attending exercises feel right?

Nathifa: Now that I tore all those pages [looks around at all the scraps of paper on the floor and proudly smiles] . . . I feel like being still. That sounds good.

Lorre: That sounds delightful. I have my Tibetan bells here. I'll ring them for you, as we've done before . . .

Nathifa: And I'll listen to the sound as it comes in and out, right? Just follow the sound as it helps to calm my NS and clear my mind a bit . . .

Lorre: Yep, just like we did before. [Nathifa closes her eyes and is in a relaxed seated position, breathing naturally as we do three bell ringing rounds together.]

Nathifa: [opens her eyes and wiggles a bit] I love how those bells tune me up [laughs heartily] — pun intended!

Lorre: Are you ready for an alignment practice?

Nathifa: Yep. Let's do the Inner Straw visualization from my menu. Like I really need to strengthen the connection between my inner and outer worlds. It's so helpful to do this with my Haelan Nurse crew when we get together. It's like the more we explore and share, the more we heal together.

Lorre: Oh, that is so lovely to hear! You all are co-healing and co-regulating together. My heart is overflowing!

Nathifa: I'm not going to lie. It felt a little awkward at first. But, we thought, "If we keep doing the same things, we'll keep getting the same results." So, we trusted the process and one another. That awkwardness disappeared once we got going.

Lorre: That's wonderful. [I facilitate the Inner Straw alignment practice.] How was your experience?

Nathifa: Well, I created a safe inner space. Everything was going along fine, and then as I started to bridge to my outer space, it was like I got gut punched. And then it's like . . . like . . . my energy . . . my inner world kinda . . . collapsed, like a house of cards.

Lorre: Would you like to lean into this sensation and gently explore?

Nathifa: Sure, it's not like you're going to gut punch me! [laughs tentatively]

Lorre: No gut punches here! Go ahead and get comfortable and close your eyes, if that feels good.

Nathifa: Eyes closed always feels good. I'm ready.

Lorre: Gently circle back to that gut punch feeling. Go only as far as is comfortable and let me know if you experience any signs of overwhelm or discomfort, OK?

Nathifa: OK. I know I need to lean in a little, but there's a part of me that doesn't want to . . .

Lorre: Is it OK with that part if you lean into it?

Nathifa: [nods yes] It's like I'm resisting. Like I want to lean in, but on the other hand, I'm . . . like . . . afraid . . .

Lorre: You're doing great. Welcome the resistance, for it is part of you in bodymindessence. Ask this resistance what it's feeling. Or if it's afraid of something. You may or may not get a response, so just lovingly open and welcome whatever comes in.

Nathifa: [takes a few moments in noble silence] It's like I'm afraid of this move. Not the moving part itself, but everything else. Finding a new place, filling out applications, packing, utilities, all the expenses, it's all just too much! [She reaches for a facial tissue and dabs her eyes.]

Lorre: It is a lot and it's certainly understandable that you might feel resistance around this uninvited move. Let's spend another moment or two with this resistance. Is it connected to that gut punch feeling?

Nathifa: It sure is! [She closes her eyes and visualizes leaning into the resistance within.] I feel so overwhelmed. Like . . . like my mom used to feel every time we had to move. [opens her eyes] Where did *that* come from?! [chuckles knowingly]

Lorre: It looks like you might have the answer to that question. Go on . . .

Nathifa: I'm betting it's an unhealed bit of wisdom! [She asserts with an a-ha awareness.]

Lorre: Good work — take a moment to explore how that unhealed bit feels today, in this present moment.

Nathifa: It feels like a sense of dread. Impending doom, even. I never wanted to move as a kid, and I certainly don't want to move now. [She dabs her eyes again as her voice softens.]

Lorre: What are your thoughts surrounding this unhealed bit and present-day move?

Nathifa: I don't want to do it. I just don't!

Lorre: Good, keep going. What emotions are you experiencing around this move?

Nathifa: I'm mad as hell, that's what.

Lorre: We can work with "mad as hell." Good work. Let's lean into that anger to see what's underneath it, if anything.

Nathifa: [after a moment or two] At first, there wasn't anything underneath it, but now there is . . . [opens her eyes, becomes verklempt] . . . I'm feeling afraid, but I don't know why. It's only a move . . .

Lorre: Beautiful. Sometimes, those unhealed bits bring with them the sensations, thoughts, and feelings that were stored at that time. We don't need to turn back the clock and relive the past, but let's see how what you described as a gut punch, an internal house of cards toppling, feeling resistance, overwhelmed, mad as hell, and fear from your inner world are manifesting in your external world today.

Nathifa: [sits more upright, leaning in slightly] Oh boy, I think I know where this is headed. [grabs the clipboard]

Lorre: You absolutely know where this is headed! Take a moment and complete the Making the Alignment Connections Worksheet. [Nathifa is familiar with the worksheet, so she takes several moments to complete the first column. Nathifa talks through her responses with me as she completes the next two columns, and then she hands me the completed worksheet.

***

Making the Alignment-Balance Connections Worksheet
Name: *Nathifa*

Step 1. After completing a YICP Flow Practice, jot down whatever inner world thoughts, emotions, sensations, or unhealed bits emerge here: *gut punch, house of cards falling down, rug pulled out from under me, resistance, mad as hell, afraid, fearful.*

Step 2. In Column #2, note how your inner world is being reflected in your outer world balance components now. Each inner world insight can be listed once or multiple times. Some balance components may not be reflected in your inner world, which is fine. This is just a small snapshot of where your inner-outer alignment is now.

Step 3. In Column #3, reframe what you wrote in the second column as a safety cue to your Threat Detector. These cues are supporting your brain's neuroplasticity and helping you to repattern, heal, and move toward feeling increasingly safe, secure, and supported.

Step 4. Align your Columns #2 and #3 into Column #4: Action steps you can take for realignment and balance.

Lorre: [reads Nathifa's worksheet] Fantastic work on this! What did you notice as you completed the worksheet?

Nathifa: Well . . . I didn't realize how much my inner world was affecting me. Normally, I take on challenges and don't let them bowl me over. I usually eat a healthy diet and exercise regularly, but not now. Same with my sleep. I usually sleep great [chuckles] thanks to the modern miracle of blackout curtains, but not now.

Lorre: Excellent observations. Generally speaking, before doing this Making the Alignment-Balance Connections worksheet, would you say you felt more aligned or misaligned?

Nathifa: Definitely misaligned. [She glances at her worksheet, now on the coffee table in front of her.] Sheez, I had no idea.

Lorre: That's why this exercise is so important. Now that you've reframed those misalignments into safety cues for your Threat Detector, can you incorporate them into YICP?

Nathifa: We are practically one person right now. [chuckles] I was thinking the exact same thing! I totally see how this

Alignment-Balance Connections - Nathifa

Column #1: Balance Components	Column #2: How my Inner World Is Reflected in My Balance Components	Column #3: Reframing Column #2 - Safety Cue for my Threat Detector	Column #4: Action Steps for Realignment & Balance
Personal Responsibility: Speaks to getting into the driver's seat of your adult life and lovingly care for all dimensions of self in bodymindessence, including your NS and unhealed bits of wisdom. Facilitating your healing, with others.	Gut punch, rug pulled out from under me — I feel like I can't get in the driver's seat of this move.	I am safe, supported, and capable of navigating this challenge with ease and grace.	Each day, I use my innate care plan and practices and engage virtually or IRL with my Haelan Nurse group or community to ensure my inner foundation is strong and supported.
Body & Mind Wellness: Describes supporting our physical and mental health and wellness by engaging in health promoting ways of being and doing in your daily life while addressing health disruptions, illness, or disease that emerges over time.	Mad as hell - I'm not eating right or exercising. I feel bloated and inflamed.	I am so safe, loved, and supported exactly as I am — even when I feel mad as hell. I surround myself with trusted loved ones and my Haelan Nurse community as we all lean into our deeper layers and heal together.	Each day, I honor where I am in my NS and seek, receive, and give support as we all move towards body and mind wellness.

247

Connections & Relationships: Considers your healthy connections and relationships with your loved ones, friends, family, communities, groups, and teams while addressing any unhealed-ness, codependency, power imbalances, or disease within your social relationships.	Afraid, fearful — I just don't have any oomph to be around my friends and family.	I am loved and accepted exactly as I am, even when my energy is low. It is safe for me to be seen without my oomph and to connect with my loved ones and my Haelan Nurse group.	Each day I connect with one or more people with whom I have a healthy and meaningful relationship so I can co-regulate, co-heal, and thrive in practice and in life.
Environments & Contexts: The environments and contexts within which you live and work and are influenced by (physical, emotional, intellectual, social, spiritual, environmental, relational, occupational, ergonomic, etc.) which are ideally safe, supportive, creative, and healthy and the need to address disruptions or dynamics that interfere with bodymindessence wellbeing.	House of cards falling down, rug pulled out from under me - I can't wrap my head around needing to move.	I am safe and supported in all aspects of my life. When unexpected changes emerge, I honor my inner sensations and perceptions with compassionate inclusion and my innate care practices.	From a place of inner and outer alignment, I find safe, affordable, and comfortable housing in my kids' school district.

Financial Wellness: Speaks to your relationship with resources, money, and money management, including the ability to meet current and future financial needs in support of your optimal safety, security, health, and wellness in bodymindessence.	Gut punch, rug pulled out from under me — I wasn't anticipating a move and will have to use our vacation money to cover expenses.	I am safe, secure, and supported while being flexible with my finances as unforeseen needs emerge, knowing that I will always find a way to enjoy our family during vacation times.	I engage in financial wellness practices such as budgeting, saving, investing, and planning for today and the future.
Regulate, Relax & Recharge: Describes how we take care of our NS and regulation as foundational to relaxing and recharging our bodymindessence. This includes YICP practices, healthy sleep and screen time, relaxing alone, with trusted loved ones, and Haelan Nurse Communities, and leveraging the health and wellness properties to regulate, relax, and recharge.	Afraid, fearful - I wake up in the middle of the night fraught with fear and anxiety and can't go back to sleep.	I am safe, secure, and supported - even while I sleep. Should I experience a sleep or relaxation disruption, I will engage with my MicroDoses Matter routine and YICP Flow Practices.	I consistently practice MicroDoses and YICP with trusted loved ones and my Haelan Nurse Community knowing that every time we do, we become more regulated, more relaxed, and begin to thrive in all that we do.

Beliefs, Values & Purpose:			
Living in alignment with your perceived core values, beliefs, and life purpose, which change and evolve as you do. Showing up with and for yourself and your deepest truths while lovingly and compassionately making changes in your outer world to align with living your highest and best life, as defined by you.	Resistance - it's not like me to shy away from a challenge.	I am a strong and resilient woman who is safe, secure, and supported. I adapt to and manage life's challenges while taking good care of myself and my family.	As part of my daily YICP Flow Practice, I open within to welcome new insights that guide me toward living my best life. I note these insights in my journal and share them with others so we may all support one another in living in alignment with our beliefs, values, and purpose.

will help me realign. Maybe that's why I've been feeling so disconnected inside.

Lorre: Wonderful observation. You are way ahead by taking an inside-outside approach to healing. Most people tend to start working on the balance components externally, without much consideration for those deeper inner sensations, thoughts, and feelings.

Nathifa: It's because we're all so dang busy! It's easy to forget about yourself in the sprint from sun-up to sundown [glances at worksheet again], but I can see how important it is to lean into my layers . . . and realign.

Lorre: Yes, it's so very important. How do you feel about the action steps you've set for yourself?

Nathifa: Well, they're "right" [gestures air quotes] in that they are positive, present-focused goals. But they're not SMART goals. Shouldn't these be SMART goals?

Lorre: We work with SMART goals directly in the Balance part of YICP. Here, in the Alignment part of YICP, we're exploring the correspondence, congruence, and relationship between your inner and outer worlds. Think of these actions as precursors to the SMART goals you might set later. Some people just roll with the action steps while others prefer SMART goal setting. Do or don't do whatever feels right for you.

Nathifa: Oh, that makes sense. I was like, um, yeah . . . I'm not ready to set big goals. I feel like I'm hanging by a thread most days.

Lorre: I've been there. That's why it's important to lean into your alignment, just as you are so brilliantly doing. Let's think about the action steps as Not So SMART goals.

Nathifa: [laughing and sitting more upright] Now why in the world would I do that?!

Lorre: Remember when we talked about how the LH and RH need to collaborate effectively?

Nathifa: I do. I also remember how most people are left-shifted [moves her head and leans far to the left with animation], including me!

Lorre: [laughs heartily] I'm so using that move in the future! Excellent. Yes, most people are left-shifted, so they don't always receive the full story from their bodily neural pathways, sensations, and that beautiful, juicy, and subjective RH information.

Nathifa: Because the LH kills the RH vibe so it can create structure and order, right?

Lorre: [nods affirmatively] Exactly.

Nathifa: That really stuck with me, and now I can't unsee it. It's like my LH wants to skip over the vibes, the feels, and get right to the logical point. It feels like I lose a little piece of myself every time that happens.

Lorre: What an astute insight. I've felt similarly myself, as have many others. That's why here, in the Alignment section of YICP, we're using the reframed safety cues and action steps as Not So SMART goals. We're giving a little time and space for all of your parts, unhealed bits, and neural pathways to be seen, heard, and healed as you share and co-heal with others. Not So SMART goals are intended to provide new, safe stimulus for the limbic system and ANS to support repatterning, neuroplasticity, and a growth mindset.

Nathifa: I love that. It's like we have to tap the brakes and stop internally for a minute. Usually I push all that stuff down because I'm so busy. And . . . [hesitates and reflects] because I'm more comfortable with my left-shiftedness.

Lorre: Most people are these days — but that's a topic for another time!

Leaning Into Our Balance Layer

Terminology Refresher: Balance

Balance involves showing up for oneself with personal responsibility for and a commitment to healing of self, with others. It includes body and mind wellness, connections and relationships, beliefs, values and purpose, personal and professional contexts, financial wellness, and the all-important and frequently sacrificed regulating, relaxing, and recharging component.

Most people approach healing from an outward perspective, much like you might splint a broken bone or put a bandage on a small wound. While such approaches certainly work in some acute situations, the outward quick-fix approach doesn't get to the root cause of healing that is needed in the deeper layers of bodymindessence. We can't quick fix or bandage over the deep wounds of traumatization. As we learned in Nathifa's sessions, much of what she was experiencing in her outer balance components were secondary to misalignments in her deeper layers.

Recall that where trauma is concerned, the brain is a pattern recognition system. For Nathifa, the shock of having to move unexpectedly in the present moment was recognized by the Threat Detector as a familiar pattern as it triangulated similar experiences in Her Repository. She wasn't able to fully integrate the moving-related traumas when she was a child. The unhealed bits from these experiences were stored in her body and neural circuits. Now, as a similar pattern emerged in her adult life, the unhealed bits emerged. Present-day Nathifa *does* have the resources and the people she needs to support her as she navigates an unexpected move and emerging unhealed bits. My role, as her facilitator, is to position her in *right relationship* for healing in bodymindessence so she can repattern that which is unhealed as she moves toward healed wholeness in both her inner and outer worlds. This is exactly what you are doing by sharing your healing journey with your trusted loved ones and Haelan Nurse communities. We are all healing together.

It would have been a disservice to Nathifa if she or I focused solely on the external balance manifestations of sleep, nutrition, and exercise disruptions. Sure, sleep hygiene, optimal nutrition, and regular exercise are essential wellness lifestyles to embrace. Had we just started there and focused on sleep hygiene and behavioral changes around food and exercise choices, we would have missed the deeper healing opportunities. Had we ignored the 3As and jumped right to the B (balance) component of her innate care plan, we may have added another layer of trauma instead of co-healing and co-regulating. As it turns out, the 3As support a regulated NS and open Window of Tolerance. This is the foundation upon which all Balance nurturing and caring practices and lifestyle choices are practiced.

Nathifa, like most of us, needed to shore up the foundation (her dysregulated NS and unhealed bits) before constructing her building (stress, sleep, nutrition, and exercise strategies) on top. Without first shoring up the foundation, whatever is built on top is very difficult, if not impossible, to sustain. It's like building a house of cards on top of quicksand. No matter how many nurturing, caring, and healthy behaviors and lifestyle choices Nathifa put into place (the building), if her dysregulated or traumatized NS is the foundation (quicksand), then those practices would not be optimally productive and have potential to further traumatize her. Nathifa understood the importance of doing all aspects of YICP (3As + B → 3Rs), starting with the 3As before moving into B (balance).

Nathifa and I continued to leverage the wisdom of her NS and innate care plan. We discussed that the goal for the Balance

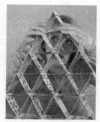

Healing Practices

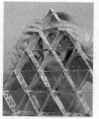

Regulated NS

Without a regulated NS
as the foundation of
YICP (3As + B → 3Rs),
healing practices aren't
optimally effective or sustainable.

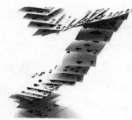

House of Cards

components is for them to be aligned and balanced, as a fully inflated bicycle wheel. The hub is our 3As from YICP, along with our Personal Responsibility from Balance. The remaining Balance components, shown in the image below, are intended to be inflated in the same manner as a bicycle tire. When Nathifa's balance components are inflated and supported by

YICP: Balance

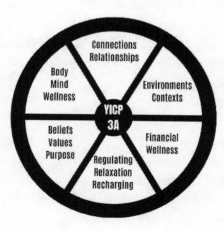

her 3As, she then glides through life with ease and grace while encountering and healing through the ruptures and repairs that are inherent with living.

Healing Gains: The 3Rs

We continued to lean into Nathifa's layers together as she moved through the home relocation process. Nathifa and her Haelan Community, which included other health professionals, really leaned into their layers together. They kept in contact via a group messaging app and met weekly. They were consistent in their MicroDoses Matter and YICP practices, which they often did together. By all accounts, they were co-regulating, co-healing, and having a lot of fun in the process. They were beginning to thrive in all aspects of their life. You are likely doing so, too, or will soon be. Trust the process. Lean into your layers while being supported by those who are sharing in this journey. Healing and co-healing are happening, and it's beautiful to behold.

Haelan Nurse Activities

Now it's your turn to lean into the layers and explore the activities and worksheets from this chapter. You can write in this book or download all of the worksheets from the Book Resources section on my website, drlorrelaws.com. Then, share your experience with your trusted loved ones and Haelan Communities. These worksheets make for lively conversation and co-healing opportunities. You can continue to add insights and practices to YICP. In the graphic, you'll find all the practices we've explored thus far.

Haelan Nurse Activity #1: Leaning In — Awareness
Below are the same two worksheets that Nathifa completed in her session. Now it's your turn. Just notice and gesture inclusion to any sensations, perceptions, or emerging unhealed bits, knowing that you are healing with so many others — including

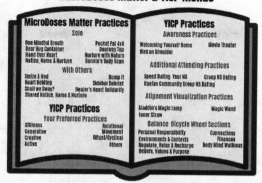

MicroDoses Matter & YICP Menus Expanded

me and our Haelan Communities. Lean into your people as often as desired.

***

Worksheet #1: How My Nervous System Feels Today (circle all that apply)

***

Circuit 1: I feel . . .

Circuit 1

Calm	Safe	Social
Connected	Relaxed	Lighthearted
Grounded	Empathetic	Settled
Rested	Relaxed digestion	Open
Capable	Breathing easy	Curious
Healthy	Engaged	Compassionate
Vital	Relatively low stress	Mindful
Present	Seeing the big picture	Relatable and relating

Number of Circuit 1 Circles: _____

***

Circuit 2: I feel . . .

Circuit 2

Frustration	Difficulty sleeping	Vigilant
Irritation	Activated	Constipated
Rage	Overly energized	Fidgety
Concern	Increased HR, BP, RR	Alert
Anger	Sweating/not sweating	Concentration challenges
Restless	Enlarged pupils	Emotionally constricted
Worry	Dry mouth	Panic
Swallowing challenges	Annoyed	Anxiety
Moderate-high stress	Appetite increase/ decrease	Not seeing the big picture

Number of Circuit 2 Circles: _____

***

Circuit 3: I feel . . .

Circuit 3

Numb	Trapped	Decreased sexual desire
Collapsed	Stuck	Depressed
Immobile	Fearful	Emotionally detached
Helpless	Decreased HR, BP, RR	Flat

Depressed	Shallow respirations	Brain fog
Disconnected	Lightheadedness	Overwhelming stress
Dissociated	Increased pain threshold	Withdrawn
Shame	Fatigue – general	Fatigue – muscle
Apathetic	Shutdown	Socially disinterested
Hopeless	Limited social interest	Can't big-picture think

Number of Circuit 3 Circles: _____

***

For sensations or perceptions not described above: I feel . . .
(Use the space below to name any other feelings or sensations that were not identified above. If what you're feeling corresponds to one of the three circuits above, add it to that list, circle it, and then adjust the tally below accordingly.)

***
***
***

Worksheet #2: Spectrum of Circuits & Hybrids
Step 1. Using the "How My Nervous System Feels Today" exploration exercise, record the number of circles for each circuit in the table overleaf.

Circuit Categories

Safety Circuit	Danger Circuit	Extreme Danger Circuit
Online circuit: Ventral vagal *I am and we are safe*	Online circuit: SNS *All hands on deck*	Online circuit: Dorsal vagal *No hands on deck*
# of Circuit 1 Circles from How My Nervous System Feels Today (above) _____.	# of Circuit 2 Circles from How My Nervous System Feels Today (above) _____.	# of Circuit 3 Circles from How My Nervous System Feels Today (above) _____.

Note any sensations, feelings, and perceptions here:

***

***

***

Refer to YICP Menu and list which practices feel right for where you are in your NS right now:

***

***

***

Step 2. Using the number of circles for each circuit in Table 1 above, explore if your NS is in one of the hybrid states now. Recall that the circuits and hybrids are like dimmer switches that can come online in varying degrees. It is possible for one or more circuits or hybrids to be online at a time.

Hybrid Categories

Play Hybrid	Stillness Hybrid	Freeze Hybrid	Fawn Hybrid
Online circuits: Ventral vagal SNS	Online circuits: Ventral vagal Dorsal vagal	Online circuits: SNS Dorsal vagal	Online circuits: SNS Dorsal & ventral vagal
I am safe, engaged, and joyful.	*I am safe, open, curious, and still.*	*I can't. I just can't.*	*I can't escape, so I'll please and appease.*
# of Circuit 1 __ & Circuit 2 ___ Circles.	# of Circuit 1 ___ & Circuit 3 ___ Circles.	# of Circuit 2 __ & Circuit 3 ___ Circles.	# of Circuit 2 ___ & Circuit 3 ___ Circles.

Note any sensations, feelings, and perceptions here:

***

***

***

Refer to YICP Menu and list which practices feel right for where you are in your NS right now:

***

***

***

Haelan Nurse Activity #2: Leaning In — Attending

Explore some of the physical grounding activities listed overleaf. Add them to YICP and have fun playing with them in your Haelan Communities. What other physical grounding activities can you add to this short list?

Physical Grounding Activities

☐ Slowly open and close your jaw several times.

☐ Rub your palms together as fast as you can, feel the heat.

☐ Sway, swan dive, or dance.

☐ Stomp or jump up and down.

☐ Tear pages out of a phone book, newspaper, or magazine.

☐ Yell or scream into a pillow.

☐ Do some stretching exercises.

☐ Get some exercise — even 10 jumping jacks or pushups will do!

☐ Mindfully make a hot or cold beverage and feel every sensation as you drink it.

☐ Any other physical movement that feels safe and supportive.

Haelan Nurse Activity #3: Leaning In — Alignment & Balance
As individuals and then together with trusted loved ones and Haelan Community members, reflect, note, and discuss how you are realigning and reframing to optimize your Balance components.

***

Making the Alignment-Balance Connections Worksheet
Name:
Step 1. After completing a YICP Flow Practice, jot down whatever inner world thoughts, emotions, sensations, or unhealed bits emerge here:

***
***
***

Alignment-Balance Connections - Blank

Column #1: Balance Components	Column #2: How my Inner World is Reflected in My Balance Components	Column #3: Reframing Column #2 - Safety Cue for my Threat Detector	Column #4: Action Steps for Realignment & Balance
Personal Responsibility: Speaks to getting into the driver's seat of your adult life and lovingly care for all dimensions of self in bodymindessence, including your NS and unhealed bits of wisdom. Facilitating your healing, with others.			
Body & Mind Wellness: Describes supporting our physical and mental health and wellness by engaging in health promoting ways of being and doing in your daily life while addressing health disruptions, illness, or disease that emerges over time.			

Connections & Relationships: Considers your healthy connections and relationships with your loved ones, friends, family, communities, groups, and teams while addressing any unhealed-ness, codependency, power imbalances, or disease within your social relationships.

Environments & Contexts: The environments and contexts within which you live and work and are influenced by (physical, emotional, intellectual, social, spiritual, environmental, relational, occupational, ergonomic, etc.) which are ideally safe, supportive, creative, and healthy and the need to address disruptions or dynamics that interfere with bodymindessence wellbeing.

Financial Wellness: Speaks to your relationship with resources, money, and money management, including the ability to meet current and future financial needs in support of your optimal safety, security, health, and wellness in bodymindessence.

Regulate, Relax & Recharge: Describes how we take care of our NS and regulation as foundational to relaxing and recharging our bodymindessence. This includes YICP practices, healthy sleep and screen time, relaxing alone, with trusted loved ones, and Haelan Nurse Communities, and leveraging the health and wellness properties to regulate, relax, and recharge.

Beliefs, Values & Purpose: Living in alignment with your perceived core values, beliefs, and life purpose, which change and evolve as you do. Showing up with and for yourself and your deepest truths while lovingly and compassionately making changes in your outer world to align with living your highest and best life, as defined by you.

Step 2. In Column #2, note how your inner world is being reflected in your outer world balance components now. Each inner world insight can be listed once or multiple times. Some balance components may not be reflected in your inner world, which is fine. This is just a small snapshot of where your inner-outer alignment is now.

Step 3. In Column #3, reframe what you wrote in the second column as a safety cue to your Threat Detector. These cues are supporting your brain's neuroplasticity and helping you to repattern, heal, and move toward feeling increasingly safe, secure, and supported.

Step 4. Align your Columns #2 and #3 into Column #4: Action steps you can take for realignment and balance.

Deeper Dive Resources

Henson, C., Truchot, D., & Canevello, A. (2021). "What promotes post traumatic growth? A systematic review" in *European Journal of Trauma & Dissociation, 5*(4), Article 100195. https://doi.org/https://doi.org/10.1016/j.ejtd.2020.100195.

Hershler, A., Hughes, L., Nguyen, P., & Wall, S. (Eds.) (2021). *Looking at trauma: A tool kit for clinicians.* The Pennsylvania State University Press.

Schwartz, A. (2021). *The complex PTSD treatment manual: An integrative, mind-body approach to trauma recovery.* Pesi.

Substance Abuse and Mental Health Services Administration (SAMHSA). (n.d.). *Creating a healthier life: A step-by-step guide to wellness.* https://store.samhsa.gov/sites/default/files/d7/priv/sma16-4958.pdf.

Section III

Thriving in Practice & in Life

Chapter 7

Transcending the Shame Layer

We are making incredible progress in our *haelan*, or healing, journey. You are no doubt seeing and experiencing post-traumatic growth, and those gains will continue, and these practices will support your regulation, reconnection, and restoration of your innate wellbeing and healer's heart. As we embark on this last section of the book, you may be wondering how leaning into the shame layer can help you shift from survival to thriving mode. That is because shame is almost always imperceptible. It's a slippery and pervasive state of unhealed-ness that often goes unnoticed. It is easily mistaken for other things or other layers. If you've been making gains in YICP and NS health but keep encountering a wall, barriers, or feel like this *haelan* process isn't always working for you, chances are that you've met your shame layer and either didn't know it existed or didn't know how to navigate it. Or you bumped into it and shoved it down or locked it away because the magnitude and intensity of it was too much.

That is the nature of the shame layer, and it can be a doozy for many people. Once you're primarily living in your regulated Window of Tolerance, the biggest barrier to thriving in practice and in life is the shame you carry or embody. In this chapter, we'll ever so gently explore, navigate, heal, and transcend some of our shame layers. You'll learn how to expand YICP practices to address the unique needs of the shame layer. Shame will lose its silent hold on you as you put a beacon of healing light on it and blaze a new neuroplastic thriving pathway. Over time, the old shame-related neurons will not fire much — they'll become like old dirt roads filled with weeds and rock because of the infrequent travel. Instead, you'll have a thriving neural network that will be a smooth ride, with ease and grace in all that you do.

Let's get started by recalling the ways in which nurses are traumatized and subsequently experience shame at work. Consistent with Foli's middle range theory of nurse psychological trauma, we'll classify these traumas as *unavoidable* (those which are inherent with the nurse role) and those that are secondary to healthcare system inadequacies as *avoidable*.

There may have been times in your career when things didn't go to plan. Perhaps you made a medication or medical error. Or, you may have experienced near misses, adverse events, or even sentinel events. Maybe you weren't able to be as compassionate as you'd otherwise be if you were practicing without the daily dose of *avoidable* nurse trauma. You may harbor regrets, embarrassment, compassion fatigue, moral injury, or shame as a consequence of these devastating experiences. Most of us carry these unhealed bits deep, deep within. Through YICP and MicroDoses Matter routines, you may have encountered some shame-related unhealed bits. Perhaps you didn't know what to do with it, or the discomfort was so great that you shoved it down even further within. My shame-related unhealed bits were always stored in my gut region, locked away from the light of day under the most rigorous of inner security systems. So overwhelming were my shame-related unhealed bits, that I

Avoidable & Unavoidable Nurse Traumas

Unavoidable traumas	Avoidable traumas
Inherent with the nurse role	Secondary to healthcare system inadequacies
Vicarious or secondary trauma	Workplace violence
Historical trauma & disasters	Insufficient resource trauma
System-induced (treatment) trauma	Second-victim trauma

couldn't bear to acknowledge them, let alone lean into them as part of my healing process.

I didn't have the resources or the people I needed when I encountered my shame-related unhealed bits years ago, but you do. It was for me to discover for myself and share with you, as has been the case for this entire book. Everything has been in service to my, yours, and every nurse's liberation and healing. Now there is language and a framework to guide us through our deepest layers as we move toward healed wholeness in the fullest sense of the word. For this to be fully realized, we must lean into the deepest layer of shame that is often embodied and unknowingly transmitted from generation to generation through family, nurse, and healthcare systems. If you are getting a "hard no" of resistance as you read this, know that resistance is expected. Allow it to be as it is as you come to understand that shame, known or unknown, may be ready to emerge as an unhealed bit. Trust that you're in the right place. If you are feeling like you want to close this book and never open it again, you're in the right place. If you're feeling like you don't have any shame and there's nothing for you to heal in this deepest layer, you, too, are in the right place. This can be a very heavy and dense topic for most of us, so let's ever so gently and tenderly explore the shame layer together. You can move as fast or as slow as desired. Shame is a complex and often painful experience. So, with ease and grace, let's prepare ourselves for the journey from embedded shame that has you stuck in survival mode to liberation, inner peace, and thriving in all that you do.

Slow the Pace Speed Bump: YICP for Leaning into the Layers of Shame Practice

At the time that the perceived shameful event occurred, it is likely that your safety or professional wellbeing *was* threatened. Our first step, as always, is to signal signs of safety to the Threat Detector so we may lean into this very deep layer.

Your Threat Detector may be recognizing your emerging shame-related unhealed bits as a threat to your safety. You may be noticing that different circuits or hybrids are coming online. All of these responses to shame-related unhealed bits are natural and expected. I and our community are with you in noble, unconditional love and acceptance. You are safe.

This practice is intended to be done with your trusted loved ones and Haelan Community. Co-healing is how the shame layer is transcended. Below are the steps for you to explore and practice now — and use in your co-healing practice later.

Awareness:
Let's start with a bear hug to give ourselves a container in which to be felt, seen, and healed. Give yourself and one another a few loving squeezes and deep breaths. If you feel like moving to another area that may feel safer, go ahead and do so now.

Should you experience the emergence of shame-related unhealed bits, gesture inclusion, love, care, and healing by placing one hand, then the other, over your belly. It is an act of tremendous courage to welcome these unhealed bits. They would not be emerging if you weren't ready to heal and co-heal through them.

With one hand on your heart and the other on your belly, breathe naturally for several moments. Observe and welcome whatever sensations you may be experiencing, from utter despair to shutdown or collapse, to anger or rage, or to the stream of tears that are beginning to cover your face.

You have been through so much. Love and welcome those unhealed bits, for they are the parts of you that had to be stored until conditions were more favorable for healing. Now is your time. It's just you, me, our trusted loved ones, and our beloved Haelan Community. You are safe and loved beyond measure, no matter what happened.

Attending: Power Hara Breath with gratitude to Amy Weintraub.

Please check with your healthcare or wellness provider if you recently had abdominal surgery, have untreated high blood pressure, or if you are pregnant.

- Stand or sit with your feet a little wider than hip width apart.
- Bring your left hand to left shoulder, right hand to right shoulder, elbows pointed out like chicken wings.
- Inhale, filling your lungs halfway while twisting to the left.
- Inhale fully as you twist to the right
- In one motion, extend your right arm powerfully as you twist to the left and exhale with a vigorous "haaaa" sound.
- Return to center, hands still touching each shoulder with elbows out, deep inhale and hold.
- In one motion, extend your left arm powerfully as you twist to the right and exhale with a vigorous "haaaa" sound.
- Do 5-10 rounds.
- When you are done with your rounds, return to your starting position (standing or seated).

- With your eyes closed or with soft eyes, sense deeply your face, your neck, your arms, the palms of your hand. What sensations, such as tingling, are you experiencing? Notice and gesture inclusion as your unhealed bits are transformed into regulated parts of your true self.

All aspects of me are safely held and loved. All is forgiven.

- While standing, bring both hands to the dantian, about two fingers below the navel. Bring your thumbs and forefingers together in a triangle shape. Say aloud (preferable) or to yourself, "My hands are safely held and loved. All is forgiven."
- Gently bounce on your feet for 30 seconds and notice any sensations. Say aloud (preferable) or to yourself, "My feet are safely held and loved. All is forgiven."
- Move into a comfortable seated or reclined position. Prepare to repeat this exercise through your entire body.

Left side of the body
- Start with the left foot. Say aloud (preferable) or to yourself, "My foot is safely held and loved. All is forgiven."
- Move from the left foot towards the crown of your head. Let your inner wisdom guide you. As you move to each new location in your body, say aloud (preferable) or to yourself, "My — is safely held and loved. All is forgiven."
- When you reach the crown of your head, place your hands such that your little fingers are at the border of your forehead and hairline; index fingers at your crown. Say aloud (preferable) or to yourself, "All aspects of me are safely held and loved. All is forgiven."

Right side of the body

Repeat the steps for the right side of the body, culminating in the crown of your head.

Torso

Move through your torso, gently touching each part as it is comfortable and nurturing. Include your chest, spine, breasts, back, belly, genitals, and buttocks. Say aloud (preferable) or to yourself, "My — is/are safely held and loved. All is forgiven."

Close practice at the heart

End this self-acceptance and forgiveness practice by placing your right hand on your heart, left hand over the right, thumbs linked in a garuda mudra. Say aloud (preferable) or to yourself, "All aspects of me are safely held and loved. All is forgiven."

"All aspects of me are safely held and loved. All is forgiven."

"All aspects of me are safely held and loved. All is forgiven."

And so it is.

When you are ready, which could be at some later time, you may (or may not) complete the Alignment & Balance segments for YICP. Trust your intuition, inner wisdom, and the wisdom of your NS.

Healing is happening.

You did great in this exercise. Please return to it often, for sometimes shame shows up in many different ways. Now, let's explore together the nuances of embodied shame and how it can affect us all.

Transcending Shame

Scientist and author, Dr. Brené Brown, defines shame as "an intensely painful feeling or experience of believing we are flawed and therefore unworthy of acceptance and belonging." Participants in her grounded theory study used other words to describe their sense of shame, such as devastating, excruciating, rejected, separate from others, isolated, and *the worst feeling ever*. People who are experiencing shame often feel trapped, powerless, and isolated — like a web of layered and conflicting expectations regarding who we "should be" based upon (a) *our identity* (for example, gender, race, age, religion, sexual orientation, religious identity, etc.); (b) *our role* (for example, nurse, partner, spouse, adult child, parent, group member, etc.); (c) *our social context* (for example, how we are viewed by ourselves, family, partners, coworkers and colleagues, community members, etc.). Dr. Brown describes the complexity of shame as "The Shame Web" to highlight how pervasive and limiting this experience is to us all. The burden of shame is devastating to all aspects of our bodymindessence.

Where trauma and recovery are concerned, shame closely corresponds with the dorsal vagal circuit and corresponding hybrids. Gabor Maté describes shame as a loss of contact with oneself — that dorsal vagal sense of inner disconnection or disassociation — and corresponding limiting beliefs such as "I'm not good enough" or "There's something wrong with me." Trauma visits us all over the course of our lifetimes. Each of us carries our own Repository of shame in the form of unhealed bits, limiting beliefs, and false narratives. We carry this stored Repository of trauma, guilt, and shame individually and collectively. Left unhealed, it is unknowingly passed down from one generation to the next, including generations of nurses.

We all have experienced shame, for it is inherent with the human experience and with both the avoidable and unavoidable nurse-specific traumas. Recall the unavoidable traumas we experience, shown in the table along with descriptions.

Shame and Unavoidable Nurse Traumas

You may be able to recall a time when you or someone you know experienced **vicarious or secondary trauma** while caring for a patient. Hearing about and witnessing the patient's suffering may activate the nurse's unhealed bits, thoughts, and feelings surrounding their own trauma. Perhaps you have been on the giving or receiving end of **historical trauma** that manifests as subtle workplace incivilities such as eye rolling, muttering, sighing, gossiping, being sarcastic, avoiding colleagues, giving the silent treatment, or rudely using your mobile device. If you were the one unconsciously transmitting a workplace incivility, you likely felt embarrassment or shame when you became aware of the behavior. If you were on the receiving end of workplace incivility, you likely felt shame — like you didn't belong or were somehow less worthy than your colleagues. Or, you might have been a first responder during a **natural disaster** or pandemic where many patients died or had poor outcomes. You may have felt shame, knowing that you did everything you could, but it still "wasn't enough." Many nurses experience **system-induced or treatment trauma** that occurs secondary to a treatment intervention or protocol. This type of trauma often overlaps with vicarious or secondary trauma.

These experiences will influence which of a nurse's unhealed bits, circuits, and hybrids will come online. When the patient's trauma touches the nurse's trauma, it may be difficult to stay fully regulated and present in the Window of Tolerance in these circumstances. Accordingly, nurses might feel a sense of shame, that they aren't a "good nurse," or that "there's something wrong with me" in turn. It's a vicious cycle of trauma and shame that is pervasive in many healthcare contexts. Add that

Shame and Unavoidable Nurse Traumas

Unavoidable traumas	Description
Vicarious or secondary trauma	Often described as "the cost of caring." We witness and listen to our patients' accounts as they experience physical or mental health challenges, pain, fear, violence, traumatization, abuse, or death. Many nurses feel shame because, despite our best efforts, we weren't able to fix, heal, cure, etc.
Historical trauma	How trauma is passed down from one generation to the next, rendering the new generation vulnerable to the original trauma. Given the dynamics of nurses being a historically oppressed group, the legacy of our collective traumas is transmitted to other nurses through many subconscious manners such as lateral violence, bullying, and workplace incivilities. Many nurses feel shame because, despite our best efforts, we knowingly or unknowingly transmitted the legacy of nurse-specific trauma to our colleagues or the next generation of nurses.
Trauma from disasters	Trauma resulting from natural or global disasters that require nurses to serve as first responders, thereby placing them at direct and/or secondary trauma. Many nurses feel shame because, despite our best efforts and following trauma and triage protocols, we were not able to fully care for those in their greatest time of need.

System-induced trauma (treatment trauma)	Often overlapping with vicarious/secondary trauma, this medically induced trauma occurs as part of the treatment process. For example, during the pandemic, nurses experienced their patients' traumatization secondary to the strict isolation requirements. Residents in assisted living or skilled nursing facilities were denied contact with their loved ones or hospitalized patients died alone. Many nurses feel shame because, despite our best efforts, we were not able to fully address the suffering being experienced by our patients and their families.

to any shame that may have resulted from individual traumas (acute, chronic, complex, developmental, or neglect) and it can be a lot to experience and manage.

Shame and the Dorsal Vagal Circuit

The first order of business is to destigmatize the concept of shame, which gets a bad rap in most cultures. Shame, like most emotions, has varying degrees of intensity from mild to excruciatingly intense. People tend to perceive the intensity of their shame as commensurate to the degree that they feel they messed up or how inadequate they are — when, in fact, *shame is actually a metric of how deeply we care*. So, let's officially gesture inclusion and welcome any shame-related unhealed bit that emerges as a perfectly natural response to how our Threat Detector signaled and our NS adapted to keep us safe. Let's be curious with shame and open to what we can learn from it.

Like our fluctuating circuits and hybrids, shame is a natural human experience. From an evolutionary mammalian perspective, we absolutely need our family, tribe, or community to survive. None of us can survive childbirth, infancy, or childhood without the support of others. We are social creatures who depend upon one another — directly or indirectly — for our health, wellbeing, and survival. Shame is a high-stakes, three-part phenomenon, described in detail below, that is in service to our social acceptance, and therefore, our short- and long-term survival. It is so very pervasive and often presents with harsh self-judgment or self-criticism. Unhealed shame grows stronger over time, strong enough to be passed on through generations. Shame can be a little pesky to work with.

Most people feel sensations of shame in the organs below the diaphragm, which is home to the dorsal vagus nerve. It can feel like a punch in the gut, inner collapse, dread, or mortification. It can feel overwhelmingly painful, invasive, burdensome, or heavy. Shame and guilt are frequently confused. Guilt signals that "I did something bad or wrong" and may motivate you to rectify or correct an action or behavior. There are two types of guilt: helpful and unhelpful. **Helpful guilt** is healthy — this psychological discomfort nudges us with the message that something we've done was objectively wrong. It leads to healing and a positive outcome when we change our behavior, right a wrong, or seek forgiveness. **Unhelpful guilt** is unhealthy — this psychological discomfort is centered on something that we've done against our very unrealistic and high standards. It leads to negative and unhealthy outcomes because it emphasizes self-punishment instead of behavioral change, thereby keeping us stuck in the unhelpful guilt.

Shame is an intense and painful feeling of being flawed, worthless, or inherently defective. People who experience shame see themselves as deeply flawed and unworthy. Shame has negative outcomes because it causes us to fear that we will be rejected. It tempts us to disconnect within and with others and to avoid whatever is causing the shame. It signals through the dorsal vagal circuit that "I am bad," which in turn leads to a freeze, helplessness, hopelessness, and inaction.

Shame can be a paralyzing experience because the SNS fight-or-flight response isn't available, so the body reflexively shuts down. That's why we used our breath, movement, and gestures in the Slow the Pace Speed Bump above. These voluntary movements of SNS mobilization counter the initial dorsal vagal circuit and help to keep that shut-down response at bay. Continue to engage with YICP Shame Layers Practice as you move through this chapter and then as part of YICP general practice. Shame can be sneaky, so let's shine a healing spotlight on it and keep it in our field of awareness.

Does This Shame Fit the Facts?

Shame, like all emotions, has a function that brings value to it. So, we must ask, what is shame's evolutionary value? You might be thinking, "Wait, WHAT?! Shame has value?!" Yes. Because of its pervasive, gut-wrenching nature, many people overlook that shame has important functions in service to our survival. The reason shame has value is because it protects us from being kicked out of our life-sustaining family, social circle, tribe, village, profession, workplace, or community. Shame protects us from being ostracized and cut off from life-sustaining relationships and resources. It makes you want to disappear, hide, or become invisible so that no one finds out about what you've done lest you be kicked out of the community.

For nurses, there is shame connected to keeping our life-sustaining jobs or licenses. For us, it's a super high stakes situation. Just as it has been for people throughout the millennia. Back in the day, historically speaking, if you were booted out of your tribe or community, you'd likely perish soon thereafter. In modern times, you'd probably not die, but you'd have to start over, build another life, or embark upon a new career role. In

Does this Shame Fit the Facts?

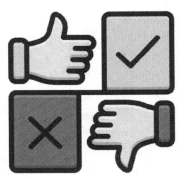

It is TRUE.

You have been or will be
rejected from a
life sustaining group

It is FALSE.

You were not or are not rejected
from a life-sustaining group.

short, shame's job is to make sure that you don't let people find out what you did "wrong" to prevent you from getting kicked out of the life-sustaining group. But shame can be pesky to detect and address, so we'll use Dr. Marsha Linehan's "Does It Fit the Facts?" test to assess whether or not shame is supporting your survival or if it is an outdated narrative or unhealed bit that is ripe for healing.

When Shame Has Value

Shame has value when it is in service to your survival. It does this by helping you to self-modulate and adapt to the ever-changing conditions of your life so that you can retain membership in the social system(s) that are directly or indirectly keeping you alive. When it is *true* that you're going to be rejected or ostracized from a group, then shame fits the facts. Therefore, shame DOES NOT fit the facts when it is *not true (false)* that you're going to be rejected or ostracized from a group. For those of us who carry the burden of shame, which is most of us either knowingly or unknowingly, it is mission critical to do Dr. Linehan's "Does It Fit the Facts?" litmus test. In the table below, you will find examples of when shame does and does not fit the facts:

Does It Fit the Facts?

YES	NO
Shame fits the facts when it is TRUE that you'll be rejected from a life sustaining group.	Shame DOES NOT fit the facts when it is FALSE and you WILL NOT be rejected from a life sustaining group.
Engaging in child sexual abuse.	Stealing a candy bar from the corner market when you were six years old.
Disclosing a mental health condition on a job application (you won't get hired because the people making the hiring decision don't want to hire you - they want you out).	When you cannot be fully present with a patient's trauma because your own circuits are coming online while otherwise giving excellent nursing care.
Being grossly negligent, neglectful, or incompetent in nursing practice.	During a natural disaster or pandemic, an increased number of patients in your care died or had poor outcomes through no fault of yours.

Most cultures have social norms that prohibit mistreatment of minors. Sadly, there are systemic stigmas, prejudices, discriminations, and biases where mental health conditions are concerned. It's pretty clear that when shame fits the facts, that you'll be rejected from the group. It gets a little murky when shame does not fit the facts because we don't want to take any chances where group rejection is concerned. We tend to view our mistakes and misgivings through a unitary lens — meaning that *every* mistake or misgiving can get us rejected. Even when the shame DOES NOT fit the facts and we WILL NOT be rejected from a life-sustaining group, we still hold onto the shame . . . just in case.

Let's take a look at how this affects nurses. Let's say you had a very long shift and one of your patients was really, *really* traumatized. Their trauma touched on your own, and perhaps some unhealed bits emerged. Or perhaps you felt slightly dysregulated or your Window of Tolerance was very small. You took very good care of your patient, but you couldn't really connect with them as you usually would. You may have been a little less socially engaged (a natural response when the ventral vagal tone is diminished as the SNS or dorsal vagal circuits come online). On your way home from work, you keep replaying all the interactions with this patient and their family. You start mentally "beating yourself up" with the shame narratives uttered by your inner critic who is incessantly reminding you that you're not a good nurse, that you better watch out or you'll get written up. Or fired. Or lose your license. Without your job, you won't be able to pay your rent or mortgage payment. You'll be homeless. You'll lose everything and live on the streets for the rest of your life. You get the idea. Shame narratives can subconsciously take you from thriving to destitute in the blink of an eye. We can go from "I wasn't able to be fully present" or "I made a minor mistake" to "My career is over and my life is ruined" in a matter of seconds. This happens, despite the fact that excellent nursing care was provided overall. Shame is so very pervasive that most people don't even recognize it. When presented with a shame narrative or unhealed bit, ask yourself, **"Does it [the shame narrative] fit or *not* fit the facts?"** In this example, "Does not being fully present with a patient or making a minor mistake while providing otherwise excellent nursing care fit the facts?"

The answer is no. You WILL NOT be rejected from a life-sustaining group, such as your employing or licensing organization. You provided excellent nursing care while also managing how your NS was touched by your patient's trauma. You will not get fired from your job or lose your license. You will not lose your housing arrangement. You will not be homeless. Your life is not over. *But the shame narrative FEELS like you will.* Hence, the three-part phenomena of shame:

The Shame Narrative

Part 1: The inner critic is telling you that you're worthless, like garbage.

Part 2: An aspect of self that believes Part 1 to be true.

Part 3: The behavioral response to the false shame narrative.

Staying with our example, Part 1 is your inner critic telling you that you're a bad nurse and that you're going to lose your job (shame-reinforcing narrative). Part 2 is an aspect of self that believes this shame narrative to be true (believing the shame-reinforcing narrative). Part 3 is you feeling anxious, depressed, or so hopeless that you start applying for other jobs because you know this one will soon be gone (shame-reinforcing behavior),

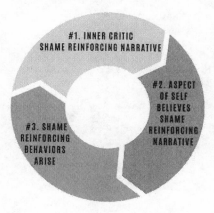

SHAME
A THREE-STEP VICIOUS CYCLE

#1. INNER CRITIC
SHAME REINFORCING NARRATIVE

#2. ASPECT OF SELF BELIEVES SHAME REINFORCING NARRATIVE

#3. SHAME REINFORCING BEHAVIORS ARISE

Shame Cycle

even though there is no evidence to support the notion that your job is in jeopardy.

What you then have is a vicious cycle of shame . . . **and this event doesn't even fit the facts.**

Whew. That was a lot of information to take in. Let's take a moment to notice any thoughts, perceptions, or sensations that may be arising. Perhaps you are experiencing some shame-related unhealed bits or outdated shame narratives. Whatever you may or may not be experiencing, know that you are safe. I feel you and have my healer's heart wrapped around yours, as do your trusted loved ones and Haelan Community members. Let's take a moment to co-heal as we do a YICP Shame Layers Practice together. Refer to the above Slow the Pace Speed Bump or the summary graphic. Healing and co-healing are happening.

You are doing great while navigating the heavy yet essential shame healing process. Fine tune your awareness and monitor for the emergence of unhealed bits, dysregulation, or a diminished Window of Tolerance. Step away from this chapter and lean into YICP as often as desired. There's no rush

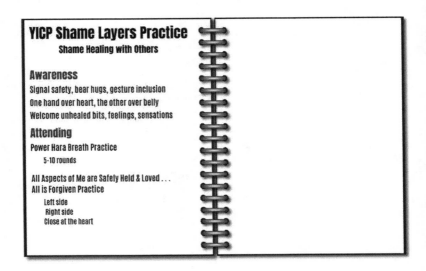

YICP Shame Layers Practice
Shame Healing with Others

Awareness
Signal safety, bear hugs, gesture inclusion
One hand over heart, the other over belly
Welcome unhealed bits, feelings, sensations

Attending
Power Hara Breath Practice
5–10 rounds

All Aspects of Me are Safely Held & Loved . . .
All is Forgiven Practice
Left side
Right side
Close at the heart

to get to the end of the book, and there will be resources for you after you finish reading it. For now, read and experience at your own pace, knowing that you are so richly supported, valued, and appreciated. In the next section, I'll discuss how to address both avoidable and unavoidable nurse traumas and how to work with your inner critic to transcend the vicious cycle of shame.

Shame and Avoidable Nurse Traumas

These nurse traumas are those which create the most angst for most nurses and are the reason that many nurses are burning out, leaving the profession, or experiencing presenteeism. It's one thing to carry the burden of shame related to *unavoidable* nurse traumatization, but the shame associated with *avoidable* nurse traumatization is unbearable for most, and it shatters the healer's heart. In the *Escape Fire* documentary, healthcare quality improvement leader, Don Berwick, asserts that there are excellent healthcare professionals who, along with their patients, are needlessly suffering in poorly designed healthcare systems. This perspective of good people in these bad systems is reflected in Dr. Paul Batalden's famous quote, "Every system is perfectly designed to get the results it gets." It stands to reason, therefore, if we have healthcare systems that are so poorly designed that they create multiple types of nurse-specific traumas, then we need to redesign those systems to ensure a sufficient number of healthy, thriving nurses.

As traumatized nurses who are retraumatized frequently in our professional roles, we don't have time to wait for the system redesigning process. That's why we're here — in this book and in our Haelan Communities — now. We're not waiting for anyone, nor are we willing to be further traumatized by healthcare system inadequacies. No one should have to bear the agonizing shame secondary to these system shortcomings. And so, we shall persist now by leaning into and healing the *avoidable* shame that so many of us carry or embody. Let's review the *avoidable* nurse traumas in the table on page 291.

Chances are that you have experienced one or more of these *avoidable* nurse traumas and corresponding shame during your career. I personally have experienced the full spectrum of workplace violence in my (gasp) forty-year career. I've been hit, scratched, hair pulled, spat upon, verbally abused, bullied, and the list goes on. I suspect that you have, too. It's not OK for anyone to be abused or traumatized while delivering nursing care.

I remember one example from when I was a nursing student. We had all just passed our clinical skills testing and were going out to our clinical sites. I was eager to apply everything that I had learned and didn't anticipate that the nurses working at the unit wouldn't want to precept me. I endured the eye rolls, the sighs, and the dismissive body language as no one wanted to be a preceptor. I knew it wasn't personal. I knew that it was because the nurses had too many patients with too few resources. But it *felt* personal. The vicious cycle of shame ran nonstop. My inner critic constantly told me that I wasn't good enough, smart enough, or skilled enough. That's why no one wanted to precept me, insisted the inner critic. My unhealed bits and vulnerable nursing student self-believed the inner critic's narrative despite my logical brain telling me otherwise. I was able to self-modulate and respond with appropriate behavioral actions, but after my shift I was self-medicating with junk food.

In other words, my limbic system was in the driver's seat every time the precepting nurses argued over who would "have to" take the nursing student that day — grousing among themselves as though I weren't standing right in front of them. Later, and despite my best efforts to the contrary, my behaviors became more shame-based during the morning huddle. I avoided eye contact and felt nauseous, anxious, and internally collapsed as the dorsal vagal circuit came more prominently online. During the shifts with the precepting nurses, I felt unworthy and incompetent despite being an excellent student. These feelings and behaviors fueled my inner critic, and the vicious cycle of shame perpetuated.

My story is like so many others. Nearly every nursing student I've educated in the past decade has similar stories to

Shame and Avoidable Nurse Traumas

Avoidable traumas Like sentinel events, these *avoidable* nurse-specific traumas should never occur.	Description
Workplace violence	Any form of nurse-directed verbal, emotional, written, or physical abuse or assault from patients, their visitors, or colleagues. This includes lateral/horizontal violence and workplace incivilities in the form of disrespectful gestures, attitudes, actions, words and/or behaviors. Shame can result for nurses who find themselves on either the giving or receiving end of workplace violence.
Insufficient resource trauma	This type of trauma occurs when nurses don't have the tangible or intangible resources they need to deliver ethical, professional nursing care or meet organizational responsibilities. Shame can result when patient safety, quality of care, or outcomes are compromised despite an under-resourced nurse's best efforts.

Second-victim trauma	Often secondary to insufficient resource trauma. Second-victim trauma occurs when an avoidable or unavoidable medical error, adverse or sentinel event happens. The patient experiences the trauma first-hand while the nurse is traumatized secondarily.
	Shame can result from being under-resourced, careless, or negligent in a health culture with a shame and blame culture. It can also result from a patient experiencing an unexpected adverse outcome while receiving excellent care.

share. It's a cluster situation of nurse traumatization. Students experience workplace incivilities secondary to the nurse traumas experienced by their preceptors. This is how "nurses [unintentionally] eat their young" and how systemic embedded trauma and shame passes from one generation of nurses to the next (historical trauma). Traumatized and under-resourced nurses don't have bandwidth in a climate of limited time and resources (insufficient resource trauma) to train a student nurse. Both the student and the precepting nurse experience workplace trauma and, likely, shame. Let's put this scenario to the "Does it fit the facts?" test on page 293.

Let's explore a couple of other examples before you reflect upon the shame you may be carrying or embodying.

Engaging the Shame to Break Its Power

In each of the scenarios in the table, shame resulted that may or may not have fit the facts. But each nurse was profoundly impacted and whatever shame-related unhealed bits in their Repository

Avoidable Nurse Trauma: Does This Shame Fit the Facts?

Type of *Avoidable* Trauma	Scenario & Point of View (POV)	Does this shame fit the facts?
Workplace violence or incivility	POV: The precepting nurse doesn't have time or bandwidth to train a student nurse due to insufficient resources and feels ashamed that they talked disrespectfully in front of the student.	It *feels* like this shame fits the facts, but it does not. This shame DOES NOT fit the facts. It is false. The precepting nurse will not be rejected from their job, which is a life sustaining professional group.
	POV: The student nurse feels ashamed, unwanted, and unworthy. They must be a bad student if nobody will train them.	It *feels* like this shame fits the facts, but it does not. This shame DOES NOT fit the facts. It is false, but it's a little more complex. The student nurse needs to complete their clinical hours to graduate from nursing school. The student nurse would not necessarily be rejected from their nursing program or a current or future life

sustaining group. The
nursing school and
the clinical partner
would likely resolve
the issue to ensure
the nursing student
had a preceptor. But
the student doesn't
always know this.

emerged, their Threat Detector responded accordingly. So
how do you move through the real or perceived vicious cycle
of shame? Trauma experts Drs. Joan Borysenko and Marsha
Linehan recommend engaging the shame to break its power.
First, give that inner critic a silly name. I named my inner
critic Endora after the entertainingly, always critical mother-
in-law in the 1960s TV series *Bewitched*. Listen to the inner
critic. What are they saying? Engage the inner critic's story,
the shame narrative, by doing the "Does it fit the facts test"
exercise. This will help you to determine if your life-sustaining
membership in a particular group is *actually* or just *feels like* it's
being jeopardized. This distinction will de-escalate any shame
scenarios that (a) don't fit the facts, (b) are false, and (c) will
not result in you being rejected from a life-sustaining group. In
some cases, when the facts *do* fit the test, we experience being
kicked out of a life-sustaining group. The same course of action
can be taken to heal and transcend shame that does or does not
fit the facts. Sharing our shame stories through YICP Shame
Layers Practice is how we align our inner and external worlds.
By sharing these stories with trusted loved ones and Haelan
Community members, we experience support and inclusion
instead of real or perceived threat of expulsion. As it turns out,
this is mission critical information for the Threat Detector to
consider and is essential for co-healing our shame layers.

Does This Shame Fit the Facts?: Example

Type of Trauma	Scenario	Does this shame fit the facts?
Insufficient resource trauma	Hospital acuity is high and the nurse is required to admit a complex patient whose needs exceed that unit's capacity to safely deliver care. The nurse must spend most of their time with the new complex patient and doesn't have time to fully meet the needs of their other patients. After work, the nurse breaks down and cries in their car, feeling guilty and ashamed that they couldn't do everything they were supposed to do for every patient.	It *feels* like this shame fits the facts, but it does not. This shame DOES NOT fit the facts. While it is sad and frustrating that this nurse was prevented from fully caring for their patients due to insufficient staffing, there were no near misses, medical errors, adverse events, or other egregious oversights that warrant this nurse being rejected from their job and the life sustaining professional group.

Second-victim trauma	The same nurse in the above scenario made a medication administration error that caused an anaphylactic response that was quickly resolved with no additional health consequences for the patient. After work, the nurse hits their steering wheel several times in frustration and feels ashamed. Several hours later, the nurse feels despair, hopelessness, shutdown, and shame.	It *feels* like this shame fits the facts, but we can't tell for sure. This is a borderline case that is contingent upon multiple factors, including the nurse's work history, organizational policies, and licensing requirements. At minimum, this nurse could be at risk for current or future dismissal from the job (and/or life sustaining professional group).

Sharing Our Shame Stories through YICP Practices

Building upon YICP Shame Layers Practice from the previous pages, we're going to align outdated shame stories with the present-day reality. In our Haelan Community, everyone is safe and supported. Sharing our shame stories will be celebrated, for we are liberating ourselves from the mental and emotional chains that bind us to outdated narratives. Recall from earlier in this chapter where we are in this YICP practice:

YICP Awareness

Signal safety, bear hugs, gesture inclusion. Place one hand over our hearts, the other over our bellies as we welcome any unhealed bits, feelings, or sensations.

YICP Attending

Power Hara Breath (5-10 rounds) followed by All Aspects of Me are Safely Held & Loved . . . All is Forgiven Practice.

YICP Alignment

In this step, we nurture ourselves a little differently. Within each of us are outdated shame narratives that either don't fit the facts or used to fit the facts but are no longer relevant. A few of us may be moving through a shameful situation that *does* fit the facts. Regardless of the status of our shame stories, the remedy is the same: love, compassion, acceptance, inclusion, and forgiveness. We love ourselves. We have compassion for ourselves. We accept all the parts of ourselves and one another. We forgive ourselves and others. We heal together. Over and over and over again. It is mission critical that we tell our stories. Start first by sharing the shame story with yourself through journaling or other creative expressions. While this is a start, it doesn't provide the social feedback you need from others that signals safety (you're not being kicked out of a life-sustaining group), acceptance, and inclusion. Your Threat Detector needs this feedback to signal differently for our circuits and hybrids. Share your stories with your trusted loved ones and your Haelan Community — over and over and over again. The repetitive nature of sharing our shame stories reinforces the truth of the situation. **The truth is that you are safe. You are NOT being rejected for your shame story.** Here's how to start breaking the shame cycles by leaning into them with YICP Alignment Practice.

1. **Recall & tell** a low-stakes shame story to yourself through journaling or other creative expression.
2. **Notice & welcome** any sensations, feelings, or perceptions that emerge with radical self-acceptance.
3. **Signal safety** to the Threat Detector, which is receiving new data from which to make this and future assessments. Engage whatever creature comforts or activities that help you to feel safe and supported, including nature.
4. **Share** a low-stakes shame story with a trusted loved one or Haelan Community member. This is where we show up for one another with our healer's hearts overflowing with compassion, support, nurturance, and acceptance. Together, we are breaking the shame cycles and replacing them via neuroplasticity as new neural pathways are being formed. Here, we are all experiencing exponential healing.
5. **Repeat** this process with shame stories that emerge for healing over time. Go low and slow so as not to overwhelm your NS. Give plenty of time and space to integrate the healing gains as we liberate one another and step into our empowerment together.

We all have *a lot* of shame neurons that are wired and are firing together. We don't have nearly as many love, compassion, and forgiveness neurons firing in the context of an outdated shame story. By repeatedly telling our shame stories and experiencing

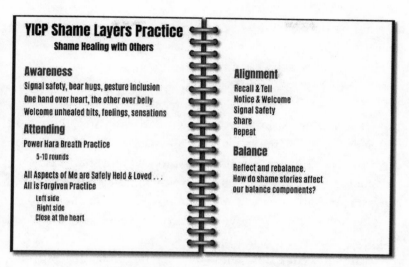

YICP Shame Layers Practice
Shame Healing with Others

Awareness
Signal safety, bear hugs, gesture inclusion
One hand over heart, the other over belly
Welcome unhealed bits, feelings, sensations

Attending
Power Hara Breath Practice
   5-10 rounds

All Aspects of Me are Safely Held & Loved ...
All is Forgiven Practice
   Left side
   Right side
   Close at the heart

Alignment
Recall & Tell
Notice & Welcome
Signal Safety
Share
Repeat

Balance
Reflect and rebalance.
How do shame stories affect
our balance components?

YICP Shame Layers Practice FULL

acceptance by our trusted loved ones, we're leveraging the properties of neuroplasticity to eradicate the shame story and replace it with radical acceptance. The shame highway will become overgrown and impassable as the acceptance superhighway is built and traveled over time.

It can be very scary to tell our shame stories the first few times. It takes tremendous courage and bravery to share shame in seemingly high stakes social contexts. Know that your trusted loved ones are not rejecting you when you share your deepest, most vulnerable truths. I am not rejecting you. I am celebrating you. Our Haelan Community is not rejecting you. We are embracing you with unconditional support and acceptance. As we experience the truth surrounding our shame stories, we also experience the support and acceptance of our trusted loved ones. This is essential feedback for the Threat Detector. The shame story comes to light and we are being accepted. This new information is being stored in Our Repositories. This radical acceptance will be accessed by the Threat Detector, which — going forward — will begin to signal safety instead of an extreme danger. We are breaking the shame cycles. We are liberating ourselves from the shackles of shame.

Healing, very deep healing, is happening for us all.

YICP Balance

Now that you've explored your inner landscape and discovered where and how shame is being expressed and healed, you can use any YICP Balance practice to explore where shame is being reflected in your body and mind wellness, relationships, social contexts, and any financial implications. You'll see how shame may be interfering with your ability to regulate, relax, and recharge. Or, you may discover how shame has steered you off the path that is consistent with your beliefs, values, and purpose. Either way, you are shifting the shame narrative and integrating the healing you've experienced and will continue to experience.

Liberation: Our Thrive Neural Networks Are Established

Now that we have an understanding of how shame works and how to manage it, we can continue to heal through our shame, with trusted loved ones and our *Haelan Community*. Return to this chapter frequently to continue the shame liberation process. The more time we experience thriving through acceptance, regulation, and connection within our inner and outer worlds, we'll find that our healer's heart and wellbeing are flourishing. In the next chapter, we'll explore some archetypal and resistance challenges you may encounter while growing and thriving in practice and in life. For now, savor and celebrate the healing gains made in this chapter. Then, let's continue our healing and liberation journey through the following activities.

Haelan Nurse Activities

Let's continue to lean into our shame layers. As we become proficient in navigating our very mild, low-stakes shame stories, continue to lean into those less mild, higher-stakes shame stories. As always, pause for YICP practices as needed and connect with your trusted loved ones and our *Haelan Community* often. If your inner wisdom is guiding you to seek the support of a health professional, please heed that wisdom and get the support you need. There is no shame in getting shame support — I've certainly benefited from professional support and I'm betting that you can, too. Shame. It's a tricky one.

Let's gently expand our shame story list to include those that are a little more intense or have slightly higher stakes.

***

My mild, lower-stakes shame stories:

1.
2.
3.

***

Now, refer back to the latter part of this chapter to complete YICP Shame Layers Practice. Start with one less mild, higher-stakes shame story until you've experienced self-acceptance

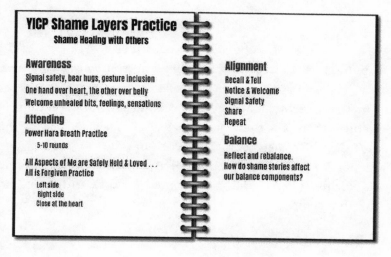

301

and the acceptance of others. Every time you transcend one of these shame stories, you've added new thrive neural pathways and diminished the outdated shame ones.

Then, continue with the other two shame stories, similarly. When you're ready, repeat this exercise to include:

***

My more intense, higher-stakes shame stories:

1.
2.
3.

***

Take one shame layer at a time, steady as you go — with others. It is very common to move through some shame layers quickly while other layers may take a longer time. Let your inner wisdom and NS guide you. Stay in your Window of Tolerance. Should a shame layer lead to difficulty in maintaining your Window of Tolerance, that is a signal that additional time, support, perhaps professional support, is needed. Remember, there's no shame in getting shame support. We are healing and liberating ourselves from our shame stories. We're breaking and releasing the shame cycles and replacing them with our neoplastic thrive superhighway.

Deeper Dive Resources

DeYoung, P. A. (2021). *Understanding and treating chronic shame: Healing right brain relational trauma.* Routledge.

Goffnett, J., Liechty, J. M., & Kidder, E. (2020). "Interventions to reduce shame: A systematic review" in *Journal of Behavioral and Cognitive Therapy,* 30(2), pp.141-160.

National Institute for the Clinical Application of Behavioral Medicine. (2023). *How to work with shame.* https://www.nicabm.com/.

Chapter 8

Archetypes & Resistance Patterns

You are likely becoming more proficient in navigating your inner and outer worlds now. You may be seeing signs that your worldview is shifting from "What's wrong with me?" to "Oh, this is what happened and/or is happening to me." Your understanding of how your NS adapted to keep you safe then, may have resulted in patterns, beliefs, perceptions, feelings, or behaviors that may not be serving you well now. You have learned so much, and I am so proud of you and happy for you. I'm sending you a virtual bear hug, from my healer's heart to yours. Well done!

As you grow increasingly more regulated and spend more time in your Window of Tolerance, you may be noticing collective patterns of unhealed-ness in coworkers, colleagues, friends, and family. If so, embrace this insight as a testament to your growth and healing. Humanity is experiencing unprecedented challenges, and the state of this macrocosm is being reflected in our microcosms across all dimensions of life. Although you can't, as one nurse, fix the global healthcare and nursing crises, you *can* be a beacon of wayshowing and healing light. You *can* consistently embrace your MicroDoses Matter routine, YICP practices, and 3Rs of regulation, reconnection, and restoration. As you continue to thrive instead of survive, you *are* facilitating co-regulation and co-healing with every person you encounter. You don't have to do anything to "fix" another. There's nothing to fix, for what you are encountering are the collective trauma patterns that have been unknowingly transmitted through generations of nurses and individuals. While there's nothing to fix, there is a lot to navigate as you bump up against these collective patterns of humanity's trauma NS adaptations, which I refer to as The Archetypes.

Archetypes Defined

Where trauma is concerned, the brain and NS are pattern recognition systems. Your ever-vigilant Threat Detector is on duty 24/7, continually assessing for threats and cross-checking with the repository containing all your lived experiences. As safety or danger patterns are detected, signals are sent to the ANS, which prompts the circuits (ventral vagal, SNS, dorsal vagal) and their hybrids (stillness, play, fawning, freeze) to come online. This influences your inner world and outer world responses, as well as adaptations to safety and danger. As humans, we are inextricably linked to and embedded within the contexts and systems in which we live and work — even those that are traumatizing or fraught with emerging unhealed bits.

It makes sense, then, for us to explore how traumatization of the masses and their emerging unhealed bits may externally manifest in recognizable collective patterns or archetypes. Recognizing these archetypal patterns helps us to navigate through the ruptures and repairs inherent with daily living. Collectively, our traumatic experiences and unhealed bits contribute to the archetypal patterns. Each traumatic experience has its own root cause(s) and was incompletely integrated at the time. The unhealed bits were uniquely stored in our individual and collective repositories. These unhealed patterns and bits are unknowingly passed on to others through ancestral, cultural, spiritual, religious, societal, systemic, organizational, and professional lineages and legacies. As such, the archetypes are general depictions of traumatic residues across time, contexts, and cultures.

"Archetypes are longstanding collective NS adaptations and unhealed bits that are unknowingly transmitted and embedded within the structures and systems that form the tapestry of our daily lives."

Lorre Laws, PhD RN

An archetype is a recurring symbol or depiction of dispositional thoughts and behaviors, which are shaped by events, circumstances, and situations. They tend to have the same foundation but express themselves in different patterns of emotions and behaviors. Archetypes commonly pop up through many generations (including nursing generations) and can be passed down or transmitted through ancestral (workplace and educational) lines. When these patterns of traumatization and unhealed bits manifest internally or externally, they may seem out of time or context and can be disproportionate to, or misaligned with, the present-day challenge. In short, archetypal patterns are longstanding collective NS adaptations that are unknowingly transmitted and embedded within the structures and systems that form the tapestry of our daily lives. They can feel messy, unpredictable, or perplexing as they emerge. Archetypes (yours and those of others) live in the blind spot of your awareness and are subconscious barriers that can impede healing progress at the individual and collective levels.

It's important to gesture inclusion when you detect an archetypal pattern rather than judge, minimize, or ignore it. Although it's natural to meet the archetypes with denial, resistance, judgment, shame, or blame, strive to gesture inclusion. For, as you learned with emerging unhealed bits, pushing archetypal patterns away is like pushing a part of yourself away. This exacerbates the inner sense of disconnectedness. Instead, gesture inclusion to the archetypes that we all embody and explore what lessons and healing opportunities are shrouded within them. Archetypes are simply collective NS adaptations from the past that may be maladaptively manifesting now. Leaning into the archetypes provides tremendous opportunities in transcending systemic, embodied traumas from the past at the individual and collective levels.

Each of us embodies some or all of the archetypes from time to time. Sometimes, like unhealed bits, they lay dormant within. They can awaken spontaneously or emerge when a person's Threat Detector signals danger and recognizes all similar experiences in our repositories. It can be challenging to interact with an archetypal manifestation, whether it is yours or somebody else's. It is easy to judge or blame oneself or another in the heat of an archetypal moment. If that happens, take a mental step back. Breathe. Gesture inclusion to the archetypal pattern as a NS adaptation from the past that may be maladaptive in the present. Do a perspective shift from "What is wrong with me/you/us/them?" to "I wonder what happened to me/you/us/them?"

Recognizing and welcoming archetypal patterns for what they are (collective trauma conditioning) is far more helpful than resisting, blaming, shaming, ignoring, deflecting, or denying them. Remember, the archetypes are adaptations. They are not conscious choices. The limbic system may be temporarily in the driver's seat. Various circuits and hybrids come online that may be contextually misaligned with what is happening in the present moment. Thoughts, feelings, and behaviors may be incongruent with the present situation or overblown. The person exhibiting the archetypal pattern is likely unaware of its existence. What's needed is your regulated NS and for you (within healthy boundaries and parameters that support you staying within your Window of Tolerance) to be the co-regulating, inclusive, and supportive person who can be with the archetypal pattern before, during, and/or after its emergence. You don't need to fix or do anything right now other than to stay in *your* Window while compassionately and implicitly helping to position the other person (or people) in *right relationship* for their healing through gestures of inclusion and co-regulation.

That's it. You don't have to diagnose anything. You don't have to explain or describe what is happening to the person through whom an archetype is being expressed. Nurture your

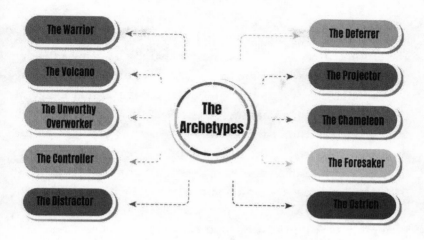

NS as you encounter an archetype. Do several MicroDoses Matter rounds. As soon as practical, do a YICP practice. Signal safety by connecting internally through bodily sensations, connecting to the stimuli in the external environment, and co-regulating with others. Depending upon which circuits and hybrids are online for the archetype, there are other strategies to consider. But first, I'll introduce the ten archetypes, which can appear alone or together, in response to inner or outer, real or perceived, threats to safety or security. They are: The Warrior, The Volcano, The Unworthy Overworker, The Controller, The Distractor, The Deferrer, The Projector, The Chameleon, The Foresaker, and The Ostrich.

Common Archetypes

These ten archetypes can arise depending upon a person's circumstances, context, NS navigation literacy, and Repository. There is a mixology to the archetypes, which is determined by how that person's Threat Detector signals for the various circuits and hybrids to come online. Each archetypal pattern is a protective adaptation, not a conscious choice. Over time, circuits and hybrid patterns formed, like the grooves in an old vinyl record. These patterns were "wired and fired" together initially. Each time the archetypal pattern emerged, the wiring and firing patterns, thanks to neuroplasticity, became a deeper groove. After a while, the circuits and hybrids came online in predictable ways, as though our collective Threat Detector were a mixologist, signaling for a shot of this, a splash of that, with a dash of the other. Each archetype has its own unique mixology comprising the three circuits. The mixology scheme is hierarchical: a dash is the smallest unit of measure, the shot is the largest measure, and a splash is somewhere in between. In the table, you'll find each archetype's mixology and a general description of how their NS adapted to keep them safe over time.

Each archetype is unique in regard to which circuit is dominant, comprising a spectrum of archetypes that range from SNS to dorsal ventral dominance, as shown in the image.

The Archetypes & Their Mixology

The Archetype	Mixology	NS Adaptation Over Time
The Warrior	3 shots SNS	The Warrior protects themselves by turning everything into a battle, argument, or aggressive overture as they swiftly move towards the stressor in SNS activation.
The Volcano	2 shots SNS, a dash each of ventral and dorsal vagal	The volcano protects themselves by erupting, spewing harmful or gaslighting words, or responding or behaving aggressively.

The Unworthy Overworker	2 shots SNS, a dash of ventral vagal with a dash of dorsal vagal	The Unworthy Overworker protects themselves by overachieving and accomplishing goals that are often rewarded by societal norms.
The Controller	1.5 shots SNS, a splash of ventral vagal with a dash of dorsal vagal	The Controller feels inwardly out of control and protects themselves by outwardly controlling people and situations.
The Distractor	1 shot SNS with a splash each of ventral and dorsal vagal	The Distractor protects themselves through distractions and procrastination. From daydreaming to endless social media scrolling to starting but not completing new projects.
The Deferrer	1 shot SNS with a splash of dorsal vagal with a dash of ventral vagal	The Deferrer protects themselves by insisting that inner and outer conditions must be perfect at all times. This manifests as chronic just-as-soon-as-it-is.
The Projector	1 shot SNS, 0.5 shot ventral vagal with a dash of dorsal vagal	The Projector protects themselves by projecting their stress, dysregulation, or unhealed bits onto others. Unlike The Volcano, The Projector uses more socially accepted passive or passive aggressive approaches.

The Chameleon	5 shots each of SNS, ventral and dorsal vagal	The Chameleon protects themselves by recognizing that fight, flight, and freeze are not viable survival options, so instead, they please and appease to stay safe.
The Foresaker	0.5 shots each of SNS and dorsal vagal with a dash of ventral vagal	The Foresaker protects themselves through self-sacrifice or self-punishment, often unknowingly so, to retain their membership in a life-sustaining group or social context. This archetype is frequently associated with systemic oppressions such as structural racism, or marginalization of women, persons of color, indigenous persons, members of the LGBTQIA+ community, among others.
The Ostrich	1 shot of dorsal vagal with a splash of ventral vagal and a dash of SNS	The Ostrich protects themselves by putting their head in the sand to avoid or ignore discomfort, conflict, or confrontation. The Ostrich is a master of denial.

Mixology: Shot > splash > dash

Archetypal Resistance Patterns

Just as the archetypes are collective adaptive patterns, our collective resistance to their emergence is similarly adaptive

Archetypes & Circuits

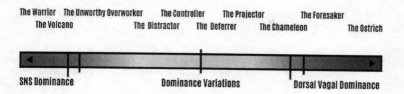

| The Warrior | The Unworthy Overworker | | The Controller | The Projector | | The Foresaker | |
| The Volcano | | The Distractor | | The Deferrer | The Chameleon | | The Ostrich |

SNS Dominance   Dominance Variations   Dorsal Vagal Dominance

and patterned. Once we bring these resistance patterns to the field of awareness, then we can begin to see how we can heal through them. Resistance patterns, like archetypes, operate subconsciously and are not choices. Once we are aware of the archetypes and their resistance patterns, we can position ourselves in *right relationship*, with others, to regulate and use YICP practices to blaze new, more adaptive neuroplastic pathways and responses. There are three common resistance patterns that protectively emerge when the archetypes are online and are perceived as danger cues by the Threat Detector.

Hamster Wheel Resistance

The Hamster Wheel protects by trying to outrun the archetypal pattern. It is built from concern, worry, fear, and anxiety. Its mantra is from the classic movie *Forrest Gump*: "Run, Forrest, run!" Its protective mechanism is to move away from the archetypal patterns.

Brick Wall Resistance

The Brick Wall protects by being a barrier between you and the archetype. Your NS is signaling for you to fight the archetype (figuratively speaking) and is fueled by frustration, annoyance, irritation, anger, and rage. Every time you run toward the archetype, the brick wall of resistance appears, and you are stopped in your tracks. Its mantra is: "Stop trying to make it happen." Its protective mechanism is to move towards the archetypal pattern.

Break Down Resistance

The Break Down is a last resort, protective mechanism when the Hamster Wheel and Brick Wall patterns fail. You're exhausted from running on the hamster wheel or hurling yourself against the brick wall. Your energy stores are depleted. Its mantra is: "Nope. Not happening." Its protective mechanism is to shut you down to keep you safe.

What Happened to Us? Jordan's Story Continues

Before we continue with our case story, it's important to point out a potential pitfall or trap. As nurses, we're highly trained to assess and make nursing diagnoses as the first two steps of the nursing process. It would be easy for us to take The Archetypes and their corresponding Resistance Patterns and subconsciously make assumptions or judgements about others using a "What is wrong with you?" perspective. It would be very easy to unknowingly judge, criticize, or take a them-versus-us, or a divide-and-conquer approach, in response to the archetypes and their resistance patterns. Stay open and observant. Notice when the archetypes tend to come online and under what circumstances. Be the beacon of co-regulation and co-healing. Strive for a heal-and-harmonize approach, where the goal is to position ourselves, as individuals, teams, and a profession in *right relationship* for healing. As Haelan Nurses, our overarching goal is to usher forth *Nursing 2.0: The Nurse Safety and Professional Wellbeing Edition*. We do this by reflecting upon our workplaces and our healthcare systems and asking, "What happened to us?"

My work with Riley's team continued, as did their flourishing and growing Haelan Nurse group. I met with some of the team members individually and as a group when their schedules aligned. I met with Jordan weekly to support her while she navigated particularly difficult circumstances and coworkers. Jordan was engaged in her MicroDoses Matter routines while at and away from work. She was a consistent YICP practitioner and regularly used the tools in this book to navigate her NS, which vacillated between the fawn and freeze hybrid states.

Jordan noticed YICP misalignments and other imbalances in her domains of Financial Wellness (overspending), Regulate, Relax & Recharge (re-emergence of insomnia symptoms), and Beliefs, Values & Purpose (uptick of adverse events and one sentinel event secondary to insufficient resources and personnel). With that information in mind, let's sit in on one of Jordan's sessions:

***

Jordan: I can't believe I'm right back where I was before — the same patterns. Here they are again, like a bad remake of [the movie] *Groundhog Day*.

Lorre: I, too, am seeing some parallels between what was happening when we last met and what is happening now. What do you see in the big picture that is contributing to the recurring patterns?

Jordan: Well, it's like a cliche of idioms. [chuckles] Like "The grass is always greener on the other side" meets "Wherever you go, there you are." I thought for sure that everything would get better after I left my former toxic workplace. And it did, for a few months. As it turns out, that was just a honeymoon phase. Now it's [laughs] a recurring nightmare of same sh*t, different day.

Lorre: I hear that a lot from different clients. What are some of the particulars in this recurring nightmare at work?

Jordan: So, it's the same sad story. We have more patients with more complex comorbidities and not enough nurses. It's like the hits just keep coming. Over and over again. It's "Jordan, I need you to take an admit" when I'm already two patients over what is safe. Then it's "Jordan, can you come in early, stay late, or come in on your day off?" I get like 4-6 calls and messages every day off. I can't get a break from work, even when I'm taking care of myself. [eyes mist up, voice drops] And that's become the status quo. But it's not the worst of it . . . [voice trails off]

Lorre: Take however much time you need. I get that this is so very difficult.

Jordan: It's beyond difficult, honestly. I am losing a lot of sleep over it, if I'm to be honest. My work BFF, Camila, is inconsolable. She can't even bring herself to come back to work after what happened. And it's not even her fault! It's none of our nurses' fault! [voice cracks, sobs quietly into facial tissue] We're stretched so thin that we can't get everything done in a timely manner. Like, there's a rapid response, two other patients swirling the drain, and the meds and interventions — they just pile up until someone dies. [sobbing while her chest heaves and tears stream down her face]

Lorre: [moves to sit on the sofa next to Jordan, opens arms to offer a hug, which she accepts and continues to cry for several minutes] I'm so sad for you and Camila. I've got you. It's safe to let it all out now. [Jordan continues to sob for a few more moments, during which the intensity wanes.] You're doing great.

Jordan: [slowly leans out of the hug and gestures a heart mudra] Thank you. I didn't know all those feels were there. [chuckles] I guess I've been holding it all inside. I just don't know what to do. I'm not even sure if I want to be a nurse anymore. [sniffles and chuckles at the same time] None of us do.

Lorre: Everything that you're feeling is a natural response to extraordinarily difficult and trying situations. [Jordan nods knowingly.]

Jordan: Well, I don't want to lose my [nursing] license. But on the other hand, I don't know if I even want this license. What I do know ... [sitting up, eyes focused] is that I can't keep nursing in a world where near misses and adverse events happen on the regular. And now, we — specifically Camila — just had a sentinel event that could have been prevented, if only we were properly staffed and resourced.

Lorre: I totally get it. What you and your team are experiencing are *avoidable* nurse-specific traumas. [Jordan nods.] Do you remember way back at the beginning of our time together when we talked about the types of traumas that nurses experience? [hands clipboard with the nurse-specific trauma infographic to Jordan]

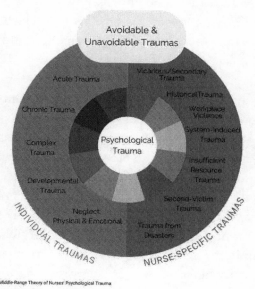

Adapted from Foli (2022). Middle-Range Theory of Nurses' Psychological Trauma

Avoidable & Unavoidable Traumas

Jordan: [nods affirmatively with animation] I do remember this! It's like there are many of these traumas every day at work right now. [tensely chuckles]

Lorre: Yes, yes, there are. It's important to keep this information in mind — you and your team are experiencing substantial nurse-specific traumas. I'm betting that many of your colleagues are traumatized as a result.

Jordan: For sure. We're all struggling. I'm on the brink of a collapse. Camila is utterly shut down. Everybody else is disrupted or dysregulated.

Lorre: That's a very astute observation. With the amount of trauma being experienced each day, compounded by frequent contact and work requests on days off, it is very difficult to maintain NS regulation or keep your Window of Tolerance widely open.

Jordan: Exactly! It's like there's no escape. I know when we were working together when I was still on Riley's team, I wasn't really ready to do any healing work. I truly thought that if I just changed jobs, everything would be better. It was, until it wasn't. [eye rolls as she laughs lightly] I'm ready to work on this stuff now.

Lorre: That's an important realization, and it's one that we all seem to make during our careers at some point. And now, given the widespread prevalence of nurse-specific traumas, it's equally important for each of us to position ourselves *in right relationship* for healing, with others. You'll discover where *your healthy* is in your practice so you can thrive and not just survive.

Jordan: That's exactly why I'm here again! There's so much nurse traumatization happening everywhere. It's not just at this unit or this setting. It's flipping everywhere! [throws hands up in the air and chuckles with exasperation]

Lorre: Yes, sadly, it is.

Jordan: And I don't want to keep changing jobs and burning out. I worked my a** off to get into and through nursing school. I have a mountain of student loan debt to pay off. I feel so trapped. I don't want to leave nursing and I can't afford to leave nursing, but it's like there's no other choice. I can't fix the system. I'm stuck. Hopeless. [puts head in hands, eyes covered]

Lorre: [scoots a little closer and side hugs Jordan, who returns the gesture] I know. It is an overwhelming feeling for so many nurses right now. I know it's been awhile since we took a big picture view of the phases we move through in response to trauma, extraordinary events, circumstances, and situations. Would it help if we did a quick refresher?

Jordan: [dabs her eyes with facial tissue] Yes, please. Anything is better than what I've been feeling . . .

Lorre: I want you to know that you are not alone. Millions of nurses are experiencing traumatization and burnout. We can heal together, as individuals and as a profession. I know it doesn't feel like it right now, but by virtue of you being

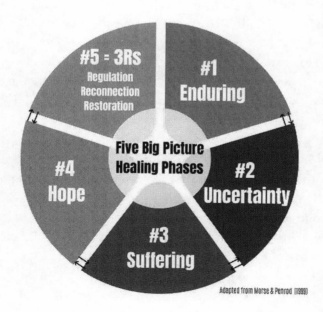

Adapted from Morse & Penrod (1999)

here, healing is happening. [places another sheet of paper on the clipboard and passes it to Jordan] Do you remember this?

Jordan: [quickly reviews the handout] Oh, yes, I do! It's been a long minute since we talked about this, but I do remember!

Lorre: Fantastic! Let's look at these phases through the lens of goals and routes.

Jordan: [with a puzzled facial expression] Um, I sort of remember, but not really. What do you mean?

Lorre: If you look to the next page of the handout, you'll see a table that shows how our goals and the routes we'll take to reach those goals are aligned with each phase. [Jordan flips to the next page and skims the table.]

Jordan: Oh, yes. I remember this table now. I'm literally living this right now. [chuckles]

Lorre: Yes, you certainly are! Remember when we first started working together? [Jordan nods yes.] You were enduring a very difficult workplace culture.

Jordan: [chuckles] If by difficult you mean a cesspool, then yes, I was!

Lorre: How about if we connect what you've experienced to these phases to help you get a sense of where you are now in the big picture? [Jordan nods affirmatively.] I'll get us started and you add in as we go along.

Jordan: Perfect.

Lorre: Let's start with our initial appointments, several months ago. When we first met, you were enduring a very challenging workplace. You said you were "overwhelmed beyond measure."

Jordan: [chuckles] That's exactly what I said! [glances at worksheet] I was in the Enduring Phase. I had no clue as to what to do — no goal and no route.

Big Picture Journey

Phase	Description	Goal Present?	Route Present?
Enduring	Getting through an extraordinary situation or trauma. Focus on making it through by suspending emotions and remaining in control.	No	No
Uncertainty	Recognizing that something needs to be done about the situation or trauma. A goal(s) is set, but the route or means by which to accomplish the goal is not yet clear.	Yes	No
Suffering	**Step 1.** Acknowledging the impact of the situation or trauma in the past, present, and future. Emotions previously suspended emerge, often overwhelmingly so, which temporarily obliterates the goal(s) previously set. Emotional tsunami described as complete blackness or a dark tunnel with no end. **Step 2.** As the emotional tsunami is processed, slowly and incrementally begin to piece together a goal and a route. Suffering, while difficult, is a process of healing and repair.	No	No

Hope	Acknowledging and accepting what has happened and its significance in one's past, altered present, and new future. The outcome isn't certain, so emotions are held in check while bracing for potential negative outcomes. Refines goals in response to internal and external conditions. Seeks and engages in supportive relationships that support positive outcomes.	Yes	Yes
3Rs: Reconnection Regulation Restoration	Transcending the trauma or event by accepting the past and embracing an altered future. Emerging with a new perspective on life and living a richer and more meaningful life. Gaining a deeper connection within and with others, increased NS regulation, and restoration in the healer's heart and bodymindessence.	Yes, until the next rupture occurs in service to our growth and resilience.	Yes, until the next rupture occurs in service to our growth and resilience.

Adapted from Morse & Penrod (1999).

Lorre: Exactly. And then, in our next sessions, you became conflicted as to whether to stay or leave the unit.

Jordan: Yes! And I decided to leave, but I didn't know where I was going then. [glances at worksheet again] So, I was in the Uncertainty Phase. I had a goal to leave, but I didn't have the route to my current position. Wow, these phases really line up!

Lorre: They sure do. How did you experience this Suffering Phase then?

Jordan: Well, that emotional tsunami came crashing down. I was all up in my feelings and was despairing over leaving my team. I loved that team. I still do. I started second guessing myself. Should I stay? Should I go ...? [voice trails off]

Lorre: And you lost sight of your goal for a minute there.

Jordan: I did. [glances at worksheet again] But then I moved into Step 2 of the Suffering Phase. I just needed some time to process everything that I was feeling and doing. I see that now. When I entered Step 2, I was then able to update my resume and start applying for positions.

Lorre: That's right. And we also talked about exploring the deeper layers of your suffering.

Jordan: That's right, we did! [sits up straight] I forgot all about that. But yes, I do remember. I just couldn't process anything else at the time.

Lorre: And your inner wisdom was spot on. Your inner plate was full. Taking on anything more — deeper layers — was too much.

Jordan: It's like that Desmond Tutu quote. Like we can only eat an elephant — or in my case, a very full plate — one bite at a time.

Lorre: [laughs enthusiastically] I love that quote! Spot on. I also remember when you were hired into your new position. What did that feel like for you?

Jordan: [moves eyes to skim the bottom of the worksheet] Well, I was hopeful and optimistic, so that looks like I was in the Hope Phase. I met my goal of leaving the unit, and the route to that goal — my new position — was clear. OMG, this is so cool to see myself in this way!

Lorre: Very cool, indeed! As you transitioned into your new role, how did you experience the 3Rs?

Jordan: I felt so clear, so rejuvenated. [glances to the bottom of the worksheet] I felt really aligned and connected inside. I stayed connected with my former team in our Haelan Group and other fun get-togethers. I connected with my new colleagues and made new friends there, too. I was definitely more regulated and felt like I was in my Window of Tolerance more than I was before. I had a sense of being restored, becoming more whole, I guess. Now I'm just rambling. Does this make sense?

Lorre: You're not rambling at all. It makes perfect sense. I don't know if you remember, but you sent me an email shortly after you started that position. [Jordan looks puzzled.] I printed it out before you came. Would you like to read it?

Jordan: Absolutely! [I hand the paper to Jordan, who reads aloud this excerpt] "Even though it's the early days, leaving that cesspool was the Best. Decision. Ever." [becomes verklempt] I was so happy then. Why is this happening? It feels like I'm right back where I started. It's so frustrating!

Lorre: [lights Jordan's favorite candle and offers a soft throw blanket] It can feel so very frustrating. Our mind, our LH, wants everything to be structured and ordered. Like we should move from one phase to another and get to some final destination. But that's not how life works. It's a much more dynamic process, with many layers. Many ruptures. Many repairs. All in service to our growth and resilience.

Jordan: Well, my mind gets it, but my emotions are like, "I just don't want to do this again."

Lorre: That's a very natural response — resistance. It's a protective adaptation to avoid what might be perceived as uncomfortable or unsafe. This is what we mean when we talk about *leaning in*. We acknowledge the resistance and lean into it so we can heal and grow in the deeper layers. You're ready now to lean into your layers.

Jordan: I am?

Lorre: Well, let's see about that. Do you remember what you said at the beginning of this session?

Jordan: [ruminates and gestures for me to go on]

Lorre: You said, "I'm ready to work on this stuff now."

Jordan: [looks surprised initially, then realizes an epiphany] Wow, that's spot on. My innate care plan in action. I would have missed it.

Lorre: You didn't miss it or you wouldn't be here. [We both laugh.] But it was not in your field of awareness just yet.

Jordan: It always amazes me how this all works. I'm so grateful. So, that means then ... that I'm in the next layer of figuring out what to do with my career.

Lorre: Exactly. You are ready now to take the next bite, the next steps. You didn't have bandwidth a few months ago to lean into this layer, but you are now. Or so it appears from my vantage point.

Jordan: I didn't see it at first, but when you put it that way — yes, I guess I *am* ready. I can't just keep changing jobs. The system is a mess. And I can't change the system . . .

Lorre: What can you change now?

Jordan: I can lean into my layers and change how I navigate the system. I guess you could say I can lean in and find where my healthy and happy is career-wise.

Lorre: Brilliant! One small bite at a time. Now, checking back to the worksheet, in which phase do you feel you are in now, in the big picture?

Jordan: [glances at worksheet, inhales and exhales deeply] Well, I guess I'm back at the Enduring Phase.

Lorre: How about reframing this to be the *next layer of enduring*?

Jordan: Oh, I like that much better! I'm not stepping back like I would on a regular staircase. It's like I keep stepping forward, like I would on a circular staircase. The steps are the phases. Enduring, Uncertainty, Suffering, Hope, 3Rs. I just keep climbing the circular staircase as I move through it all — one step at a time.

Lorre: What a beautiful way to put it. Yes, just like a circular staircase. I love that! So, as we lean into your next layers together, it might be helpful to use a systems lens to guide the navigation.

Jordan: What's a system lens?

Lorre: It's where we consider the situation through the systems and subsystems, the recurring patterns perspective.

Jordan: I guess. [looks confused] Why would we do that?

Lorre: Well, because we are all connected to the systems and contexts of our lives. We cannot separate ourselves from them. They are part of the ecosystem.

Jordan: Oh, I get it. Like I have systems in my life — like the healthcare system that I work in and the healthcare system that I use for my family's health.

Lorre: Right, and the same goes for our family, coworkers, friends, community, and other social networks. Transportation, education, technology systems — and the list goes on.

Jordan: OK, that makes sense. I'm not living in a vacuum. I'm a member of the human race, society, a daughter, a friend, a nurse, a coworker, and so on.

Lorre: Beautifully stated. So, as you lean into this next layer, let's look at some of the patterns that you are bumping into. We'll take a "What happened to us?" systems approach to see what unhealed bits are collectively emerging in your systems. Particularly those at work, since that's what brought you to this session. Does that make sense?

Jordan: It does, and I'm really curious about how all this works.

Lorre: Well, we'll delve into it fully in our next sessions. Basically, we're going to explore your systems, starting at work, to see how different NS adaptive patterns are affecting you. From there, you'll start to see how to navigate it.

Jordan: [glancing at the worksheet] Like, I'll move into the Uncertainty Phase. I'll make some goals but won't know the route yet.

Lorre: Good work! And then . . .?

Jordan: And then that Suffering Phase. That's the one that worries me the most. [dabs eyes with facial tissue]

Lorre: Most people feel that way. It can be a little uncomfortable, but being aware of the patterns and the big picture makes this phase far more manageable than being unaware. We all get more proficient in maneuvering through the Suffering Phase as we lean in.

Jordan: Yeah. It's like where my parents live — literally on the beach. If they know the storm is coming, they can board up the windows, store the outdoor furniture, and either hunker down or head inland until the storm passes.

Lorre: You have such a way with words! Yes, it's just like that. Now that you know what the Suffering Phase is, as a process of healing and repair, you can move through it with more tools and awareness. Suffering seems to be a necessary process that helps us to move past our inherent resistance to change. Most people aren't motivated, willing, or able to make internal or external changes until the pain of the suffering exceeds the discomfort of change.

Jordan: Exactly. I totally see how my suffering had to get bad enough for me to want to leave my unit. Now, my suffering is so painful that I'm motivated to lean into my deeper layers. And through this process, I'll discover my next steps — my goals and routes. I'm not stuck at all. It just feels that way because of where I'm at right now. Then I'll move into the Hope and 3Rs again. Oh, this all makes so much more sense now. I'm actually excited to do this again. Thank you for revisiting this with me. It is so very helpful to see the big picture!

Lorre: You're doing such a great job with all of this. You're ready to lean in, to take the next bite. And you have grown in your resilience and have more inner tools at your disposal. BRAVO! So, to prepare you for our next session, I have an archetypes worksheet for you to read and reflect upon. [hands Jordan the worksheet]

Jordan: [skims worksheet] Oh, this looks good. What should I do after I read it?

Lorre: I recommend reading it thoroughly a few times. You can make notes on the worksheet itself or in your journal. For now, just be with this new information, see how the archetypes and resistance patterns are manifesting in your life, and observe what comes into your field of awareness. We'll review your insights next time and go from there. How does that sound?

Jordan: That sounds great! I'm really excited to lean into my layers now. It was a little scary for me before, but now that I see it, I'm stoked!

Lorre: I'm so happy for you! You did good work today.

***

Over the next week, Jordan checked in several times with great enthusiasm. She scheduled her next appointment earlier than usual, as she was "bursting" with insights and awareness. When she arrived for her next appointment, she brought her journal along with the archetype worksheet, which you'll explore at the end of this chapter. Jordan was in good cheer and her energy level was higher than I'd seen it before. Let's sit in on part of Jordan's session:

***

Lorre: I'm so happy to see you! I appreciate you checking in with me in between sessions. How are things going for you?

Jordan: Well, honestly, things are going better even though nothing has changed. I guess you could say that I'm doing better with how I'm seeing things more clearly inside and out.

Lorre: That's wonderful! It sounds like you may have moved into the Uncertainty Phase.

Jordan: I think so, too. And you know what? I'm not really afraid of the Suffering Phase anymore. I know I might feel a lot of sensations and emotions. But I also know that it helps me to untangle and clarify all my feelings. I have had a lot of insights since last time.

Lorre: You certainly did, and that is wonderful. It's beautiful to behold, truly. Tell me about those insights!

Jordan: [laughs playfully] I thought you'd never ask! Well, after our last session, I carefully read through the archetypal worksheet before my YICP practices. Each time I did, it was like OMG, I can so see myself in some of these archetypes. And then it was like OMG, I can see my colleagues in these archetypes, too. It was like a whole new world opened up for me.

Lorre: Look how much you've grown in this exercise. It looks like you are really stepping into an expanded awareness of yourself and your situation.

Jordan: Totally! So, if it's OK, can I just do like a Show-and-Tell to catch you up?

Lorre: Absolutely! [Jordan glances at her journal and worksheet.]

Jordan: OK, so, [chuckles] there's a lot! What I noticed first is how nuanced my NS adaptations are. It's not like a black-or-white kind of thing. There are a lot of nuances and shades of gray. It sort of gave me a sense of appreciation for all I've been through and how my NS continually adapts to keep me safe, even if I'm not aware of it in the moment.

Lorre: There are so many nuances and adaptations — and being aware of them is one big step to position yourself in *right relationship* for healing and clarity.

Jordan: I totally feel that happening now. It's like that "Who's in the Driver's Seat?" exercise. I feel like I'm in the driver's seat more and my NS is more regulated just by virtue of what we're doing. Nothing has changed on the outside, but I'm feeling more stable and connected inside.

Lorre: So beautifully stated. Healing is definitely happening, cheers to that! [We toast with our teacups.]

Jordan: So, what I noticed, in both my last workplace and this one, is that my NS adaptations are most like The Unworthy Overworker, The Distractor, and The Foresaker. Like, we're so busy at work, that I just push the override button on my basic needs — like food, water, and restroom breaks. It's like I push myself aside and treat myself like a robot. Going as fast as I can to get everything done while also trying to be compassionate toward my patients, their visitors, and my colleagues. But it's just not sustainable to do this for 12-14 hours [chuckles] because a girl needs to eat, drink, and pee!

Lorre: I totally get that, and I see The Unworthy Overworker archetype a lot. How did you translate awareness of this archetype into your daily living?

Jordan: Well, I'm still wrapping my head around it, honestly. I'm probably not all the way there yet [chuckles], but I'm trying. I went back to the Leaning into the Layers of YICP Menu and ramped up my [Mind Your] Transition Gaps. I gave myself permission — and I know this sounds silly — but I'm striving to do a MicroDoses Matter practice at as many transition gaps as possible. Like while my coffee brews, when at a stop light, in the parking garage, every time I wash my hands or start charting. Like that.

Lorre: It doesn't sound silly at all. That is exactly how we can embed and thread MicroDoses and YICP lightning round practices throughout the day. Brilliant!

Jordan: So, that is helping. I feel like I matter. Like it's OK for me to take air into my body and fuel myself with healthy food — not the crap I get in the cafeteria or drive through. I'm eating better, but not great.

Lorre: So, is it fair to say that you are taking your awareness of these archetypes and making Alignment-Balance Connections?

Jordan: [laughs with animation] Well, now that you mention it, I think that I am! I'm being kinder to myself. [She pauses then looks upward in contemplation.] From my inner healing, I am seeing gains in my outer balance. Wow. I had no idea. Again. But I am making gains. I see more personal responsibility, better physical and mental wellness, and I'm doing better with regulation and relaxation. It's not perfect, but it's a start!

Lorre: You are making gains, leaps, and bounds! I see what you're describing all the time. Most people start working on the externals, the balance components, without addressing the internals. But you're doing the inner work and seeing how it flows to your outer world. I marvel at how much you've learned and grown since our last session. What else did you notice?

Jordan: Well, I noticed that I slip into The Foresaker archetype, putting everyone else's needs ahead of my own — at home and at work. On my days off [looks downward, slumps slightly], I see The Distractor, The Projector, and sometimes The Ostrich.

Lorre: That must be a lot to take in and feel . . .

Jordan: [voice drops] It is. I mean, I know I need to see this, but it's hard. I didn't realize how much my work life was affecting my home life. I thought I was just two people — the Work Jordan and the Home Jordan. But that's not the case. [chuckles, sitting more upright and talking in her normal speaking voice] As if I could split myself into two people! It sounds ridiculous when I say it out loud, but that's how it felt. But now I see it. I am constantly distracting myself — numbing myself — scrolling through social media, online shopping, ordering take out. I see myself as The Projector sometimes, and I don't like that one little bit. Sometimes I just can't hold everything inside and I just explode. It hurts everyone's feelings when this happens. I just feel unlovable when it does. [dabs eyes with tissue] Other times, it's all just too much. Work, family, maintaining my house, car, finances, health and dental care. I just need everything to stop so I can just breathe and rest. That's when The Ostrich archetype is online — I just can't, so I just don't! Whew. [inhales deeply then exhales] That was a lot to unpack.

Lorre: You are doing such a great job with navigating it all. You have gained so much insight and clarity. Remember, we're only taking one bite at a time here. Low and slow is the way to go. [Jordan chuckles as she rolls her eyes with animation.]

Jordan: I know, I know! [laughs heartily]

Lorre: Now that you've had some time to sit with these archetypes, how are you feeling about them?

Jordan: Honestly, I feel better when I see the archetypes as adaptive patterns rather than defects in myself. I'm so hard on myself. I was always blaming myself for this, that, and the other. I would make myself feel guilty about everything. I wasn't good enough. I should have done this, could have done that. All that negative self-chatter. The archetypes help me to see how my NS has adapted — there's nothing wrong with me — I've been through a lot. I mean *a lot*. My body adapted and these patterns emerged over time. It's not a bad thing. It's actually a good thing. These adaptations, these patterns . . . [looks upward, eyes misting] . . . they kept me safe then. But they aren't working for me now. They're like old friends who have overstayed their visit.

Lorre: Fantastic insights. Would it be accurate to say that being aware of your archetypes, these patterns, has led you to be more compassionate and kinder with yourself? With others?

Jordan: You could definitely say that. Like, it's not perfect, but seeing these patterns takes some of the blame and the shame away. I can see which circuits and hybrids tend to come online under certain conditions, and then I can help myself through it by doing my MicroDoses and YICP practices. It's like I have a clearer internal road map with an inner GPS now.

Lorre: That's terrific. I see that in you, too. You are so courageous, so consistent with navigating your NS and healing practices. As you continue leaning into your layers, you'll gain more clarity and navigate your inner landscape with more compassion and certainty. As you keep using these tools, you'll spend less time in the Suffering Phase and the intensity will lessen over time. You'll begin to anticipate how you may suffer and will proactively lean into your healing and layers. You'll position yourself to be *in right relationship* for healing before the suffering intensifies into a tsunami that feels like it's wiping you out internally.

Jordan: Totally. I get it! So, if I'm understanding correctly, then I can cross the bridge from Suffering to Hope and the 3Rs more quickly with less disruption?

Lorre: Yes, exactly. Every journey is unique unto itself. But we become very proficient in navigating it all with practice. This reminds me of a handout we talked about when you

Your Innate Care Plan (YICP)™
3A + B → 3R

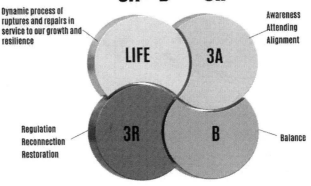

Dynamic process of ruptures and repairs in service to our growth and resilience

LIFE 3A

Awareness
Attending
Alignment

Regulation
Reconnection
Restoration

3R B

Balance

YICP Connection

first learned about YICP. Do you remember this one? [passes Jordan the clipboard]

Jordan: I sure do! This has been a game changer for me. So, is this what I use when the archetypes come online, just like the circuits and hybrids?

Lorre: Fantastic question. The archetypes are simply patterns, and patterns can be changed. We work with archetypes in the same way as our circuits and hybrids. Everything you've learned and practiced to this point can be applied to the archetypes when they emerge.

Jordan: Oh, that's good to know! [gestures mind blown while laughing] Because my brain is full!

Lorre: [laughs] Understandable! Let's see if looking at it this way helps. [passes a handout to Jordan] Sometimes it's helpful to think of YICP as a pyramid that supports you in all dimensions of bodymindessence.

Jordan: [looks over the image] So . . . my foundation is the 3As. Nurturing my inner world.

Lorre: Yes, exactly.

Shoring Up Our Foundation

YICP = 3A + B ⟶ 3R

3R
Regulation
Reconnection
Restoration

B - Balance
Traditional Self Care
Body & Mind Wellness
Personal Responsibility - Contexts
Connections - Financial
Recharge - Purpose

3A - Inner Self Nurturance
Starts with the NS
Awareness + Attending + Alignment
MicroDoses Matter
Co-Healing with Others

Jordan: And before we move to our outer world — the Balance layer of the pyramid — we make the Alignment, or the inner-outer connections. Right?

Lorre: Perfect, and beautifully stated. Then, once we've shored up the foundation with our NS, we're ready to draw from there to manage our outer life in the Balance layer. The goal is to have the inner world wellbeing align with and flow into all aspects of our outer wellbeing.

Jordan: And, violá! Just like that. I'm at the 3Rs!

Lorre: Indeed! Though this is a dynamic process, with some steps forward and others backward, as we go through our journey. We're always moving toward and more frequently experience the 3Rs — regulation, reconnection, and restoration.

Jordan: I get it now! The pyramid example really makes sense. It's like, without taking care of my NS, my inner foundation isn't as strong as it could be . . . [voice trails off, pauses for a moment] . . . OMG, which means it is easier for outside forces to knock me off my center! [gestures another mind blown emoji] No wonder it feels like the tiniest bit of stress or disruption makes me feel like I'm getting bowled over internally!

Lorre: Jordan, you are so brave and insightful. Look at you, leaning into your layers and discovering such rich insights. Amazing! So, with this awareness in mind, how do you suppose the archetypes come into play?

Jordan: That's a really good question . . . [pauses to reflect] . . . so let me externally process this if I can.

Lorre: Absolutely! Keep going!

Jordan: Well, the archetypes are adaptive patterns that developed over time while my NS was keeping me safe. So, it's like they're those . . . what do you call them . . . the parts? No, that's not it. Help me out here. [chuckles]

Lorre: Your unhealed bits?

Jordan: Yes! My unhealed bits developed into patterns . . .

Lorre: That wired and fired together.

Jordan: Oh, hold on now! I'm starting to get it. So, when I become aware of and attend to my unhealed bits and archetypes, then healing starts happening.

Lorre: BINGO! Keep going. You're doing brilliantly!

Jordan: And as I heal through my unhealed bits and archetypes, then they are — what's the word — transformed? Transmuted?

Lorre: Either word works well here.

Jordan: They get transformed into the 3Rs. What?! [animatedly flops back into the sofa cushion] And I get even more regulated, more connected, and restored? Is that the gig?

Lorre: [chuckles] I never thought about it that way! Essentially, that's the gig. Becoming aware of the archetypes — just like your unhealed bits — and then attending to them through your MicroDoses Matter and YICP is how you position yourself in *right relationship* for healing and co-healing with others as you move into the 3Rs.

Jordan: This is so helpful. Seriously. I don't feel like a lost puppy right now. I hope I can hold on to all of this later . . . [voice trails off, looks doubtful]

Lorre: We're just applying what you've learned thus far to the archetypes, that's all.

Jordan: That makes so much sense. So, what do I do about these? [She holds up The Archetypes & Mixology Handout with her colleagues' archetypes noted.] What do I do with the archetypes I keep bumping into at work?

Lorre: That's a really good question. I'm assuming you are seeing many of the archetypes coming online in your colleagues while at work?

Jordan: It's raining archetypes at work! It's like I can't unsee them, in the best sense of the word. I see them in my patients, their families, my coworkers, my leaders. They're everywhere! [laughs]

Lorre: And how did you experience these archetypes? How did they feel?

Jordan: If I'm to be honest, it was a little overwhelming at first. But then, it was oddly comforting. Knowing that their archetypes were online made me feel like it wasn't personal. My mind knows that everybody is doing the best they can, but there's just so much going wrong that it gets overwhelming sometimes. Make that a lot of the time.

Lorre: What happens when you feel overwhelmed?

Jordan: Well, at work, it's like we have amazing people — nurses — in poorly designed systems. We're all doing our very best. I know it. I feel it. I see it. But, as the system malfunctions and we get stretched even thinner, it's like we're stuck in the Suffering Phase. We devolve. We all start playing the blame game. Everybody is blaming something or someone. It's counterproductive. And exhausting. It drags the morale down.

Lorre: So, what can you do when this happens? I'm not trying to put you on the spot — we're just exploring here.

Jordan: [laughs] I know. Thank goodness I'm not in nursing school anymore or that question would freak me out! So, what I'm *tempted to do* is try and fix everything and everyone. I just want to make it stop. Go away. I just want everything to get better . . . [inhales sharply as shoulders shrug] And, sorry to say this, but I just don't see how working with the archetypes is going to help. [A lone tear trickles down her cheek.]

Lorre: Thank you for sharing your truth. That took a lot of courage and self-compassion. [reaches over to squeeze Jordan's hand, who returns the gesture] Just to confirm, I'm hearing that your desire — your goal, even — is to try to fix everything, everyone; to make it go away or just stop.

Jordan: Yes. [eyes cast downward] I don't know how much longer I can go on like this . . .

Lorre: That's fair and true. These are very challenging times for all nurses, and what you're feeling is perfectly natural. You are so brave, strong, and perceptive. I'm wondering if your desire or goal to make everything better — is it realistic, attainable?

Jordan: What do you mean?! [laughs loudly in epiphany] That I can't fix *everything and everyone*?!

Lorre: Exactly. [chuckles] Instead of looking outward to see what needs to be fixed from a system or personnel perspective, let's work from your point of empowerment in the present moment. What can *Jordan* do to help *Jordan* feel safer and more supported while working?

Jordan: Oh, that's a good one! Give me a minute. [eyes grow soft in contemplation] Well, I can't fix the healthcare system. So that's out. And I can't fix anyone because no one is broken. [looks directly into my eyes with a knowing nod] They, too, have been through a lot. Their NSs adapted just like mine did. That's where the archetypes come in. No one is broken. There's no fixing I can really do on the outside ... so it must start on the inside. Just like it does in my MicroDoses and YICP practices.

Lorre: Very astute insights. So, if the point of empowerment is on the inside before the outside, what then would that desire or goal look like?

Jordan: Well, I guess it would look like how to find my healthy — dare I say, happy — within a poorly-designed and under-resourced system. [pauses, eyes look upward as tears emerge] I would find my healthy and work from there . . . when interacting with my coworkers and their archetypes when they come online . . . ? [chuckles] I guess I'm more asking than telling here!

Lorre: That sounds like a far more attainable goal. So, we could say, "finding *your* healthy — *your* happy — within the system and drawing from that space while interacting with colleagues." How does that feel?

Jordan: [laughs while shaking her head] It sounds a whole lot more manageable! I was literally trying to solve world hunger by myself for a minute there! I get it. I have to work from my inner space of empowerment first. Then create my healthy space within the system and find my edges and boundaries as I go through the day. Like, for example, not guilt tripping myself for needing to [feigns being shocked] step away to hydrate, nourish, breathe, support my NS, or relieve myself!

Lorre: That's a great place to start while keeping Maslow's Hierarchy of Needs on the radar. As you know, at the base of that pyramid are . . . [passes handout to Jordan, who glances at it before responding]

Jordan: Yep. I remember this! Physiological needs first. Then safety.

Shoring Up Our Foundation

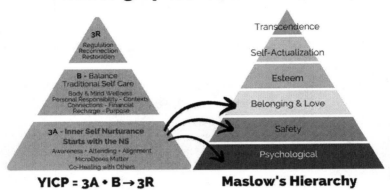

YICP = 3A • B → 3R   **Maslow's Hierarchy**

Shoring Up Our Foundation & Maslow's Hierarchy

Lorre: Right, and this connects to the YICP pyramid. There, at the base of the pyramid, are the 3As — awareness, attending, and alignment. Caring for our NS is an essential part of Maslow's physiological needs, right along with nutrition, hydration, and relieving yourself. It also is an essential part of Maslow's safety level.

Jordan: There you go again. [She does yet another very animated mind blown gesture.] OK, got it. And our Threat Detectors, they're always surveilling for our safety. Neuroception. It's all coming back to me. [chuckles] So, then how do the archetypes in others help me with my new goal of finding *my healthy* at work?

Lorre: It is so insightful of you to ask! This is a very common question. There are two basic practices to employ when you encounter an archetype: You can be a beacon and/or a mirror. [passes Jordan the next handout]

Jordan: This is so helpful. Taking the Beacons & Mirrors approach will help me stay in my Window. I'm excited to share these practices with my Haelan Group.

Lorre: Yes, please do!

Beacons & Mirrors
What to Do When An Archetype Comes Online

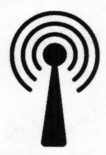

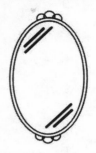

YICP Beacon of Coregulation Practice   Mirror of Reflection, Learning & Growth

Jordan: So, [pauses for a moment] as I think this through, I'm thinking of a particularly challenging colleague whose Projector or Volcano archetype comes online. A lot. And when I say a lot, I mean constantly. I go out of my way to avoid her, but there are some times that I just can't. Even if I use the Beacons & Mirrors, I think she'd be exhausting. She literally sucks all the air from the room — no offense — but that's what happens. What then?

Lorre: This is just another layer to lean into. But we can't lean into someone else's layer — we can only lean into our own. In these instances, where there's a pervasive online archetype, continue with the Beacons & Mirrors practice to support your Window, your regulation. When time allows, which may be during or after work, you can lean into *your* resistance patterns.

Jordan: [laughs] Great. More layers! Do they ever end?!

Lorre: In our dynamic world of ruptures and repairs, there are plenty of layers. But navigating the layers — just like navigating your NS — gets easier over time. As you put more tools in your toolkit and spend increasingly more time in

Beacons & Mirrors

Strategy	What to Do When You Encounter an Archetype
YICP Beacon of Co-regulation Practice	During the encounter, be a Beacon of Co-regulation by attending to *your* NS in the present moment so other NSs co-regulate in kind. Depending upon the circumstances, you can do a MicroDoses Matter or YICP Lightning Round at the moment. **MicroDose Beacon Practice** (solo or with others depending upon context) • Private space, if possible, if not then connect with your private inner space • Ground and center with a 4x4 breathing round • Signal safety to your NS: connect with your five senses, feel your pocket pal or nature artifact • Either physically or in your mind's eye, place your hand(s) over your healer's heart **YICP 16-Second Lightning Round** (solo or with others depending upon context) Here's an example that can be done during one round of 4x4 breathing: • Long inhale to the count of four: Bonnie's Body Scan (Ground & Center) • Hold inhale to count of four and visualize Bird on Shoulder or Movie Theater (YICP Awareness)

	• Long exhale to the count of four: Gesture inclusion to any arising sensations or unhealed bits, physical or virtual bear hug, notice and name something you can see, hear, and feel (YICP Attending) • Hold exhale to the count of four and visualize your healer's heart opening with compassion for whatever happened to the other person's NS that patterned as an archetype. • Compassionately respond to the person whose archetype is online. Respond to the situation from your Window of Tolerance instead of reacting from your adaptations, archetypes, or resistance patterns. Allow innate and unspoken co-regulation to occur without driving the process. This is a process of allowing. Human-being, not human-doing.
Mirrors of Reflection, Learning, and Growth	After the encounter, use the archetype you encountered as a mirror to gain deeper awareness, insight, and compassion toward yourself and those for whom archetypes are online. Reflection or conversation prompts to consider as you lean into the deeper layers: When does this archetype come online for me? What does it feel like? What unhealed bits of wisdom are emerging to be healed? Which MicroDose or YICP practices are most helpful when one of your or another's archetype is online?

your regulated Window, you develop a buffer — resilience — when archetypes come online.

Jordan: OK, bring on the resistance patterns! What do *those* look like?

Lorre: [passes the next handout to Jordan] There are three collective resistance patterns that correlate with our NS adaptations. The resistance patterns follow how our NSs adapt over time to move away from or toward the stress, or when the dorsal ventral circuit comes online and we feel a little freezy.

Jordan: [after skimming the handout] This is all so connected — how my NS adapted to what happened to me. How other people's NSs did the same. How, by virtue of these experiences, our NSs were wired and fired together over time. Now, those neuroplastic superhighways are showing up as archetypes and resistance patterns. We're all so interconnected, aren't we?

Lorre: Indeed, we are! And just as the principles of neuroplasticity brought us our adaptations, archetypes, and resistance patterns . . . that same neuroplasticity can facilitate our healing, from which thriving follows. Individually and collectively. But it starts within, first, to embrace our personal responsibility for healing, growing, and engaging with YICP.

Collective Archetypal Resistance Patterns

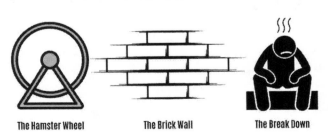

The Hamster Wheel　　　　The Brick Wall　　　　The Break Down

Collective Archetypal Resistance Patterns.

Collective Archetypal Resistance Patterns

Resistance Pattern in Response to Archetype in Others Coming Online	How Our NSs Adapted to the Archetypes Over Time	Collective Protective Mechanism
Hamster Wheel	The Hamster Wheel protects by trying to outrun the archetypal pattern. It is built from concern, worry, fear, anxiety, etc. Its mantra is from the classic movie *Forrest Gump*: "Run, Forrest, run!"	Protective resistance to move away from archetypal patterns.
Brick Wall	The Brick Wall protects by being a barrier between you and the archetype. Your NS is signaling for you to (figuratively) fight the archetype and is fueled by frustration, annoyance, irritation, anger, and rage. Every time you run toward the archetype the protective brick wall of resistance appears. Your Threat Detector is signaling that fighting this archetype is futile. You are being guided to lean into *your* layers instead of fighting a losing archetypal battle with another. Its mantra is from the movie *Mean Girls*: "Stop trying to make fetch happen."	Protective resistance to move toward the archetypal pattern.

| Break Down | The Break Down is a last resort protective mechanism when Hamster Wheel and Brick Wall patterns can no longer sustain the resistance. You're exhausted from running on the hamster wheel or hurling yourself against the brick wall. Your energy stores are depleted and you may feel like you're emotionally breaking down. Its mantra is "Nope. Not today." | Protective resistance that starts to shut you down in response to feeling overwhelmed, shamed, or trapped by the archetypal pattern. |

Jordan: Just like YICP formula. We start with inner self-care and our 3As. We address our misalignments. Where our once adaptive responses are maladaptive now. [laughs loudly] Like it used to be adaptive when I threw a temper tantrum as a toddler, but I can't exactly do that now at work.

Lorre: [laughing with Jordan] My grandchildren are about that age — and yes — a toddler meltdown is definitely a maladaptive NS adaptation in the workplace! But recognizing our adaptations, archetypes, and resistance patterns and caring for them as the foundation upon which all other healing and thriving activities are built . . . now that's positioning ourselves in *right relationship* for healing, transcendence, and the 3Rs.

Jordan: This gives me a lot of hope. I can see how to navigate my archetypes and I know what to do when others come online. Leaning in and doing my healing work, with others, so I can be the person my colleagues, family, and friends need before, during, and after their hardships.

Lorre: You've done such great work here today. I'm so impressed with your growth and where you're going in your big picture journey. [gives Jordan a big hug which she returns as we bring the session to a close]

***

Jordan, like you, is learning so much about how to address collective patterns of NS adaptations (The Archetypes) and resistance patterns when they emerge. We can't control another person's NS adaptations, but we can stay within our field of awareness and *respond rather than react* to The Archetypes of collective conditioning. As you do so, you will get clarity about what *your* "healthy and happy" looks and feels like at work. Like Jordan, you'll notice and experience that healing is happening. You'll start living from your scars instead of your wounds. Let's continue practicing compassionate responses to The Archetypes and Resistance Patterns in the Haelan Nurse Activities.

Haelan Nurse Activities
Big Picture Journey Exploration

Reflect upon where you are, either as an individual or as a group, in the big picture of a challenge, trauma, or unhealed bit that is emerging in your personal or professional life. Briefly describe or discuss in your Haelan Group the situation and symptoms you are experiencing. Then, map what you are experiencing onto the Five Big Picture Phases. You can annotate, circle, and mark up this table however desired!

My/Our Big Picture Journey Now

My situation(s):

***
***

My symptom(s) are:

***
***

Responding to The Archetypes With Radical Compassion and Co-regulation

It would be natural and easy to fall into the pattern of unknowingly judging or shaming someone when one of their archetypes is online. Doing so would further perpetuate the collective conditioning of trauma *reactions* instead of regulated

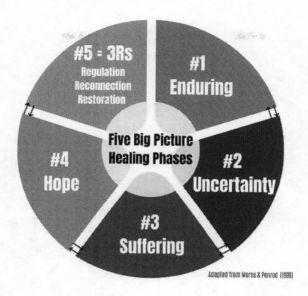

Adapted from Morse & Penrod (1999)

responses from our Window of Tolerance. To prepare us to be beacons of co-regulation and radical compassion when archetypes come online, let's proactively frame how we'll respond by completing the table below. In the last column, you'll find an example. Below that example, jot down and then discuss with your Haelan Group how you will compassionately respond to the archetype when it comes online while availing your NS for regulation, assuming you're in the Window of Tolerance.

Archetypes & Circuits

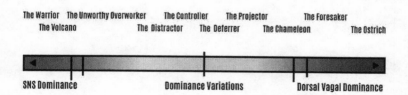

Big Picture Journey Exploration

Phase	Description	Goal Present?	Route Present?
Enduring	Getting through an extraordinary situation or trauma. Focus on making it through by suspending emotions and remaining in control. *My/Our notes about the enduring experience:*	No	No
Uncertainty	Recognizing that something needs to be done about the situation or trauma. A goal(s) is set, but the route or means by which to accomplish the goal is not yet clear. *My/Our notes about the uncertainty experience:*	Yes	No
Suffering	**Step 1.** Acknowledging the impact of the situation or trauma in the past, present, and future. Emotions previously suspended emerge, often overwhelmingly so, which temporarily obliterates the goal(s) previously set. Emotional tsunami described as complete blackness or a dark tunnel with no end. **Step 2.** As the emotional tsunami is processed, slowly and incrementally begins to piece together a goal and a route. Suffering, while difficult, is a process of healing and repair. *My/Our notes about the suffering experience:*	No	No

Hope	Acknowledging and accepting what has happened and its significance in one's past, altered present, and new future. The outcome isn't certain, so emotions are held in check while bracing for potential negative outcomes. Refines goals in response to internal and external conditions. Seeks and engages in supportive relationships that support positive outcomes. *My/Our notes about the hope experience:*	Yes	Yes
3Rs: Reconnection Regulation Restoration	Transcending the trauma or event by accepting the past and embracing an altered future. Emerging with a new perspective on life and living richer and more meaningful lives. Gaining a deeper connection within and with others, increased NS regulation, and restoration in the healer's heart and bodymindessence. *My/Our notes about the 3Rs experience:*	Yes, until the next rupture occurs in service to our growth and resilience.	Yes, until the next rupture occurs in service to our growth and resilience.

The Archetypes & Their Mixology Responses

The Archetype	NS Adaptation Over Time	How I/We Will Compassionately Respond to the Archetype
The Warrior 3 shots of SNS	The Warrior protects themselves by turning everything into a battle, an argument, or aggressive overture as they swiftly move toward the stressor in SNS activation.	*I understand that this archetype is a NS adaptation because this person experienced real hardship or trauma in their life. I hold compassionate space for their healing while professionally communicating my needs and boundaries.* Your response:
The Volcano 2 shots SNS, a dash each of ventral and dorsal vagal	The volcano protects themselves by erupting, spewing harmful or gaslighting words, responding or behaving aggressively.	*I understand that this archetype is a NS adaptation because this person experienced real hardship or trauma in their life. I hold compassionate space for their healing while proactively protecting my safety and seeking support through personal and professional channels and resources, including the employee and human resources department, supervisors, and other leaders.* Your response:

The Unworthy Overworker 2 shots SNS, a dash of ventral vagal with a dash of dorsal vagal	The Unworthy Overworker protects themselves by overachieving and accomplishing goals that are often rewarded by societal norms.	*I understand that this archetype is a NS adaptation because this person experienced real hardship or trauma in their life. I hold compassionate space for their healing while knowing that I am not bound by the Unworthy Overworker's goals. I communicate, collaborate, and advocate for reasonable, attainable goals that support all nurses to thrive within their Window of Tolerance.* Your response:
The Controller 1.5 shots SNS, a splash of ventral vagal with a dash of dorsal vagal	The Controller feels inwardly out of control and protects themselves by outwardly controlling people and situations.	*I understand that this archetype is a NS adaptation because this person experienced real hardship or trauma in their life. I hold compassionate space for their healing, while articulating my need for autonomy and productive collaboration while practicing to the full scope of my license. I seek the support of coworkers, leaders, and professional resources to establish healthy working parameters.* Your response:

| The Distractor
1 shot SNS with
a splash each
of ventral and
dorsal vagal | The Distractor protects themselves through distractions and procrastination. From daydreaming to endless social media scrolling, to starting but not completing new projects. | *I understand that this archetype is a NS adaptation because this person experienced real hardship or trauma in their life. I hold compassionate space for their healing while proactively engaging with the task, goal, or deadline. Should The Distractor archetype become a barrier to meeting the objective, I will proactively communicate with team members and leaders to harmonize our collective efforts.*
Your response: |
| The Deferrer
1 shot SNS with
a splash of dorsal
vagal with a dash
of ventral vagal | The Deferrer protects themselves by insisting that inner and outer conditions must be perfect at all times. This manifests as chronic just-as-soon-as-it-is. | *I understand that this archetype is a NS adaptation because this person experienced real hardship or trauma in their life. I hold compassionate space for their healing while holding my own alignment in response to the ruptures and repairs that are inherent with living.*
Your response: |

The Projector 1 shot SNS, 0.5 shot ventral vagal with a dash of dorsal vagal	The Projector protects themselves by projecting their stress, dysregulation, or unhealed bits onto others. Unlike The Volcano, The Projector uses more socially accepted passive or passive aggressive approaches.	*I understand that this archetype is a NS adaptation because this person experienced real hardship or trauma in their life. I hold compassionate space for their healing while safeguarding my energy, physical, mental, and emotional fields. I choose not to receive that which is not mine to carry, and send The Projector energy to the earth where it can be absorbed and transmuted into light and love.* Your response:
The Chameleon 0.5 shots each of SNS, ventral and dorsal vagal	The Chameleon protects themselves by recognizing that fight, flight, and freeze are not viable survival options, so instead, they please and appease to stay safe.	*I understand that this archetype is a NS adaptation because this person experienced real hardship or trauma in their life. I hold compassionate space for their healing while staying aligned in my truth, knowing that I do not need to shapeshift every time that The Chameleon does. I choose to stay regulated and thrive within my Window of Tolerance.* Your response:

The Foresaker 0.5 shots each of SNS and dorsal vagal with a dash of ventral vagal	The Foresaker protects themselves through self-sacrifice or self-punishment, often unknowingly so, to retain their membership in a life-sustaining group or social context. This archetype is frequently associated with systemic oppressions such as structural racism, or marginalization of women, persons of color, indigenous persons, members of the LGBTQIA+ community, among others.	*I understand that this archetype is a NS adaptation because this person experienced real hardship or trauma in their life. I hold compassionate space for their healing while supporting myself and others in living their highest and best life, as each defines it for themselves. I choose my words and actions with loving care, knowing that they matter so much to those who receive them. When it resonates to do so, I advocate for and support The Foresaker in their efforts to be liberated from the legacies of suffering and oppression.* Your response:
The Ostrich 1 shot of dorsal vagal with a splash of ventral vagal and a dash of SNS	The Ostrich protects themselves by putting their head in the sand to avoid or ignore discomfort, conflict, or confrontation. The Ostrich is a master of denial.	*I understand that this archetype is a NS adaptation because this person experienced real hardship or trauma in their life. I hold compassionate space for their healing while staying rooted in my truth and alignment. I choose to live and work within the issness of each present moment, knowing that change, growth, and healing are always possible.* Your response:

Beacons & Mirrors
What to Do When An Archetype Comes Online

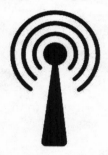 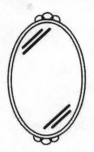

YICP Beacon of Coregulation Practice   Mirror of Reflection, Learning & Growth

Beacons & Mirrors: Reflection and Discussion

In the above activity, we framed how we intend to respond to an archetype when it comes online. This framing will evolve over time. You may encounter the same archetype in different people. When this happens, you can nuance your framing to meet that archetype as they are in their NS regulation.

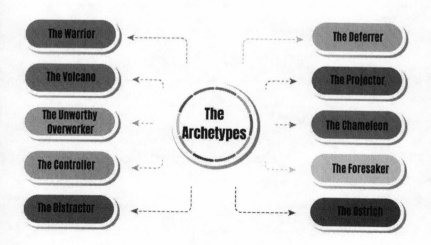

Reflect on and discuss these questions:
1. When does the _____ archetype (fill in the blank with the name of each archetype as you explore all ten of them) come online for me? What does it feel like? What unhealed bits of wisdom are emerging for healing and co-healing?
2. What might the _____ archetype feel like for the other person who is portraying it? How can I support them while staying regulated and thriving in my Window of Tolerance?

Archetypes & Resistance Responses

Archetype & Resistance Patterns	MicroDose and YICP Responses to Archetype & Resistance Patterns
The Warrior	
The Volcano	
The Unworthy Overworker	
The Controller	
The Distractor	
The Deferrer	
The Projector	
The Chameleon	
The Foresaker	
The Ostrich	
The Hamster Wheel	
The Brick Wall	
The Break Down	

Practices to Use When Archetypes & Resistance Patterns Come Online

Now it's time to explore the MicroDose and YICP Beacon of Co-regulation Practice that was described earlier. Do a few rounds solo and then with others. What resonated with you? What didn't? How can you tailor that practice to best meet your needs?

Now explore the full menu of MicroDoses Matter and YICP practices you've learned thus far. Which practices will best support you in responding to the archetypes and resistance patterns when they come online? What new practices can you envision and explore? Note your insights and inspirations in the table.

Deeper Dive Resources

Joye, M. (2021). *Codependent discovery and recovery 2.0: A holistic approach to healing and freeing yourself.* Simon and Schuster.

Williamson, M. (1992). *A return to love: Reflections on the principles of "A Course in Miracles".* HarperCollins.

Wilson, J. P. (2006). "Trauma archetypes and trauma complexes" in J. P. Wilson (ed.), *The posttraumatic self: Restoring meaning and wholeness to personality.* Routledge.

Chapter 9

Thriving in Practice & in Life

Congratulations on reaching the last chapter of this book! Although our time together in this book is coming to an end, our journey continues in the Haelan Academy & Community, where you'll find a wealth of resources and a safe, supportive community with which to engage as we heal together. You ARE transcending nurse traumatization, and so much healing has been happening! You're finding more moments of regulation and thriving in practice. And you're probably wondering how you can transition fully to thriving in your practice . . . and in life. Sometimes, we can feel growing pains or a bit wobbly as we transcend where we were and flourish in our next steps or life chapter. Sometimes the internal, conditioned mental chatter might tell you that you're not ready and not good enough, strong enough, or fill-in-the-blank enough. When I hear outdated and untrue mental chatter, I refer back to one of my favorite quotes from Maryanne Williamson, which I refined in bold to be as inclusive as possible:

"Our deepest fear is not that we are inadequate. Our deepest fear is that we are powerful beyond measure. It is our light, not our darkness, that most frightens us. We ask ourselves, 'Who am I to be brilliant, gorgeous, talented, fabulous?'

Actually, who are you not to be? You are a part of **Life**. Your playing small does not serve the world. There is nothing enlightened about shrinking so that other people won't feel insecure around you. We are all meant to shine, as children do.

We were born to make manifest the glory of **Life** that is within us. It's not just in some of us; it's in everyone. And as we let our own **healing** light shine, we unconsciously give other people permission to do the same.

As we are liberated from our own **trauma**, our **healing** presence automatically liberates others."

Maryanne Williamson

Knowing that each one of us is rising up together as we heal and become leaders and wayshowers for other nurses, we'll explore how to really thrive in practice. In this chapter, I'll also discuss launching off approaches should you care to be an advocate, change agent, or leader in ushering out *Nursing 2.0: The Nurse Safety and Professional Wellbeing Edition*. In our *Nursing 2.0* chapter, the end goals are: (a) to do our part to end nurse traumatization; (b) to facilitate healing (directly or indirectly) for nurses experiencing traumatization; (c) to be safe and regulated at work so we can provide optimal patient care as we thrive in our Window of Tolerance, and; (d) to promote safe working conditions and professional wellbeing for all nurses and healthcare professionals.

These goals start with each of us, as individuals and nursing communities. By virtue of the fact that you are reading this chapter, you are already engaged in this process through your increasingly regulated NS. This is huge. Without your regulation and ability to co-regulate with others, we'd be spinning our tails. You've done and will continue to do the hardest part — healing the inner layers. Positive gains are being realized by everyone you encounter, though you may not be aware of them. I thank you, from the bottom of my healer's heart, for your healing engagement. Doing the inner work is paramount and difficult, and you're doing it! I feel you and I appreciate you beyond measure. I'm reminded of Eckhart Tolle's famous quote that speaks to the importance of our inner healing:

"If you get the inside right, the outside will fall into place. Primary reality is within; secondary reality without."

Eckhart Tolle

By the end of this chapter, you'll have even more resources should you care to advocate for and lead the *Nursing 2.0* changes that are needed in your practice, unit(s), organization(s), and healthcare delivery system(s). Let's start by describing what thriving in practice means and how we can leverage neuroplasticity principles as we individually and collectively envision the future of nursing.

Thriving in Practice: Visualization and Neuroplasticity

As any nurse can attest, being resilient in and of itself does not lead to thriving in practice. Resilience is a combination of traits (personality, psychological, physical, etc.) that support nurses in maintaining equilibrium after hardship. Well, we've endured the hardship. Equilibrium, NS regulation, and a wide Window of Tolerance are difficult to attain and maintain in largely unsafe nurse practice environments that repeatedly inflict *avoidable* trauma through healthcare system inadequacies. Resilience is a personal journey, one of self-development. It underpins but does not, in itself, translate to thriving in practice.

Thriving describes how we are vital and are learning in our personal and professional roles. Thriving is based upon positive experiences. Let's read that again, just to make sure our brains are retaining that information: **Thriving is based upon positive experiences**. Many nurses have, and are having, positive experiences, perhaps less so in recent years, but they are there. These positive experiences are often obliterated in the wake of *avoidable* traumatization that happens over and over and over again. Thriving can result from overcoming adversity, but please know that hardship, suffering, or adversity are NOT prerequisites for thriving. When nurses are thriving, it is because they and the wider teams feel that they have agency, are empowered, and are able to maintain NS regulation within their Window of Tolerance, from which the ability to deliver safe, high-quality nursing care is optimally delivered in a sustainable manner over time.

Terminology Refresher: Thrive

Thriving describes how we are vital and always open to learning in our personal and professional roles. It is based upon positive experiences, even those that emerge after overcoming adversity or hardship. Thriving is connected to improved health and wellbeing across all dimensions of bodymindessence.

Despite the ever-changing healthcare systems and contexts, nurses who feel safe, seen, heard, supported, and valued — with the autonomy to fully practice within the full scope of their license — tend to thrive professionally. When nurses have this autonomy, along with trust and a sense of agency or control over their work, it positively impacts wellbeing, as well as a sense of empowerment, commitment, and overall vitality. It should be a no-brainer to support nurses so they can thrive in their practices, but that's usually not the case. Leaders who support thriving in practice usually embrace a relationship-driven approach and create an environment where nurses experience professional safety, NS regulation, positive experiences, and positive emotions and behaviors. Thriving, therefore, is connected to better health and wellbeing of the nurse workforce, improved patient outcomes, quality of care, engagement, improved stress and mental health, and decreased attrition, burnout, and presenteeism. The time to start thriving in practice is now. Thriving is one of the end goals for *Nursing 2.0: The Nurse Safety and Professional Wellbeing Edition.* You know where you're heading — to thrive in your practice. Let's, as my Mom always says, "Start as we intend to go" by first envisioning what thriving looks and feels like for you.

Using the Principles of Neuroplasticity
to Visualize Thriving

You've experienced the importance of feeling safe, grounding and centering, becoming aware of your NS, and then attending to its needs through various attending and alignment exercises — many of which include visualization techniques. Through practicing YICP, Leaning Into the Layers, and Transcending Our Shame Layers, you've created new neural pathways that have resulted in tangible gains in your outer world experiences (balance step of YICP). You are beginning to thrive in many areas of life.

It's time to level up the degree to which you are thriving by ramping up the existing thriving neural pathways into Thrive Superhighways. The process starts in YICP during your Attending and Alignment steps. During YICP and assuming you're within your Window of Tolerance, visualize what it looks and feels like to thrive in your nursing practice (or in other areas of your life, as desired). Use your senses to experience it in your mind's eye. What does it look like, feel like, and smell like? How does your energy feel? How does the energy in your workplace feel? Who are the people around you? What music is playing, if any? What does your workstation look like? The break room? Bring as much detail and sensory information into your Thriving in Practice visualization as possible.

Where are your hydration, nutrition, and MicroDose moments woven into the day? They matter immensely, even when you're regulated and in your Window of Tolerance. It's like keeping your cell phone battery charged by continually topping it off with MicroDoses and lightning YICP rounds throughout the day. As you do so, your Threat Detector is being bathed in signals of safety. Your emotional state, energy levels, and vibrations are elevating. Stress hormones and catecholamine levels are decreasing while endorphins, oxytocin, serotonin, and dopamine levels increase. Your body is responding to the

Threat Detector's sense of safety as you blaze the Thriving in Practice Superhighway by strengthening these neural networks and adding to them each time you engage in YICP practice.

When Visualization Doesn't Work

I can almost hear some of you saying, "I've already tried visualization and it doesn't work!" I hear this frequently from my students and clients — they've tried visualizing, they've tried meditation practices, and they're convinced that they don't work. The reason that they don't work is usually because they weren't in a regulated state or in their Window of Tolerance at the time. If their Threat Detector was signaling for the SNS circuit to ramp up or the dorsal vagal circuit to come online, then it's very difficult, if not impossible, to engage with visualization techniques. Most people haven't learned the language of their NS or how to navigate it as you have done. So, they tried visualizing a new job, a new car, a new partner, or a winning lottery ticket without results. Why? Because they probably (a) were dysregulated and outside of their Window, (b) unaware of their inner state, (c) lacking tools to address their dysregulation and inner state, and/or (d) misaligned in their inner and outer experiences. Chances are their limbic systems were in the driver's seat and their circuits and hybrid states were such that the old survival pathways were engaged. Visualization alone cannot get the job done. The NS must be regulated in order for them to create the new thrive neural pathways that they seek.

When Visualization Works

Visualization works when your NS is regulated — when you feel safe, present, calm, and connected. In other words, when your ventral vagal circuit is online, the more ventral vagal tone, the easier it is to visualize. When we are within our Windows of Tolerance, it is easier to get an inner picture and a better sense or feel of our desired outcome. As we do so, those new thrive neural pathways are created and reinforced with every visualization exercise. Like a muscle, the more we engage with it, the more it grows. These strong neural pathways, in our case, the Thrive Superhighway, support us in actually shifting our experience. Surviving in Practice becomes a distant rearview mirror image as Thriving in Practice becomes the new normal. Neuroplasticity. It's a beautiful process. Your thriving visualization is best practiced in the Alignment phase of YICP. Here's what you can do:

1. **Use your breath as a bridge between your inner and outer worlds.** Visualize what it looks and feels like to thrive in practice and in life. Use your five senses as a launching off strategy. Really sense, feel, and get into the thrive vibe as you lay down those new neurons and your Thrive Superhighway.

2. **Include Thrive Visualization in the Welcome Home Inner Sanctuary Practice.** Welcome yourself to your new thriving practice and life through this practice. Feel all the feels, visualize in as much detail as you can.

3. **Incorporate Thrive Visualization in the Aladdin's Lamp or Magic Wand visualization.** There are no limits or boundaries to how you can thrive in practice and in life. Ask "What else is possible?" Visualize beyond your wildest dreams as you lay down that neural Thrive Superhighway to bring it to your outer world.

4. **Add Thrive Visualization to your Inner Straw visualization.** Wherever you encounter a kink or bend in your inner straw, or when you encounter sluggish flow, this is where new neurons and your Thrive Superhighway are needed. Keep visualizing until your inner straw is aligned and flowing with your thriving energy.

End each alignment practice by saying aloud (if possible, if not, say it internally) this affirmation for your thriving future: **All of**

Life comes to me with ease, grace, glory, light, love, intimacy, laughter, health, wellness, abundance, and prosperity. Edit this affirmation to align with whatever words resonate with living your highest and best life, as you define it. End it with whatever closing remark feels right for you, such as And So It Is, Amen, It Is So, Namaste, etc. Repeat this affirmation frequently throughout every day. Weave it into your MicroDoses and YICP routines. Every time you do so, you're recruiting more neurons to construct your Thrive Superhighway. Enjoy reaping the bounty of these Thrive Visualization seeds as they come to fruition.

Slow the Pace Speed Bump: Thrive Visualization

This is our last speedbump together, so let's make it the most glorious one yet! You're going to start building your Thrive Superhighway. Take a few moments to reflect on where you've been and where you are now as relates to our time together in this book. If you can feel or imagine my healer's heart giving yours a virtual hug, then you're right where you should be at this moment. Let's do one last YICP round together, adding a rich Thrive Visualization to the Alignment step. Here we go, together!

- Settle into a safe, comfortable, and private space.
- Do your favorite grounding and centering exercise.
- Enjoy your favorite awareness practice.
- Engage in your favorite attending exercise for where your NS is right now.
- Scan for any layers or shame layers that may need your support. Make a self-care date to attend to those layers soon.
- Choose an alignment practice that feels best for your first Thrive Visualization. See yourself thriving in all that you experience. Bathe yourself and your budding Thrive

Superhighway in all the sights, sounds, tactile sensations, tastes, and energies in this scene. Notice the weather, the setting, and any nature or animals that may be with you. Notice any people and ancestors in this earthly dimension or beyond. Notice all the non-earthly beings that may be with you. Notice yourself as so very, very loved and valued in wholeness and oneness with the grand systems and contexts. Feel yourself in glorious regulation. Feel how internally connected and aligned you are. Feel your Healer's Heart — the passion, the hope, and the yearning to serve and make a difference however you feel called to do so. Allow the veil of duality to lower and experience the miracle that YOU are in bodymindessence across all dimensions of time and space.

- Speak your affirmation (substitute yours in for the ones below, as desired), your truth, with earnest three times:
  All of Life comes to me with ease, grace, glory, light, love, intimacy, laughter, health, wellness, abundance, and prosperity.

  All of Life comes to me with ease, grace, glory, light, love, intimacy, laughter, health, wellness, abundance, and prosperity.

  All of Life comes to me with ease, grace, glory, light, love, intimacy, laughter, health, wellness, abundance, and prosperity.
- End it with whatever closing remark feels right for you.

Take a few moments to bask in the truth, light, love, and unlimited potential that you are, always have been, and always will be. Healing has happened. It has REALLY happened.
Healing has happened.
Healing is happening.
Healing will continue to happen, always.

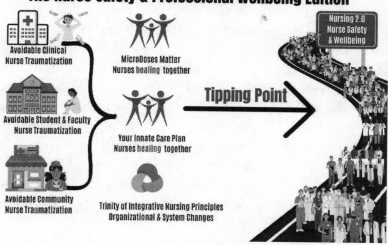

Road to Nursing 2.0 plus INPs

As your new thrive neurons grow and prosper into your Thrive Superhighway, continue blazing that trail into your workplace. In this next section, I'll present a roadmap of the Trinity of Integrative Nursing Practices that you can use to advocate for and lead unit, organizational, and system change. Now that we know how to navigate our NSs, use our MicroDoses and YICP practices, transcend shame, and address The Archetypes and their resistance patterns, we are well-prepared to facilitate and support other nurses similarly to affect the *tipping point* of massive change as we usher in *Nursing 2.0* together.

The Trinity of Integrative Nursing Principles to Guide Nursing 2.0

Each of us has a unique nursing perspective that is informed by our education, practice, and lived experiences in a myriad of social and cultural contexts. To get us all on the same page when it comes to ushering forth *Nursing 2.0: The Nurse Safety and Professional Wellbeing Edition*, let's start by taking a holistic, integrative approach. In recent years, nurse scholars, Mary Jo Kreitzer and Mary Koithan, introduced integrative nursing as a roadmap to guide holistic, person-centered nursing care. Integrative nursing is defined as a way of being, doing, and knowing, that advances a whole health perspective to optimize wellbeing. Integrative nurses use evidence-informed strategies to support the whole person (including self), systems, and planetary healing. Integrative nursing prioritizes nurse health and wellness through self-reflection, self-responsibility, and self-care — all of which you are doing in YICP practices. All said, and consistent with Jean Watson's *Theory of Human Caring*, the integrative nurse is an instrument of healing and a healing process facilitator — for their patients and for themselves as individuals, teams, and members of a global profession. At the end of the day, integrative nursing *is* nursing, which we can frame using three sets of principles.

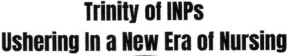

Trinity of INPs
Ushering In a New Era of Nursing

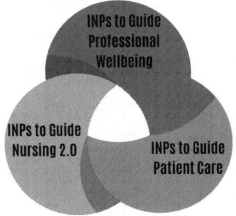

INPs to Guide
Professional
Wellbeing

INPs to Guide
Nursing 2.0

INPs to Guide
Patient Care

The three sets of principles are The Trinity of Integrative Nursing Principles (INPs): Part 1 of the Trinity are those that guide patient care; Part 2 are those that guide nurse professional wellbeing; and Part 3 are those that guide organizational and system changes. Application of The Trinity of INPs is how we can usher in *Nursing 2.0*, through which our collective healer's hearts are coveted as essential to nursing care. The Trinity of INPs represent a dynamic and iterative process that can be used by nurses worldwide to lead change and innovation efforts. It is my hope that *Nursing 2.0* becomes the future of nursing, and each of us will have done our parts, starting with the point of empowerment within, and moving the healing gains made into every dimension of our personal and professional lives.

The Trinity Part 1: INPs to Guide Nursing Practice

Before I introduce Kreitzer & Koithan's seminal INPs to guide nursing practice, it bears mentioning that integrative nursing's meta-theoretical perspective aligns with the complexity of our healthcare systems. Integrative nursing draws from systems science as a framework for the complex adaptive systems that are ever-changing as new information is added to or removed from them. For example, in one moment you might be administering Medication A to a patient. Then the lab

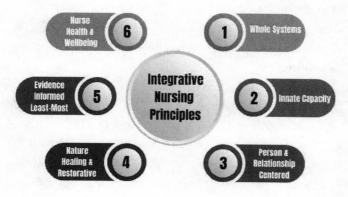

results come in, followed by new orders for Medication B to be administered. Why? Because new information was added to the system. The system, and your nursing care, is adapting in response to that system. With this system perspective in mind, let's explore how the six seminal INPs that guide patient care may already be incorporated into your practice.

INP #1: Human beings are whole systems inseparable from their environments.

All of us, including our patients, are whole people — whole bodymindessence systems. We are inextricably connected to, and influenced by, the contexts and environments within which we live and work. As nurses, we can't fully care for our patients or one another if we reduce them to a disease or chronic condition. Those in our care are whole people with a life story, hardships, and traumas of their own. We understand that the patient cannot separate themselves from the traumas they've experienced or the unhealed bits that may be emerging in response to illness, injury, chronic conditions, or hospitalization. The healthcare system, in itself, can be overwhelming to our patients. It can even be recognized by the patient's Threat Detector as a threat to safety or outright danger. Knowing this, we can be ever so compassionate when our patients or their loved ones aren't in their Window of Tolerance while in our care. Their NS may become dysregulated, and unhealed bits of wisdom may emerge. We compassionately care for them, in the entirety of their being, including but not limited to their diagnoses and symptoms.

INP #2: Human beings have the innate capacity for health and wellbeing.

In response to an ever-changing, whole-person-whole-system world, humans are continually striving for *haelan*, or healing, and moving toward wholeness in bodymindessence. You can see evidence of INP #2 everywhere. From your first skinned knee that healed as a child, to recovering from the first heartbreak as a teenager, to grieving the death of a loved one.

Or, as you're experiencing in this book, YOUR innate care plan (YICP), which accesses and leverages YOUR innate capacity for health and wellbeing. You're moving from burned out and traumatized to more regulated and beginning to thrive in a wide Window of Tolerance. Life is a process of deconstruction and reconstruction; pain and suffering give way to healing and restoration.

As a nurse, you've probably been using this principle without being aware of doing so. We are intentional about facilitating healing and wholeness for our patients. We care for and nurture them, leveraging their strength, capacity, and resources to optimize the healing process. We do this for individual patients, families, groups, communities, and the public. In short, in all that we do, we support and facilitate every person's innate capacity for health and wellbeing — along with our own.

INP #3: Integrative nursing is person-centered and relationship-based.

Most nurses practice patient-centered care for their patients and relationship-based care with the patients' care partners and loved ones. We partner with our patients, their loved ones, and various communities as we deeply listen and position them in *right relationship* for healing and co-healing. As a profession, we really shine in meeting the holistic needs of every patient and meet them wherever they are in their bodymindessence and life story.

INP #4: Nature has healing and restorative properties that contribute to health and wellbeing.

I could wallpaper your home and mine with the evidence in support of using the healing and restorative properties of nature and its utility in supporting the NS, mental health, overall wellbeing, addiction, anxiety, depression, stress, symptom management, spiritual distress, workplace wellness, among others. Forest bathing, nature bathing, and versions of the ancient Japanese practice of shinrin-yoku are popular and can be practiced anywhere, including virtually. Through practicing YICP, you've connected with nature and experienced what you probably already knew — nature makes everything feel a little better!

The healing and restorative properties of nature need to be integrated into patient and family spaces, healthcare facilities, nurses' stations, break rooms, etc., to the full extent that is feasible for the particular setting. Natural light, biophilia, intentional use of color, photographs, artwork, artifacts of nature, music, and soothing sounds are just a few ideas to consider. As often as possible, integrate and connect with nature in all aspects of your life. Enjoy the gardens, greenbelts, potted plants, labyrinths, parks, hiking trails, and nature walks that are near you, and incorporate nature into your MicroDoses of self-care throughout every day.

INP #5: Integrative nursing practice is informed by evidence and uses the full range of therapeutic modalities to support/ augment the healing process, moving from least intensive/ invasive to more, depending upon need and context.

Whew! This INP is a mouthful, as it should be. As facilitators of *haelan,* or healing, our goal is to position our patients in *right relationship* for healing in the entirety of their being, using a whole person/whole system at the individual, family, and community levels. Through our nursing care and interventions, we introduce change into the system as we meet our patients where they are in their healing process. We use the full spectrum of therapies, healing modalities, and interventions at our disposal. We draw from traditional healing practices that include ancient wisdom and practices, energy healing, healing foods, eastern and indigenous healing traditions, therapeutic communication and touch, aromatherapies, chakra and reiki healing, mindfulness practices, meditation — and that's just the short list. We also draw upon western and biomedical interventions, such as pharmacologics, and surgical and medical interventions.

Importantly, and differentiating us from other healthcare disciplines, we draw from multiple sources of valid evidence. You may have learned about these types of evidence in nursing school as patterns of knowing: empirical, ethical, aesthetic, socio-political, personal, organizational, technological, and spiritual. As nurses, we hold open and curious space for that which is not yet known to us — unknowing. Through the nursing process, we consider our patient as a whole person who is inseparable from their contexts and environments. We assess our patients and consider all relevant levels of evidence to inform and subsequently implement care plans. Our care plans reflect the patient's whole personhood while considering the full spectrum of traditional and integrative therapeutics available. We move from least intensive/invasive to more *depending upon their needs and contexts*. This is how we position them in *right relationship* for healing in bodymindessence.

You may be thinking something like, "Yeah, right. Like I'm going to give a post-operative person a visualization exercise first for their excruciating post-op pain during those initial few hours . . ." This is a very natural way to think, so let's unpack it using a surgical patient and see how we draw from the full evidence base to inform our care. Let's start in the pre-op phase. That nurse notices that the patient is restless and anxious. It's too early to give the pre-op meds, so the nurse takes a moment with the patient to facilitate therapeutic communication and a short visualization exercise, guiding the patient to a safe inner space where they can retreat amid the hustle and bustle of the operating room milieu. The nurse extends their hand, and the patient gives it a squeeze. Co-regulation is happening. Therapeutic communication and touch are helping the patient's NS to regulate. Visualization gives the patient a regulating activity so they may attend to their NS. All of these are evidence-informed, integrative nursing interventions that can be delivered in 90-120 seconds. This is appropriate to the patient's needs and their contexts. Healing happened in those moments.

Now, it's time for the patient to receive their pre-op meds and, shortly thereafter, transfer to the operating room where they undergo anesthesia. In this context, the patient's needs have shifted. Careful attention is being paid to their physiological systems, with all the appropriate anesthesia and surgical interventions being delivered with caring precision. These biomedical interventions are prioritized in this context, rightly so. Integrative interventions are also used, such as the OR tech/nurse gently whispering words of encouragement and using therapeutic touch while they reposition the patient. In the middle of an operation, invasive care is prioritized, as is contextually and clinically appropriate.

After the surgery is successfully completed, the patient is moved through the post-anesthesia phase and soon transfers to their room on the floor. The anesthesia begins to wear off and the post-operative pain lands like a ton of bricks. Here, the nurse considers the full range of evidence and therapeutic options. The nurse knows that a pharmacological agent is the contextually appropriate intervention given the patient's post-op state and pain level. Note that the nurse doesn't start with, say, aromatherapy for post-operative pain. There may come a time later in the patient's recovery process where aromatherapy will be an appropriate, less intensive/invasive intervention to consider. It all comes down to the patient's need and their context across the care continuum.

INP #6: Integrative nursing focuses on the health and wellbeing of the caregivers, as well as those they serve.

When I was first introduced to this INP, it was a mind-blowing experience in the best sense of the phrase. OF COURSE we all know that for us to give the best nursing care, we ourselves need to be regulated and optimally well ourselves. I view INP #6 as the "permission slip" for us to take care of ourselves. This permission slip is grounded in nursing philosophy, theory, and evidence. INP #6, along with the integrative nursing perspective and the plethora of evidence in support of nurse health and wellness, is our springboard into living in and leading all nurses into *Nursing 2.0: The Nurse Safety and Professional Wellbeing Edition.*

The Trinity Part 2: INPs to Guide Nurse Professional Wellbeing

Given what we now know about the importance of (a) eradicating avoidable nurse-specific traumatization from healthcare systems, (b) facilitating healing and co-healing for traumatized nurses, (c) NS regulation and a widely open Window of Tolerance, and (d) the INPs, especially INP #6 that focuses on the health and wellbeing of caregivers, we need a set of INPs that guide Nurse Professional Wellbeing as the foundation upon which all nursing care is subsequently delivered. Think of these as the prologue to the seminal INPs put forth by Kreitzer & Koithan. We now know that a regulated NS is the foundation upon which all other self-caring activities are practiced. To support that knowledge, INPs that guide Nurse Professional Wellbeing should have a regulated NS as a central theme, as shown here.

INP to Guide Nurse Professional Wellbeing #1: I am a whole person who is inseparable from the systems, contexts, and environments within which I live and work. I am also inseparable from the traumas I've experienced and the unhealed bits of wisdom that I embody. My NS and its regulation add value and quality to my life systems (including my workplace) and similarly does so for all I encounter.

INP to Guide Nurse Professional Wellbeing #2: I access and engage with my innate capacity for regulation, health, and wellbeing. I position myself in *right relationship* to access my innate capacities for health and wellbeing. I regularly do my MicroDoses Matter and YICP practices, for doing so is a foundational strategy through which I position myself, solo and with others, to be in *right relationship* in bodymindessence for professional wellness.

INP to Guide Nurse Professional Wellbeing #3: I am at the center of my professional wellness and collaborate with my colleagues through healthy, balanced relationships. I hold tender compassion for my colleagues when they exhibit stress responses, experience emerging unhealed bits of wisdom, present as one of the archetypes, or react with resistance patterns. As these trauma-related adaptations arise in the present moment, I compassionately view their experience through the lens of "What happened to you?" instead of "What is wrong with you?" I support my own NS and regulation, knowing that co-regulation is one of the many ways in which we all leverage our innate capacities for healing and professional wellbeing.

INP to Guide Nurse Professional Wellbeing #4: I use the healing and restorative properties of nature to support my regulation, health, and wellbeing. Nature provides unconditional and unlimited opportunities for grounding, centering, and NS regulation when I am alone or with others.

INPs to Guide
Nurse Professional Wellbeing

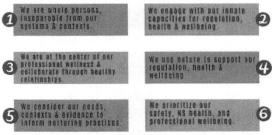

1 We are whole persons, inseparable from our systems & contexts.

2 We engage with our innate capacities for regulation, health & wellbeing.

3 We are at the center of our professional wellness & collaborate through healthy relationships.

4 We use nature to support our regulation, health & wellbeing.

5 We consider our needs, contexts & evidence to inform nurturing practices.

6 We prioritize our safety, NS health, and professional wellbeing.

Adapted from Kretzer & Kretzer (2010)

I integrate workplace artifacts of nature on my person and in my work station, as are safe, suitable, and supported by my organization.

INP to Guide Professional Wellbeing #5: I use a full range of patterns of knowing, evidence, and therapeutic modalities to support my regulation, health, and wellbeing, moving from least to more invasive, depending upon my needs and changing contexts. I am open, curious, and receptive to new individual and group practices as I lovingly care for my NS and myself in all dimensions of bodymindessence.

INP to Guide Professional Wellbeing #6: I prioritize my regulation, health, and wellbeing, along with those in my care. I weave MicroDoses Matter and lightning YICP practices throughout the day. When I'm away from work, I expand these practices to MacroDoses that support me to thrive in all aspects of my life, and make sure to include plenty of fun and laughter each day.

By keeping your NS and bodymindessence health and wellbeing at the forefront of each day, you are positioning yourself solidly in the driver's seat of your life. From there, you can live your highest and best life, as you define it. You are positioning yourself to thrive instead of just survive in your practice. So much healing is happening — and will continue to do so for us all.

The Trinity Part 3: INPs to Guide Nursing 2.0 Organizational & System Changes

My hope and intention are that this book will serve as a common frame of reference for us to think about, talk about, and use as we lead the changes we need to see in our profession. To help build a bridge between nurses who are advocating for these changes and their leaders, the INPs to Guide Nursing 2.0 are a launching point for nurses, leaders, administrators, and the C-suite executives to converse, brainstorm, and collaborate.

INPs to Guide Nursing 2.0
Organizational & System Changes

① Nurses are whole people whose regulation, health and wellbeing are influenced by their environments, including organizational environments.

② Nurses have innate capacities for professional health & wellness. Organizations position nurses in optimal work conditions to promote their regulation, safety, and professional wellbeing.

③ Nurses are central to patient-centered care that is relationship-based. Together, nurses and leaders co-create safe, diverse, equitable, and inclusive workplaces to promote wellbeing for all.

④ Nature has healing and restorative properties that support nurse professional health & wellbeing. Nature & biophilia should be reflected in workspaces to the full extent possible.

⑤ Nurses and leaders use a full range of evidence and patterns of knowing to inform innovative policies and practices that facilitate nurse safety, regulation, and professional wellbeing.

⑥ Prioritizing nurse safety, regulation, & wellbeing leads to decreased attrition, presenteeism, burnout, AND higher care quality, better patient outcomes, and improved fiscal outcomes for the organization.

Adapted from Keehan & Kallhan (2023)

The INPs to Guide Nursing 2.0 conversations are intended to complement the existing evidence base with practical, actionable ideas to seed and grow the changes that you and your leaders will implement as we move forward together. To get you started, I listed a couple of articles in the Deeper Dive Resources. Partner with your team members and leaders to locate the many excellent articles and studies, including those referenced at the end of the book, to support us in co-creating safe working conditions that promote professional wellbeing in your unique setting and circumstances.

***

Here are the Trinity of INPs and how they link together to usher in *Nursing 2.0*.

Trinity of INPs to Usher in a New Era of Nursing

INP #	INPs to Guide Patient Care (Kreitzer & Koithan)	INPs to Guide Professional Wellbeing	INPs to Guide Nursing 2.0 Organizational & System Changes
1	Human beings are whole systems inseparable from, and influenced by, environments.	We are whole persons, inseparable from the systems and contexts within which we live and work.	Nurses are whole people whose regulation, health and wellbeing are connected to, and influenced by, their environments, including organizational environments.
2	Human beings have an innate capacity for healing and wellbeing.	We engage with our innate capacities for regulation, health, and wellbeing.	Nurses have innate capacities for professional health and wellness. Organizations position nurses in optimal work conditions to promote their regulation, safety, and professional wellbeing.

| 3 | Integrative nursing is person-centered and relationship-based. | We are at the center of our professional wellness and collaborate through balanced and healthy relationships. | Nurses are central to patient centered care that is relationship based. Together, nurses and leaders co-create safe, diverse, equitable, and inclusive workplaces to promote professional wellbeing for all. |
| 4 | Nature has healing and restorative properties that contribute to health and wellbeing. | We use the healing and restorative properties of nature to support our regulation, health, and wellbeing. | Nature has healing and restorative properties that support nurse professional health and wellbeing. Use of nature biophilic designs should be reflected in the workplace to the full extent possible. |

Thriving in Practice & in Life

5	Integrative Nursing is informed by evidence and uses a full range of conventional and integrative approaches, employing the least intensive intervention possible depending on the need and context.	We consider the full range of evidence and patterns of knowing to guide our safety, NS regulation, and professional wellbeing.	Nurses and leaders use a full range of evidence and patterns of knowing to inform innovative policies and practices that facilitate nurse safety, regulation, and professional wellbeing.
6	Integrative nursing focuses on the health and wellbeing of caregivers as well as those they serve.	We prioritize nurse safety, regulation, and professional wellbeing in service to the best possible care quality and outcomes for our patients.	Prioritizing nurse safety, regulation, and wellbeing leads to decreased attrition, presenteeism, burnout, AND higher care quality, better patient outcomes, and improved fiscal outcomes for the organization.

Thriving Is Happening

You have learned and grown and planted so many thriving seeds through our work together in this book. We've made quite a journey together, haven't we?! It's been one of profound magnitude as you held up the Mirror of Truth and leaned into all your layers and shame, shattering the veil of disillusionment. You lovingly and compassionately nurtured your healer's heart, which was overgrown with old wounds, patterns, conditioning, and unhealed bits. You delicately attended to your heart and perhaps other chakras with steadfast care. What was once an overgrown inner forest, in dire need of thinning and pruning, is now a fertile garden into which the seeds of thriving were planted and are growing. You've connected with your deepest truths and are now experiencing the regeneration of your beautiful inner forest as a result. Many of the old narratives are broken, for they no longer serve you in this Thrive Chapter of Life. Let the old, stale, and outdated mental chatter fade away like a distant cloud as new life-giving, thriving narratives emerge.

Your vessel, your bodymindessence, has survived everything that you have experienced or endured to date. It has and will continue to heal as the old trauma patterns, narratives, and embodiments give way to the unlimited potential of your aligned and balanced self, always moving toward *haelan* or healed wholeness. **Healing will continue to happen in response to the ruptures and hardships that you will experience throughout your lifespan**. Of course, you'll still encounter the challenges and the ruptures inherent with living, but they won't knock you off your center, or leave you dysregulated to the same degree. Through MicroDoses and YICP daily practices, you'll sense, feel, and recognize potentially dysregulating signals from your inner and outer worlds and your Threat Detector. You'll use the tools you've gained to nurture your NS through consistent application of Micro- and MacroDoses of thrive-centered practices, alone and with others. You have a roadmap and a full toolkit. You are equipped to navigate whatever challenges arise in your Thrive Superhighway. You, in the entirety of your bodymindessence, are transcending all that has happened in the past and are prepared for all that is happening in the present moment and beyond.

This is a good time to reflect back upon those questions from the beginning of the book, as shown in the table. Take a few moments to reflect and return to the notes you made while reading the first chapter. Take in how you felt then and how you feel now. Just be with what emerges in compassionate self-acceptance, gesturing inclusion to whatever appears. You have learned a lot and experienced so much. Let's look at each of these questions now, with the benefit of hindsight and wisdom gained.

Bookends - Your Pre/Post Book Reflections

Question #	Beginning of the Book Questions	End of the Book Questions
1	Am I living Life, or is it living me?	Am I living Life, or is my dysregulated NS living me?
2	If Life were my teacher, what would it have me learn?	In what ways have I grown by virtue of reading this book?
3	Am I thriving in my practice or being drained by it?	As I thrive in my Window of Tolerance, how can I help other nurses to do the same?
4	If my practice were my teacher, what would it have me learn?	In what ways has my practice changed as a result of reading this book?

As you ponder these questions, consider how you now have a language, a roadmap, and a system through which you can nurture your NS. Reflect upon how little the limbic system gets into the driver's seat now. You have grabbed the steering wheel of your life and are driving on your Thrive Superhighway, for all of life comes to you now with ease, grace, glory, light, love, intimacy, laughter, health, wellness, abundance, and prosperity [modify as desired and then add your closing statement here].

Take another moment to reflect on your journey and all that you've learned, felt, shifted, healed, liberated, and experienced. You and your healer's heart have reconnected, grown, and flourished. Where once there was a sense of disconnectedness, numbness, hopelessness, collapse, shut down, despair, or (fill you words here), there is now a sense of inner connection as you reclaim yourself and live through the Seat of the Heart — where we are always at home within ourselves in tender, gentle, unconditional love, self-compassion, and self-acceptance. You are loved beyond measure. Take yet another moment to feel all the love that you are in the totality of your being.

If you feel inspired to express what you are feeling, consider Kim Krans' invitation:

"Some say there is a cave at the center of the heart. Others say it's a pool with a flowering white lotus. Imagine yourself there, and draw [or create using any medium] what you see."

Kim Krans

Next Steps

You are at the end of this book and at the beginning of thriving in your practice. As with any shift or change, it is important to nurture yourself and engage in the thoughts, practices, and behaviors that support you to live your highest and best nursing practice and life. To support you in this process, I am inviting you to join the Haelan Academy and Community, if you haven't done so already. There, you'll find a structured curriculum, live and video recorded resources and practices, and a community of Haelan Nurses who are as committed to being empowered as you are. You can learn more about this opportunity on my website at www.drlorrelaws.com.

Should you feel inspired to provide feedback, I would be so very grateful. Your perspective and how you experienced this book matter to me — immensely. Use the QR Code or this link, https://forms.gle/KiU4DbhturUZwuwb7, to access a two-question survey. I will use the feedback received to develop and enhance our Haelan Academy so I can meet your needs and wants as fully as possible. Together, anything and everything is possible. How else can we thrive in practice and in life?

Until Next Time . . . Namaste

I'm so grateful for the time we've shared together, the ups and downs, and everything in between. I have personally lived through each of these chapters, many times, throughout my lifetime of trauma, ruptures, and repairs. Although they were crushing and so very painful, I am grateful for all the traumas I've experienced and the healing wisdom gained, for it led me right here to you. I cannot envision a more meaningful act of love and service to my tribe, my people, and my fellow healers

QR code

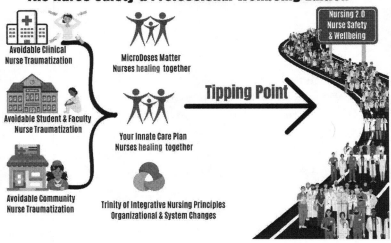

Road to Nursing 2.0 plus INPs

and nurses. I invite you to join me in the Haelan Academy & Community, on social media outlets, at speaking engagements, and on retreats. I have committed the rest of my career to the *Nursing 2.0: The Nurse Safety and Professional Wellbeing Edition* transition. It is my hope and intention that we, as Haelan Nurses, will work together, from our healed scars instead of our open wounds, to usher in *Nursing 2.0*. As we do, know that you are seen, heard, felt, valued, and loved beyond all measure. Until next time, namaste.

Deeper Dive Resources

Kreitzer, M. J., Koithan, M., & Weill, A. (eds.) (2019). *Integrative nursing* (2nd ed.). Oxford University Press.

Moloney, W., Fieldes, J., & Jacobs, S. (2020). "An integrative review of how healthcare organizations can support hospital nurses to thrive at work" in *International Journal of Environmental Research and Public Health*, 17(23), p.8757. https://doi.org/10.3390/ijerph17238757.

Russell, D., Mathew, S., Fitts, M., Liddle, Z., Murakami-Gold, L., Campbell, N., Ramjan, M., Zhao, Y., Hines, S., Humphreys, J. S., & Wakerman, J. (2021). "Interventions for health workforce retention in rural and remote areas: A systematic review" in *Human Resources for Health*, 19(1), p.103. https://doi.org/10.1186/s12960-021-00643-7.

Schlak, A. E., Rosa, W. E., Rushton, C. H., Poghosyan, L., Root, M. C., & McHugh, M. D. (2022). "An expanded institutional- and national-level blueprint to address nurse burnout and moral suffering amid the evolving pandemic" in *Nursing Management*, 53(1), pp.16-27. https://doi.org/10.1097/01. NUMA.0000805032.15402.b3.

Author Biography

Lorre Laws is a healer, teacher, and nursing leader whose scholarship and clinical practice centers on nurse traumatization, burnout, integrative health, evidence-based practice, and healthcare safety and quality. In her role as an integrative nursing professor, colleagues refer to her as a "master teacher," while students have dubbed her as "humanity's nurse". When in practice, she facilitates trauma healing for students, nurses, and health professionals.

Dr. Lorre founded The Haelan Academy & Community, a nonprofit organization where nurses across the globe can come together in a safe and nurturing virtual space to share and be supported in their healing journeys together. She is an informative and entertaining keynote speaker and retreat leader who educates and inspires. Dr. Lorre has published numerous scholarly articles and has presented her work to national and international nursing and health professional organizations.

Dr. Lorre is currently based in southern Arizona, USA, where she enjoys the love of family, friends, and community. She enjoys farm-to-table cooking, hiking, weight training, yoga, and a myriad of contemplative and healing practices, traditions, and modalities. She is attuned to her healer's heart and its calling to be of service to the global nursing community. She lives in alignment with her overarching mission: "It's not necessarily how I make a difference; I just want to be certain that I do."

References

Adams, T., Bezner, J., Garner, L., & Woodruff, S. (1998). "Construct validation of the Perceived Wellness Survey" in *American Journal of Health Studies*, 14(4), pp.212-219.

Aiken, L. H., Lasater, K. B., Sloane, D. M., Pogue, C. A., Fitzpatrick Rosenbaum, K. E., Muir, K. J., McHugh, M. D., & Consortium, U. C. W. S. (2023). "Physician and nurse well-being and preferred interventions to address burnout in hospital practice: Factors associated with turnover, outcomes, and patient safety" in *JAMA Health Forum*, 4(7), p.231809. https://doi.org/10.1001/jamahealthforum.2023.1809.

American Association of Colleges of Nursing. (n.d.). *Trauma-informed care*. https://www.aacnnursing.org/5B-Tool-Kit/Themes/Trauma-Informed-Care.

Arrogante, O., & Aparicio-Zaldivar, E. (2017). "Burnout and health among critical care professionals: The mediational role of resilience" in *Intensive Critical Care Nursing*, 42, pp.110-115. https://doi.org/10.1016/j.iccn.2017.04.010.

Badenoch, B. (2017). *The heart of trauma*. https://www.thescienceofpsychotherapy.com/the-heart-of-trauma/.

Badenoch, B. (2017). *The heart of trauma: Healing the embodied brain in the context of relationships*. Norton series on interpersonal neurobiology. W.W. Norton & Company.

Badenoch, B. (2022). *Trauma & the embodied brain: A heart-based training in relational neuroscience for healing trauma*. Sounds True. https://www.soundstrue.com/products/trauma-and-the-embodied-brain-1.

Baldwin, S. J. (2022). *How to gain control over how you feel: A Polyvagal informed approach to gaining nervous system regulation*. SarahBCoaching.

Bar-David, S. (2018). "What's in an eye roll? It is time we explore the role of workplace incivility in healthcare" in *Israel Journal of Health Policy Research*, 7(1), p.15. https://doi.org/10.1186/s13584-018-0209-0.

Bart, R., Ishak, W. W., Ganjian, S., Jaffer, K. Y., Abdelmesseh, M., Hanna, S., Gohar, Y., Azar, G., Vanle, B., Dang, J., & Danovitch, I. (2018). "The assessment and measurement of wellness in the clinical medical setting: A systematic review" in *Innovations in Clinical Neuroscience*, 15(9-10), pp.14-23.

Benazzo, M., & Benazzo, Z. (Directors). (2021). *The wisdom of trauma* [film]. Science of Nonduality.

Berlin, G., Lapoint, M., & Murphy, M. (2022). *Surveyed nurses consider leaving direct patient care at elevated rates.* McKinsey & Company. https://www.mckinsey.com/industries/healthcare-systems-and-services/our-insights/surveyed-nurses-consider-leaving-direct-patient-care-at-elevated-rates.

Berwick, D. M. (2002). *Escape Fire: Lessons for the future of health care.* The Commonwealth Fund.

Boamah, S. A., Callen, M., & Cruz, E. (2021). "Nursing faculty shortage in Canada: A scoping review of contributing factors" in *Nursing Outlook*, 69(4), pp.574-588. https://doi.org/https://doi.org/10.1016/j.outlook.2021.01.018.

Bokur, D. (2009). *Healing rituals around the world: Many of today's healing rituals draw from the wisdom of our ancestors.* Natural Awakenings. https://www.naturalawakenings.com/2009/12/01/273561/healing-rituals-around-the-world-many-of-today-s-healing-rituals-draw-from-the-wisdom-of-our-ancestors.

Brewer, K. C. (2021). "Institutional betrayal in nursing: A concept analysis" in *Nursing Ethics*, 28(6), pp.1081-1089. https://doi.org/10.1177/0969733021992448.

Brown, B. (2006). "Shame Resilience Theory: A grounded theory study on women and shame" in *Families in Society*, 87(1), pp.43-52. https://doi.org/10.1606/1044-3894.3483.

Brown, B. (2012). *The power of vulnerability: Teachings of authenticity, connection, and courage.* Sounds True.

Buchan, J., Catton, H., & Shaffer, F. A. (2022). *Sustain and retain in 2022 and beyond: The global nursing workforce and the COVID-19 pandemic.* International Council of Nurses & International Centre on Nurse Migration. https://www.icn.ch/news.

Byon, H. D., Sagherian, K., Kim, Y., Lipscomb, J., Crandall, M., & Steege, L. (2022). "Nurses' experience with Type II Workplace Violence and underreporting during the COVID-19 pandemic" in *Workplace Health & Safety,* 70(9), pp.412-420. https://doi.org/10.1177/21650799211031233.

Canadian Nurses Association. (2022). *Physicians, nurses offer solutions to immediately address health human resource crisis.* https://www.cna-aiic.ca/en/blogs/cn-content/2022/05/16/physicians-nurses-offer-solutions-to-immediately-a.

Carper, B. (1978). "Fundamental patterns of knowing in nursing" in *Advances in Nursing Science,* 1(1), pp.13-23.

Carter, C. S. (2019). "Love as embodied medicine" in *International Body Psychotherapy Journal,* 18(1).

Carter, C. S. (2022). "Oxytocin and love: Myths, metaphors and mysteries" in *Comprehensive Psychoneuroendocrinology,* 9, Article 100107. https://doi.org/https://doi.org/10.1016/j.cpnec.2021.100107.

Chinn, P., & Kramer, M. (2018). *Knowledge development in nursing: Theory and process* (10th ed.). St. Louis, MO: Elsevier.

Chmielewski, J., Los, K., & Luczynski, W. (2021). "Mindfulness in healthcare professionals and medical education" in *International Journal of Occupational Medicine and Environmental Health,* 34, 1+. https://doi.org/10.13075/ijomeh.1896.01542.

Choose Mental Health. (n.d.). *25 grounding techniques for anxiety.* https://choosementalhealth.org/25-grounding-techniques-for-anxiety/.

CMind. (2021). The Tree of Contemplative Practices [Illustration]. The Center for Contemplative Mind in Society. https://www. contemplativemind.org/practices/tree.

Complex Trauma Resources. (n.d.). *Core topics, treatment, and resources.* https://www.complextrauma.org.

Conelius, J., & Iannino-Renz, R. (2021). "Incorporating a mindfulness program in a graduate family nurse practitioner program" in *Journal of Holistic Nursing,* 39(4), pp.369-372. https://doi.org/10.1177/0898010121997303.

Conti-O'Hare, M. (2002). *The nurse as wounded healer: From trauma to transcendence.* Jones & Bartlett Learning.

Cummings, J., & Baumann, S. L. (2021). "Understanding shame as an obstacle: Toward a global perspective" in *Nursing Science Quarterly,* 34(2), pp.196-201. https://doi.org/10.1177/0894318420987186.

Dana, D. (2020). *Polyvagal exercises for safety and connection: 50 client-centered practices.* Norton series on interpersonal neurobiology: W. W. Norton & Company.

Dana, D. (2018). *The Polyvagal theory in therapy: Engaging the rhythm of regulation.* Norton series on interpersonal neurobiology. W. W. Norton & Company.

DeYoung, P. A. (2021). *Understanding and treating chronic shame: Healing right brain relational trauma.* Routledge.

Downie, R. (2012). "Paying attention: Hippocratic and Asklepian approaches" in *Advances in Psychiatric Treatment,* 18(5), pp.363-368. https://doi.org/10.1192/apt.bp.111.009308.

DuBois, C. A., & Zedreck Gonzalez, J. F. (2018). "Implementing a resilience-promoting education program for new nursing graduates" in *Journal for Nurses in Professional Development,* 34(5). https://doi.org/10.1097/NND.0000000000000484.

Dulko, D., & Kohal, B. J. (2022). "How do we reduce burnout in nursing?" in *Nursing Clinics,* 57(1), pp.101-114. https://doi. org/10.1016/j.cnur.2021.11.007.

Earl. E. Bakken Center for Spirituality & Healing. (n.d.). *Taking charge of your health & wellbeing: Wellbeing assessment.* https://www.takingcharge.csh.umn.edu/wellbeing-assessment.

Editorial Staff. (2022). *Underpaid, burnt out, and unappreciated NHS staff say they are looking to quit.* NursingNotes. https://nursingnotes.co.uk/news/workforce/underpaid-burnt-out-and-unappreciated-nhs-staff-say-they-are-looking-to-quit/.

Editorial Staff. (2022). *Understanding the nursing shortage in Australia.* Victoria University. https://online.vu.edu.au/blog/understanding-nursing-shortage-Australia.

Egnew, T. R. (2005). "The meaning of healing: Transcending suffering" in *The Annals of Family Medicine,* 3(3), pp.255-262.

Elsevier Health. (2022). *Clinician of the future: A 2022 report.* https://www.elsevier.com/connect/clinician-of-the-future.

Emmerich, N. (2018). "Leadership in palliative medicine: Moral, ethical and educational" in *BMC Medical Ethics,* 19(1), p.55. https://doi.org/10.1186/s12910-018-0296-z.

Fannin, J. L., & Williams, R. (2012). "Leading-Edge neuroscience reveals significant correlations between beliefs, the whole-brain state, and psychotherapy" in *CQ: The CAPA Quarterly,* pp.14-17.

Foli, K. J. (2022). "A middle-range theory of nurses' psychological trauma" in *Advances in Nursing Science,* 45(1), pp.86-98. https://doi.org/10.1097/ANS.0000000000000388.

Gaines, K. (2023). *2023 - This is the state of nursing.* https://nurse.org/articles/state-of-nursing-2023.

Gladwell, M. (2006). *The tipping point: How little things can make a big difference.* Little, Brown and Co.

Goddard, A., Jones, R. W., Esposito, D., & Janicek, E. (2021). "Trauma informed education in nursing: A call for action" in *Nurse Education Today,* 101, 104880. https://doi.org/https://doi.org/10.1016/j.nedt.2021.104880.

Goffnett, J., Liechty, J. M., & Kidder, E. (2020). "Interventions to reduce shame: A systematic review" in *Journal of Behavioral and Cognitive Therapy*, 30(2), pp.141-160.

Goldman Schuyler, K., Watson, L. W., & King, E. (2021). "How generative mindfulness can contribute to inclusive workplaces" in *Humanistic Management Journal*, 6(3), pp.451-478. https://doi.org/10.1007/s41463-021-00120-2.

Guo, Y. F., Luo, Y. H., Lam, L., Cross, W., Plummer, V., & Zhang, J. P. (2018). "Burnout and its association with resilience in nurses: A cross-sectional study" in *Journal of Clinical Nursing*, 27(1-2), pp.441-449. https://doi.org/10.1111/jocn.13952.

Gutowski, E. R., Badio, K. S., & Kaslow, N. J. (2022). "Trauma-informed inpatient care for marginalized women" in *Psychotherapy*. https://doi.org/10.1037/pst0000456.

Harte, S. E., Harris, R. E., & Clauw, D. J. (2018). "The neurobiology of central sensitization" in *Journal of Applied Biobehavioral Research*, 23(2), e12137. https://doi.org/https://doi.org/10.1111/jabr.12137.

Henshall, C., Davey, Z., & Jackson, D. (2020). "Nursing resilience interventions — A way forward in challenging healthcare territories" in *Journal of Clinical Nursing*, 29(19-20), pp.3597-3599. https://doi.org/10.1111/jocn.15276.

Henson, C., Truchot, D., & Canevello, A. (2021). "What promotes post traumatic growth? A systematic review" in *European Journal of Trauma & Dissociation*, 5(4), 100195. https://doi.org/https://doi.org/10.1016/j.ejtd.2020.100195.

Hershler, A. (2021). "Window of tolerance" in A. Hershler, L. Hughes, P. Nguyen, & S. Wall (Eds.), *Looking at trauma: A tool kit for clinicians*. The Pennsylvania State University Press.

Hope, T. (2017). "The effects of access bars on anxiety and depression: A pilot study" in *Energy Psychology*, 9(2). https://doi.org/10.9769/EPJ.2017.9.2.TH.

Hopper, A. (2014). *Wired for healing: Remapping the brain to recover from chronic and mysterious illnesses.* Dynamic Neural Retraining System.

Horowitz, M., & Wilcock, M. (2022). "Newer generation antidepressants and withdrawal effects: Reconsidering the role of antidepressants and helping patients to stop" in *Drug and Therapeutics Bulletin,* 60(1), pp.7-12. https://doi.org/10.1136/dtb.2020.000080.

How, L. (n.d.). *Are you empowering or enabling?* Hope Made Strong. https://hopemadestrong.org/are-you-empowering-or-enabling.

Huneke, D. (2007). "Healer's heart" in *The American Journal of Nursing,* 107(6), pp.57-57.

International Council of Nurses. (2022). *"As a profession, globally, we are asking for help." Nurses discuss ways to address the critical global nursing shortage.* https://www.icn.ch/news/profession-globally-we-are-asking-help-nurses-discuss-ways-address-critical-global-nursing.

International Council of Nurses. (2021). *The COVID-19 Effect: World's nurses facing mass trauma, an immediate danger to the profession and future of our health systems.* https://www.icn.ch/news/covid-19-effect-worlds-nurses-facing-mass-trauma-immediate-danger-profession-and-future-our.

International Council of Nurses. (2021). *International Council of Nurses COVID-19 Update.* https://www.icn.ch/news/covid-19-effect-worlds-nurses-facing-mass-trauma-immediate-danger-profession-and-future-our.

Jaeb, M. A. (2022). "Concept analysis of shame in nursing" in *International Journal of Mental Health Nursing,* 31(2), pp.295-304. https://doi.org/https://doi.org/10.1111/inm.12948.

Jarvis, J. Q., & Celani, K. (2022). "When nurses are not safe, patients are not safe" in *The Salt Lake Tribune.* https://www.

sltrib.com/opinion/commentary/2022/08/25/joseph-q-jarvis-kindra-celani.

Joye, M. (2021). *Codependent discovery and recovery 2.0: A holistic approach to healing and freeing yourself.* Simon and Schuster.

Kabat-Zinn, J. (2018). *The healing power of mindfulness: A new way of being.* Hachette UK.

Kim, E. Y., & Chang, S. O. (2022). "Exploring nurse perceptions and experiences of resilience: A meta-synthesis study" in *BMC Nursing*, 21(1), p.26. https://doi.org/10.1186/s12912-021-00803-z.

Kim, J., Chesworth, B., Franchino-Olsen, H., & Macy, R. J. (2022). "A scoping review of vicarious trauma interventions for service providers working with people who have experienced traumatic events" in *Trauma, Violence, & Abuse,* 23(5), pp.1437-1460. https://doi.org/10.1177/1524838021991310.

Kim, S., Mayer, C., & Jones, C. B. (2021). "Relationships between nurses' experiences of workplace violence, emotional exhaustion and patient safety" in *Journal of Research in Nursing*, 26(1-2), pp.35-46. https://doi.org/10.1177/1744987120960200.

Kim, J., Chae, D., & Yoo, J. Y. (2021). "Reasons behind Generation Z nursing students' intentions to leave their profession: A cross-sectional study" in *Inquiry: A Journal of Medical Care Organization, Provision, and Financing*, 58, 46958021999928. https://doi.org/10.1177/0046958021999928.

Kirmayer, L. J. (2003). "Asklepian dreams: The ethos of the wounded-healer in the clinical encounter" in *Transcultural Psychiatry*, 40(2), pp.248-277. https://doi.org/10.1177/1363461503402007.

Kohrt, B. A., Ottman, K., Panter-Brick, C., Konner, M., & Patel, V. (2020). "Why we heal: The evolution of psychological healing and implications for global mental health" in *Clinical Psychology Review*, 82, 101920. https://doi.org/https://doi.org/10.1016/j.cpr.2020.101920.

Kotera, Y., Richardson, M., & Sheffield, D. (2022). "Effects of shinrin-yoku (forest bathing) and nature therapy on mental health: A systematic review and meta-analysis" in *International Journal of Mental Health and Addiction*, 20(1), pp.337-361. https://doi.org/10.1007/s11469-020-00363-4.

Krans, K. (2019). *Archetypes guidebook*. HarperOne.

Kreitzer, M. J. (2015). "Integrative nursing: Application of principles across clinical settings" in *Rambam Maimonides Medical Journal*, 6(2), e0016-e0016. https://doi.org/10.5041/RMMJ.10200.

Kreitzer, M. J., Koithan, M., & Weill, A. (Eds.). (2019). *Integrative nursing* (2nd ed.). Oxford University Press.

Laws, L. (2022). *An integrative approach to healing the overworked, weary, or traumatized nurse*. https://www.myamericannurse.com/an-integrative-approach-to-heal-the-overworked-weary-or-traumatized-nurse/.

Laws, L. (2022). "The Great RNesignation: Shifting the paradigm from burnout to integrative nurse wellness and retention" in *International Journal of Nursing and Health Care Science*, 2(4), pp.113-115.

Laws, L. (2021). "The Great R(N)esignation: Using integrative nursing principles to promote resilience and retention" in *Arizona Nurse*, 75, p.13.

LeMaistre, C. (n.d.). *Home body: Somatic grounding exercises for coming home to your body*. https://www.carmellelauren.com/blog/2021/2/3/homebody-somatic-grounding-exercises-ebook.

Lickiss, N. (2012). "On facing human suffering" (chapter 19) in J. Malpas & N. Lickiss (Eds.), *Perspectives on human suffering*. Springer.

Lim-Saco, F., Kilat, C., & Locsin, R. (2018). "Synchronicity in human—space—time: A theory of nursing engagement in a global community" in *International Journal for Human Caring*, 22(1), pp.1-10. https://connect.springerpub.com/content/sgrijhc/22/1/29.

MacDonald, L., & Stayner, G. (2022). *Australia facing nursing shortage as more than two years of COVID takes its toll*. ABC

News. https://www.abc.net.au/news/2022-07-22/nursing-shortage-on-the-cards-due-to-pandemic/101253058.

Mareno, N., & James, K. S. (2010). "Further validation of the body-mind-spirit wellness behavior and characteristic inventory for college students" in *Southern Online Journal of Nursing Research*, 10(4).

Marie, K. S. T. S., & Cook-Cottone, C. (2022). "Mindful self-care to manage the effects of trauma, burnout, and compassion fatigue" in L. L. Douglas, A. Threlkeld, & L. R. Merriweather (Eds.), *Trauma in adult and higher education: Conversations and critical reflections*. Information Age Publishing.

Maslach, C., Jackson, S. E., Leiter, M. P., Schaufeli, W. B., & Schwab, R. L. (n.d.). Maslach Burnout Inventory (MBI). https://www.mindgarden.com/117-maslach-burnout-inventory-mbi.

Maté, G. (2021). *The myth of normal: Illness and health in an insane culture*. Penguin Random House.

McElligott, D. (2010). "Healing: The journey from concept to nursing practice" in *Journal of Holistic Nursing*, 28(4), pp.251-259. https://doi.org/10.1177/0898010110376321.

McElligott, D., Eckardt, S., Montgomery Dossey, B., Luck, S., & Eckardt, P. (2018). "Instrument development of integrative health and wellness assessment™" in *Journal of Holistic Nursing*, 36(4), pp.374-384. https://doi.org/10.1177/0898010117747752.

McElligott, D., & Turnier, J. (2020). "Integrative health and wellness assessment tool" in *Critical Care Nursing Clinics of North America*, 32(3), pp.439-450. https://doi.org/10.1016/j.cnc.2020.05.006.

McGilchrist, I. (2019). *The master and his emissary: The divided brain and the making of the Western world*. Yale University Press.

Mealer, M., Burnham, E. L., Goode, C. J., Rothbaum, B., & Moss, M. (2009). "The prevalence and impact of post traumatic stress disorder and burnout syndrome in nurses" in *Depression and Anxiety*, 26(12), pp.1118-1126. https://doi.org/10.1002/da.20631.

Miller, E. M., & Hill, P. D. (2018). "Intuition in clinical decision making: Differences among practicing nurses" in *Journal of Holistic Nursing*, 36(4), pp.318-329. https://doi.org/10.1177/0898010117725428.

Moloney, W., Fieldes, J., & Jacobs, S. (2020). "An integrative review of how healthcare organizations can support hospital nurses to thrive at work" in *International Journal of Environmental Research and Public Health*, 17(23), 8757. https://doi.org/10.3390/ijerph17238757.

Morse, J. M., & Penrod, J. (1999). "Linking concepts of enduring, uncertainty, suffering, and hope" in *The Journal of Nursing Scholarship*, 31(2), pp.145-150. https://doi.org/10.1111/j.1547-5069.1999.tb00455.x.

Morton, M. (2016). "We can work it out: The importance of rupture and repair processes in infancy and adult life for flourishing" in *Health Care Analysis*, 24(2), pp.119-132. https://doi.org/10.1007/s10728-016-0319-1.

Munhall, P. (1993). "'Unknowing' in nursing: Toward another pattern of knowing in nursing" in *Nursing Outlook*, 41(3), pp.125-128.

Murphy, G. T., Sampalli, T., Bearskin, L. B., Cashen, N., Cummings, G., Rose, A. E., Etowa, J., Grinspun, D., Jones, E. W., Lavoie-Tremblay, M., MacMillan, K., MacQuarrie, C., Martin-Misener, R., Oulton, J., Ricciardelli, R., Silas, L., Thorne, S., & Villeneuve, M. (2022). "Investing in Canada's nursing workforce post-pandemic: A call to action" in *FACETS*, 7, pp.1051-1120. https://doi.org/10.1139/facets-2022-0002.

Myers, J. E., & Sweeney, T. J. (2004). "The indivisible self: An evidence-based model of wellness" in *Journal of Individual Psychology*, 60, pp.234-244.

Myers, J. E., Sweeney, T. J., & Witmer, J. M. (2000). "The wheel of wellness counseling for wellness: A holistic model for treatment planning" in *Journal of Counseling & Development*, 78(3), pp.251-266. https://doi.org/10.1002/j.1556-6676.2000.tb01906.x

National Academy of Medicine. (2022). *National plan for health workforce well-being*. The National Academies Press. https://doi.org/10.17226/26744.

National Academies of Sciences, Engineering, and Medicine. (2019). *Taking action against clinician burnout: A systems approach to professional well-being*. https://nap.nationalacademies.org.

National Center on Domestic Violence, Trauma, and Mental Health. (n.d.). *Resources on trauma*. http://www.nationalcenterdvtraumamh.org/publications-products/resources-on-trauma/.

National Center for Integrative Primary Care. (n.d.). *Resources for patients and the public*. https://nciph.org/public.html.

National Council for Behavioral Health. (n.d.). *How to manage trauma*. https://www.thenationalcouncil.org/wp-content/uploads/2022/08/Trauma-infographic.pdf.

National Institute for the Clinical Application of Behavioral Medicine. (n.d.). *Courses, experts & continuing education*. https://www.nicabm.com/.

National Institute for the Clinical Application of Behavioral Medicine. (n.d.). *How to help your clients understand their Window of Tolerance*. https://www.nicabm.com/trauma-how-to-help-your-clients-understand-their-window-of-tolerance.

National Institute for the Clinical Application of Behavioral Medicine. (n.d.). *How to overcome the freeze response*. https://www.nicabm.com/topic/freeze.

National Institute for the Clinical Application of Behavioral Medicine. (2023). *How to work with shame*. https://www.nicabm.com.

National Institute for the Clinical Application of Behavioral Medicine. (2023). *The treating trauma master series*. https://www.nicabm.com.

National Institute for the Clinical Application of Behavioral Medicine. (n.d.). *Working with structural dissociation*. https://

www.nicabm.com/working-with-structural-dissociation/?de
l=10.1.22InfographictoFree.

Naviaux, R. K. (2020). "Perspective: Cell danger response biology — The new science that connects environmental health with mitochondria and the rising tide of chronic illness" in *Mitochondrion*, 51, pp.40-45. https://doi.org/10.1016/j.mito.2019.12.005.

Naviaux, R. K. (2023). "Mitochondrial and metabolic features of salugenesis and the healing cycle" in *Mitochondrion*, 70, pp.131-163. https://doi.org/https://doi.org/10.1016/j.mito.2023.04.003.

Naydeck, B. L., Pearson, J. A., Ozminkowski, R. J., Day, B. T., & Goetzel, R. Z. (2008). "The Impact of the Highmark Employee Wellness Programs on 4-year healthcare costs" in *Journal of Occupational and Environmental Medicine*, pp.146-156. https://doi.org/10.1097/JOM.0b013e3181617855.

Nemcek, M. A. (2003). "Self nurturance: Research trends and wellness model" in *AAOHN Journal*, 51(6), pp.260-266.

Norwich University Online. (2021). *Post-traumatic stress disorder in nursing*. https://online.norwich.edu.

Nurse.org Staff. (2021). *Nurses say violent assaults against healthcare workers are a silent epidemic*. https://nurse.org/articles/workplace-violence-in-nursing-and-hospitals/.

Online Etymology Dictionary. (2015). *Healing*. https://www.etymonline.com/word/healing.

Ozeke, O., Ozeke, V., Coskun, O., & Budakoglu, II. (2019). "Second victims in health care: Current perspectives" in *Advances in Medical Education and Practice*, 10, pp.593-603. https://doi.org/10.2147/amep.S185912.

Perkins, A. (2021). *Nursing shortage: Consequences and solutions*. Nursing Made Incredibly Easy, 19(5), pp.49-54. https://doi.org/10.1097/01.NME.0000767268.61806.d9.

Perry, B. D., & Winfrey, O. (2021). *What happened to you?: Conversations on trauma, resilience, and healing*. Flatiron Books.

Petrocchi, N., & Cheli, S. (2019). "The social brain and heart rate variability: Implications for psychotherapy" in *Psychology and Psychotherapy: Theory, Research and Practice*, 92(2), pp.208-223. https://doi.org/10.1111/papt.12224.

Poli, A., Gemignani, A., Soldani, F., & Miccoli, M. (2021). "A Systematic review of a polyvagal perspective on embodied contemplative practices as promoters of cardiorespiratory coupling and traumatic stress recovery for PTSD and OCD: Research methodologies and state of the art" in *International Journal of Environmental Research and Public Health*, 18(22). https://doi.org/10.3390/ijerph182211778.

Porges, S. W. (2004). "Neuroception: A subconscious system for detecting threats and safety" in *Zero to Three* (J), 24(5), pp.19-24.

Porges, S. W. (2022). "Polyvagal Theory: A science of safety" in *Frontiers in Integrative Neuroscience*, 16. https://doi.org/10.3389/fnint.2022.871227.

Porges, S. W. (2017). *The pocket guide to the polyvagal theory: The transformative power of feeling safe*. W. W. Norton & Co.

Porges, S. W. (n.d.). *What's happening in the nervous system of patients who "please and appease" in response to trauma?* https://www.nicabm.com/working-with-please-and-appease/.

Powley, T. L. (2021). "Brain-gut communication: vagovagal reflexes interconnect the two 'brains'" in *American Journal of Physiology-Gastrointestinal and Liver Physiology*, 321(5), G576-G587. https://doi.org/10.1152/ajpgi.00214.2021.

Prestia, A. S. (2021). "Next level self-care for nurse leaders" in *Nurse Leader*, 19(3), pp.305-307. https://doi.org/https://doi.org/10.1016/j.mnl.2021.02.006.

Purves, D., & Augustine, G. J. (2001). *The subdivisions of the central nervous system*. Neuroscience (2nd ed.). Sinauer Associates. https://www.ncbi.nlm.nih.gov/books/NBK10926.

Quinn, J. F. (1997). "Healing: A model for an integrative health care system" in *Advanced Practice Nursing Quarterly*, 3(1), pp.1-7.

Quinn, J. F. (1989). "On healing, wholeness, and the Haelan Effect" in *Nursing and Health Care*, 10(10), pp.553-556.

Quinn, J. F., Smith, M., Ritenbaugh, C., Swanson, K., & Watson, M. J. (2003). "Research guidelines for assessing the impact of the healing relationship in clinical nursing" in *Alternative Therapies*, 9(3), pp. A65-A79.

Quinn, J. F. (n.d.). *Quinn, on healing*. Saint Anselm College. https://www.anselm.edu/sites/default/files/Documents/Academics/Department/Nursing%20Cont%20Education/Handouts/6Healing_Quinn's_model.pdf.

Ra, K. (2016). *The Sophia Code* (2nd ed.). Kia Ra & Ra-El Publishing.

Rafii, F., Nasrabadi, A. N., & Tehrani, F. J. (2021). "How nurses apply patterns of knowing in clinical practice: A grounded theory study" in *Ethiopian Journal of Health Sciences*, 31(1), pp.139-146. https://doi.org/10.4314/ejhs.v31i1.16.

Rainbow, J. G. (2019). "Presenteeism: Nurse perceptions and consequences" in *Journal of Nursing Management*, 27(7), pp.1530-1537. https://doi.org/10.1111/jonm.12839.

Reed, J. (2021). *NHS in England facing worst staffing crisis in history, MPs warn*. BBC. https://www.bbc.com/news/health-62267282.

Reed, P. G. (1991). "Toward a nursing theory of self-transcendence: Deductive reformulation using developmental theories" in *Advances in Nursing Science*, 13, pp.64-67. https://doi.org/10.1097/00012272-199106000-00008.

Reese, G., Stahlberg, J., & Menzel, C. (2022). "Digital shinrin-yoku: Do nature experiences in virtual reality reduce stress and increase well-being as strongly as similar experiences in a physical forest?" in *Virtual Reality*, 26(3), pp.1245-1255. https://doi.org/10.1007/s10055-022-00631-9.

Rexroth, R., & Davidhizar, R. (2003). "Caring: Utilizing the Watson theory to transcend culture" in *The Health Care Manager*, 22(4), pp.295-304. https://journals.lww.com/

healthcaremanagerjournal/Fulltext/2003/10000/Caring__Utilizing_the_Watson_Theory_to_Transcend.2.aspx.

Rodney, T., Heidari, O., Miller, H. N., Thornton, C. P., Jenkins, E., & Kang, H. K. (2022). "Posttraumatic stress disorder in nurses in the United States: Prevalence and effect on role" in *Journal of Nursing Management*, 30(1), pp.226-233. https://doi.org/10.1111/jonm.13478.

Rushton, C. H. (2018). "Moral suffering: A reality of clinical practice" in C. H. Rushton & C. H. Rushton (Eds.), *Moral resilience: Transforming moral suffering in healthcare,* pp.10-48. Oxford University Press. https://doi.org/10.1093/med/9780190619268.003.0002.

Russell, D., Mathew, S., Fitts, M., Liddle, Z., Murakami-Gold, L., Campbell, N., Ramjan, M., Zhao, Y., Hines, S., Humphreys, J. S., & Wakerman, J. (2021). "Interventions for health workforce retention in rural and remote areas: A systematic review" in *Human Resources for Health,* 19(1), p.103. https://doi.org/10.1186/s12960-021-00643-7.

Salicru, S. (2021). *Interpersonal neurobiology, the brain, psychotherapy, brain plasticity/neuroplasticity, the mind vs the brain, and consciousness.* https://ptspsychology.com/wp-content/uploads/2021/08/Interpersonal-Neurobiology_SSalicru-PTS.pdf.

Salvon-Harman, J. (2023). *If it's not safe, it's not care*: Notes from the 2023 Global Ministerial Summit on Patient Safety. Institute for Healthcare Improvement. https://www.ihi.org/communities/blogs/if-its-not-safe-its-not-care-notes-from-the-2023-global-ministerial-summit-on-patient-safety.

Schlak, A. E., Rosa, W. E., Rushton, C. H., Poghosyan, L., Root, M. C., & McHugh, M. D. (2022). "An expanded institutional- and national-level blueprint to address nurse burnout and moral suffering amid the evolving pandemic" in *Nursing Management*, 53(1), pp.16-27. https://doi.org/10.1097/01.NUMA.0000805032.15402.b3.

Schuster, M., & Dwyer, P. A. (2020). "Post-traumatic stress disorder in nurses: An integrative review" in *Journal of Clinical Nursing*, 29(15-16), pp.2769-2787. https://doi.org/ https://doi.org/10.1111/jocn.15288.

Schwartz, A. (2021). *The Complex PTSD treatment manual: An integrative, mind-body approach to trauma recovery*. PESI Publishing.

Seay, A. (2003). "The tipping point: How little things can make a difference" in *Injury Prevention*, 9(3), p.286. https://doi. org/10.1136/ip.9.3.286-a.

Shan, G., Wang, S., Wang, W., Guo, S., & Li, Y. (2020). "Presenteeism in nurses: Prevalence, consequences, and causes from the perspectives of nurses and chief nurses" in *Frontiers in Psychiatry*, 11, 584040. https://doi.org/10.3389/ fpsyt.2020.584040.

Siegel, D. J. (2010). *Mindsight: The new science of personal transformation*. Bantam/Random House.

Siegel, D. J., & Bryson, T. P. (2021). *The power of showing up: How parental presence shapes who our kids become and how their brains get wired*. Ballantine Books.

Siegel, D. J., & Bryson, T. P. (2011). *The whole-brain child: 12 revolutionary strategies to nurture your child's developing mind*. Delacorte Press.

Spurr, S., Walker, K., Squires, V., & Redl, N. (2021). "Examining nursing students' wellness and resilience: An exploratory study" in *Nurse Education in Practice*, 51, Article 102978. https://doi.org/https://doi.org/10.1016/j.nepr.2021.102978.

Statistics Canada. (2022). *Experiences of healthcare workers during the COVID-19 pandemic*, September to November 2021. https://www150.statcan.gc.ca/n1/daily-quotidien/220603/ dq220603a-eng.html.

Stein, M. B., & Norman, S. (2023). *Psychotherapy and psychosocial interventions for posttraumatic stress disorder in adults*. UpToDate.

Stelnicki, A. M., Carleton, N., & Reichert, C. (2020). *Mental disorder symptoms among nurses in Canada.* https://nursesunions.ca/wp-content/uploads/2020/06/OSI-REPORT_final.pdf.

Stephens, T. M. (2013). "Nursing student resilience: A concept clarification" in *Nursing Forum,* 48(2), pp.125-133. https://doi.org/10.1111/nuf.12015.

Substance Abuse and Mental Health Services Administration (SAMHSA). (2022). *Addressing burnout in the behavioral health workforce through organizational strategies.* SAMHSA Publication No. PEP22-06-02-005.

Substance Abuse and Mental Health Services Administration (SAMHSA). (2014). Chapter 3 "Understanding the impact of trauma" in *In Trauma-informed care in behavioral health sciences. Treatment Improvement Protocol (TIP) Series, No. 57,* Center for Substance Abuse Treatment.

Substance Abuse and Mental Health Services Administration (SAMHSA). (n.d.). *Creating a healthier life: A step-by-step guide to wellness.* https://store.samhsa.gov/sites/default/files/d7/priv/sma16-4958.pdf.

Substance Abuse and Mental Health Services Administration (SAMHSA). (n.d.). *Find help.* https://www.samhsa.gov/find-help.

Syme, K. L., & Hagen, E. H. (2020). "Mental health is biological health: Why tackling 'diseases of the mind' is an imperative for biological anthropology in the 21st century" in *American Journal of Physical Anthropology,* 171(S70), pp.87-117. https://doi.org/https://doi.org/10.1002/ajpa.23965.

Taylor, K. (2017). *The ethics of caring: Finding right relationship with clients for profound, transformative work in professional healing relationships.* Hanford Mead Publishers.

Taylor, R. A. (2019). "Contemporary issues: Resilience training alone is an incomplete intervention" in *Nurse Education Today,* 78, pp.10-13. https://doi.org/https://doi.org/10.1016/j.nedt.2019.03.014.

The Bodymind Centre. (n.d.). *Vagal breathing technique.* https:// bodymindcentre.com/news-2/vagal-breathing-technique.

The Centers for Medicare & Medicaid Services. (2020). *Workplace violence prevention for nurses.* https://wwwn.cdc.gov/WPVHC/ Nurses/Course/Slide/Home.

Thorne, S. (2020). "Rethinking Carper's personal knowing for 21st century nursing" in *Nursing Philosophy*, 21(4), e12307. https://doi.org/https://doi.org/10.1111/nup.12307.

Tolle, E. (2006). *A new earth: Awakening to your life's purpose.* Penguin Books.

Tolle, E. (2004). *The power of now.* New World Library, New York, NY.

Toney-Butler, T. J., & Thayer, J. (2022). *Nursing process.* StatPearls Publishing. https://www.ncbi.nlm.nih.gov/books/ NBK499937/.

U.S. Department of Health and Human Services Administration — Office of the U.S. Surgeon General. (2022). *Addressing health worker burnout: The U.S. Surgeon General's advisory on building a thriving health workforce.* https://www.hhs.gov/sites/default/ files/health-worker-wellbeing-advisory.pdf.

Van der Kolk, B. A. (2015). *The body keeps the score: Brain, mind, and body in the healing of trauma.* Penguin Books.

Veterans Health Administration: Office of Patient Centered Care and Cultural Transformation. (2013). *My story: Personal health inventory.* https://www.va.gov/patientcenteredcare/ resources/personal-health-inventory.asp.

Walker, P. (2014). *Complex PTSD: From surviving to thriving: A guide and map for recovering from childhood trauma.* Azure Coyote.

Ward, K. (n.d.). *We need to urgently address the nursing crisis in Australia.* Australian College of Nursing. https://www.acn. edu.au/post/we-need-to-urgently-address-the-nursing-crisis-in-australia.

Watson, J. (2009). "Caring as the essence and science of nursing and health care" in *Mundo Saúde*, 33(2), pp.143-149.

Watson, J. (2005). *Caring science as sacred science*. F. A. Davis.

Watson, J., & Woodward, T. (2010). "Jean Watson's theory of human caring" in *Nursing Theories and Nursing Practice*, 3, pp.351-369.

Waxenbaum, J. A., Reddy, V., & Varacallo, M. (2021). *Anatomy, autonomic nervous system*. StatPearls Publishing. https://www.ncbi.nlm.nih.gov/books/NBK539845/.

Webster's New Collegiate Dictionary. Springfield, Mass: G & C Merriam Company; 1979.

Wegscheider-Cruse, S., & Cruse, J. (2012). *Understanding codependency, updated and expanded: The science behind it and how to break the cycle*. Health Communications, Inc.

Wei, H., Hardin, S. R., & Watson, J. (2021). "A unitary caring science resilience-building model: Unifying the human caring theory and research-informed psychology and neuroscience evidence" in *International Journal of Nursing Sciences*, 8(1), pp.130-135. https://doi.org/10.1016/j.ijnss.2020.11.003.

Wei, H., Roberts, P., Strickler, J., & Corbett, R. W. (2019). "Nurse leaders' strategies to foster nurse resilience" in *Journal of Nursing Management*, 27(4), pp.681-687. https://doi.org/10.1111/jonm.12736.

Weintraub, A. (2014). *Break your heart no longer: An exercise to reduce shame*. LifeForce Yoga. https://yogafordepression.com/break-heart-longer-exercise-reduce-shame.

Wheeler, K., & Phillips, K. E. (2021). "The development of trauma and resilience competencies for nursing education" in *Journal of the American Psychiatric Nurses Association*, 27(4), pp.322-333. https://doi.org/10.1177/1078390319878779.

Williamson, M. (1992). *A return to love: Reflections on the principles of "A Course in Miracles"*. HarperCollins.

Willis, D. G., & Leone-Sheehan, D. M. (2019). "Spiritual knowing: Another pattern of knowing in the discipline" in *Advances in Nursing Science*, 42(1), pp.58-68. https://doi.org/10.1097/ans.0000000000000236.

Wilson, J. P. (2006). "Trauma archetypes and trauma complexes" in J. P. Wilson (Ed.), *The posttraumatic self: Restoring meaning and wholeness to personality*. Routledge.

Wimberger, L. (2015). *Neurosculpting: A whole-brain approach to heal trauma, rewrite limiting beliefs, and find wholeness*. Sounds True.

Wolotira, E. A. (2022). "Trauma, compassion fatigue, and burnout in nurses: The nurse leader's response" in *Nurse Leader*. https://doi.org/10.1016/j.mnl.2022.04.009.

World Health Organization. (2019). *Burn-out an "occupational phenomenon"*: International Classification of Diseases. 2019. https://www.who.int/news/item/28-05-2019-burn-out-an-occupational-phenomenon-international-classification-of-diseases.

Wright, S. G., & Sayre-Adams, J. (2000). *Sacred space: Right relationship and spirituality in healthcare* (2nd ed.). Churchill Livingstone.

Zander, P. E. (2007). "Ways of knowing in nursing: The historical evolution of a concept" in *Journal of Theory Construction & Testing*, 11(1), p.7.

Zangaro, G. A., Dulko, D., Sullivan, D., Weatherspoon, D., White, K. M., Hall, V. P., Squellati, R., Donnelli, A., James, J., & Wilson, D. R. (2022). "Systematic review of burnout in US nurses" in *Nursing Clinics of North America*, 57(1), pp.1-20. https://doi.org/https://doi.org/10.1016/j.cnur.2021.11.001.

IFF
BOOKS

ACADEMIC AND SPECIALIST

Iff Books publishes non-fiction. It aims to work with authors and titles that augment our understanding of the human condition, society and civilisation, and the world or universe in which we live. If you have enjoyed this book, why not tell other readers by posting a review on your preferred book site.
Recent bestsellers from Iff Books are:

Why Materialism Is Baloney
How true skeptics know there is no death and fathom answers to life, the universe, and everything
Bernardo Kastrup
A hard-nosed, logical, and skeptic non-materialist metaphysics, according to which the body is in mind, not mind in the body.
Paperback: 978-1-78279-362-5 ebook: 978-1-78279-361-8

The Fall
Steve Taylor
The Fall discusses human achievement versus the issues of war, patriarchy and social inequality.
Paperback: 978-1-78535-804-3 ebook: 978-1-78535-805-0

Brief Peeks Beyond
Critical essays on metaphysics, neuroscience, free will, skepticism and culture
Bernardo Kastrup
An incisive, original, compelling alternative to current mainstream cultural views and assumptions.
Paperback: 978-1-78535-018-4 ebook: 978-1-78535-019-1

Framespotting
Changing how you look at things changes how
you see them
Laurence & Alison Matthews
A punchy, upbeat guide to framespotting. Spot deceptions and
hidden assumptions; swap growth for growing up. See and be free.
Paperback: 978-1-78279-689-3 ebook: 978-1-78279-822-4

Is There an Afterlife?
David Fontana
Is there an Afterlife? If so what is it like? How do Western ideas
of the afterlife compare with Eastern? David Fontana presents the
historical and contemporary evidence for survival of
physical death.
Paperback: 978-1-90381-690-5

Nothing Matters
a book about nothing
Ronald Green
Thinking about Nothing opens the world to everything by
illuminating new angles to old problems and stimulating new
ways of thinking.
Paperback: 978-1-84694-707-0 ebook: 978-1-78099-016-3

Panpsychism
The Philosophy of the Sensuous Cosmos
Peter Ells
Are free will and mind chimeras? This book, anti-materialistic but
respecting science, answers: No! Mind is foundational
to all existence.
Paperback: 978-1-84694-505-2 ebook: 978-1-78099-018-7

Punk Science
Inside the Mind of God
Manjir Samanta-Laughton
Many have experienced unexplainable phenomena; God, psychic abilities, extraordinary healing and angelic encounters. Can cutting-edge science actually explain phenomena previously thought of as 'paranormal'?
Paperback: 978-1-90504-793-2

The Vagabond Spirit of Poetry
Edward Clarke
Spend time with the wisest poets of the modern age and of the past, and let Edward Clarke remind you of the importance of poetry in our industrialized world.
Paperback: 978-1-78279-370-0 ebook: 978-1-78279-369-4

Readers of ebooks can buy or view any of these bestsellers by clicking on the live link in the title. Most titles are published in paperback and as an ebook. Paperbacks are available in traditional bookshops. Both print and ebook formats are available online. Find more titles and sign up to our readers' newsletter at www.collectiveinkbooks.com/non-fiction
Follow us on Facebook at www.facebook.com/CINonFiction